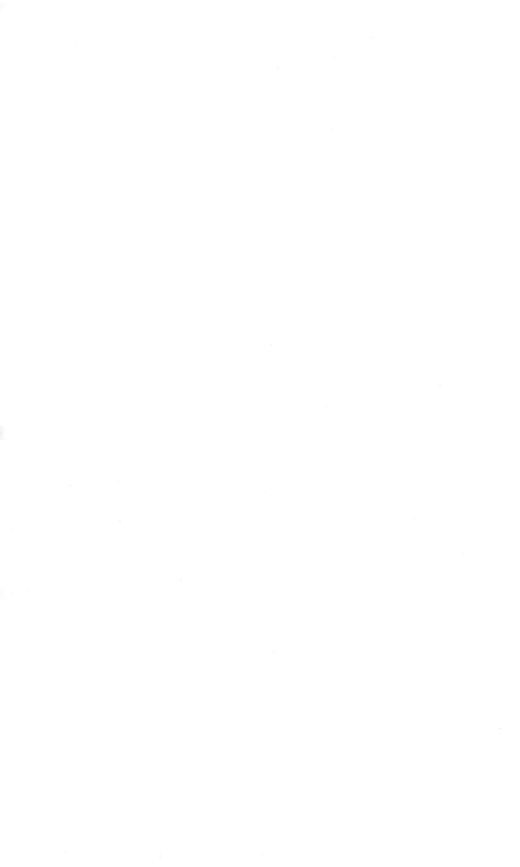

TEXTBOOK ON THE BASES OF PHARMACEUTICAL AND MEDICINAL CHEMISTRY OF ANTIBIOTICS

NAEEM HASAN KHAN

B. Pharm. (Pb.), M. Pharm. (Pb.) (Pharmacology),
Ph. D. (K.U.L. Belgium) (Pharmaceutical Chemistry), R. Ph., B.S.P.S. (Belgium)

NABILA PERVEEN

B.Sc. (Pb.), B. Pharm. (Pb) M.Phil. (Pb.) (Pharmaceutical Chemistry),
Ph. D. (U.S.M. Malaysia) (Clinical Pharmacy), R. Ph.

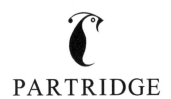

PARTRIDGE

Library of Congress Control Number:		2021909279
ISBN:	Hardcover	978-1-5437-6473-4
	Softcover	978-1-5437-6471-0
	eBook	978-1-5437-6472-7

Print information available on the last page.

To order additional copies of this book, contact
Toll Free +65 3165 7531 (Singapore)
Toll Free +60 3 3099 4412 (Malaysia)
orders.singapore@partridgepublishing.com

www.partridgepublishing.com/singapore

**"In the Name of Almighty ALLAH (ALMIGHTY GOD),
the Most Gracious, the Most Merciful"**

DEDICATED TO OUR CHILDREN

LAILA NAEEM HASAN
AAMNA NAEEM HASAN
MAHNOOR FATIMA HASAN
FAYSAL RAIHAN HASAN

FOREWORD

I am delighted to write a foreword for the book "Textbook on the bases of Pharmaceutical and Medicinal Chemistry of antibiotics" by Prof. Dr. Naeem Hasan Khan and his wife Nabila Perveen, both the authors are known to me for more than a decade, since Prof. Dr. Khan and myself were contemporaries in the two Malaysian universities, AIMST, (Kedah), and QUIP, (IPOH). During these years, I had long academic discussions with the two authors on our mutual interest, that is antibiotics.

Prof. Dr. Naeem Hasan Khan has a brilliant and enviable tract record in academics. He obtained Ph. D. Degree from Katholieke Universiteit Leuven (KUL), Belgium in the grade of "Great Distinction". His research work during his stay over Belgium was recognized world-wide. The new methods developed by him has been officially adopted as an official method for quantitative analysis of "Oxytetracycline, Tetracycline, Chlortetracycline" and their related substances in the U.S. Pharmacopeia (USP) 23, Official National Formulary Supplement 9, pages 4588-4590, November 15, 1998, in The European Pharmacopoeia (Euro. Pharm.) and in The British Pharmacopoeia (B.P.). Throughout his academic carrier, Prof. Dr. Naeem has been pursuing research and has published the number of original research articles in prestigious International journals of The U.K., The U.S.A., The Netherlands, France, Spain, Belgium, Bulgaria, Singapore and some others. He has also been invited as a keynote speaker at various International scientific conferences abroad.

Since the discovery of penicillin in early 1940, it is difficult to imagine practice of medicine without antibiotics. The problem with antibiotics is the development of drug-resistance by the microorganisms. That is why there is continuous search for newer antibiotics to bypass mechanisms of drug-resistance. Better understanding of the physicochemical properties of antibiotic chemical space is required to form new antibiotic discovery. Innovations such as the development of antibiotic adjuvants to preserve efficacy of existing drugs together with expanding antibiotic chemical diversity through synthetic biology or new techniques to develop antibiotic- producing organisms, are required to bridge the growing gap between the need for new drugs and their discovery. The book is bound to be of immense value to those involved in this field of research. Prof. Dr. Khan and Dr. Nabila deserve gratitude of the fraternity of pharmacists and pharmacologists for their singular service to the profession. I hope this book would be as popular as Prof. Dr. Khan's earlier book "New HPLC methods for quality control of tetracycline antibiotics" which was published by VDM Verlag Publishers, Germany (in English language), and printed in The U.S.A. and The U.K. in 2010.

Prof. R. K. Marya
MBBS; MD; PhD
January 2021
Former:
Professor and Head, Unit of Physiology, Faculty of Medicine, AIMST University, BEDONG
Kedah Darul Aman, **Malaysia.**
Professor and Head, Department of Physiology, Quest International University of Perak, IPOH, Perak, **Malaysia.**
Professor and Head, Department of Physiology, Postgraduate Institute of Medical Sciences, ROHTAK, **India.**

PREFACE

MEDICINAL CHEMISTRY is a science whose fundamental roots lie in all branches of chemistry and biology. The term "Pharmaceutical Chemistry" is been used for "Medicinal Chemistry". The purposes of the medicinal chemistry are the isolation, characterization, elucidation of the structure and the synthesis of the compounds which can be used in medicine for the cure/treatment of disease or a pharmaceutical agent which will benefit humanity. Moreover, medicinal chemistry is concerned with the understanding of the chemical and biological mechanisms by which the action of drugs can be explained. It also establishes the relation between chemical structure and biological activity and to link the later to the physical properties of the drugs.

The medicinal chemist is necessarily a member of a research team which usually consists the medicinal chemist, the biochemist who determine the fate of the drug in the body as an explanation of its mode of action, pharmacologist who test the drugs on animals, transposing animal experiments into clinical trials and chemical engineers/pharmacists who manufacture the tested and proved drug for general therapeutic use.

Indeed, the research area of the antibiotics has become the most important in the whole field of pharmaceutical research. Almost incredible amount of new knowledge on antibiotics involving their Chemistry, Biochemistry, Cell biology, Pharmacology is still under extensive research all over the globe.

This book is basically aimed to design for undergraduate postgraduate students of pharmacy, medical and other science disciplines, in a very simple language, as well as who might be considering a future career in academics or in the pharmaceutical industry.

The book is divided into portions. The first part deals with the antibiotics in general. Second portion covers the basic principles and techniques of medicinal chemistry. The third part is related in dealing with the chemotherapeutic properties of antibiotics while the fourth portion is composed of specific topics, within medicinal chemistry, of clinically important individual antibiotics in divided chapters.

A comprehensive description of nowadays clinically useful antibiotics is described in the book, as regards the medicinal chemistry point of view is concerned. They are the basic principles of antibiotic development, various classes of chemical compounds, difference in origin, mechanism of pharmacological actions and spectrum of activity and their structural activity relationship.

The secretarial assistance from Miss MAHNOOR FATIMA HASAN cannot be forgotten in the completion of this manuscript.

NAEEM HASAN KHAN   **AIMST UNIVERSITY**
NABILA PERVEEN   **BEDONG 08100**
2021   **KEDAH DARUL AMAN**
                             MALAYSIA

CONTENTS

CHAPTER 1

GENERAL MEDICINAL CHEMISTRY

1.1 The nature and sources of drugs in general

No.	Source	Description
1.	Plants	Numerous compounds of medicinal use have been obtained / extracted from plant sources e.g., digoxin, quinine, reserpine, morphine, vincristine and many antibiotics etc. Many plants also provide important therapeutic drugs.
2.	Animals	Medicinal compounds / drugs are obtained from animal sources (land or marine) e.g., insulin, heparin, c.v. drugs etc.
3.	Microorganisms	Bacteria and fungi which are isolated from soil are important sources of antibacterial substances e.g., β -lactam antibiotics, bacitracin etc.
4.	Minerals	Medicinal compounds / drugs have also been obtained from minerals e.g., liquid paraffin, kaolin, magnesium, silicate etc.
5.	Marine	Many medicinal compounds as c.v. drugs, cytotoxic, antimicrobials, antibiotics, anti-inflammatory etc., are obtained from this source.
6.	Synthetic	Wide variety of medicines are also manufactured synthetically or semi-synthetically that involve chemical reactions e.g., antibacterial sulphonamides, acetyl salicylic acid, procaine etc. Majority of medicinal products / drugs are synthetic.

| 7. | DNA recombinant technology | This technology is also known as genetic engineering. Drugs are also manufacture based upon this technology e.g., human insulin, human growth hormone etc. |

1.2 Pharmaceutically / pharmacologically active ingredients from plants, microbes and marine origins

1.	Alkaloids	Alkaloids are basic substances containing cyclic nitrogen and for water soluble salts with acids e.g., morphine, atropine etc.
2.	Glycosides	These are organic substances which are linked with sugar/s in ether like combination. It can be hydrolyzed with mineral acids converting into: sugar part **(glycoside)** and non-sugar component **(aglycone).**
3.	Oils	Oils also possess pharmaceutical and pharmacological activities. These are usually edibles.
		Fixed oils: These are glycerides of oleic acid, palmitic acid and stearic acid. Many of these oils are edible having pharmacological and food values e.g., coconut oil, olive oil, castor oil, palm oil etc. **Volatile oils:** These types of oils are evaporating, especially on heating, with peculiar aroma. These are also known as "essential oils "has immense medicinal importance as carminatives, antiseptics, analgesic e.g., eucalyptus oil, clove oil, olive oil etc. **Mineral oils:** the mineral oils are usually derived from hydrocarbons which are obtained from petroleum and are used as lubricant laxative e.g., liquid paraffin etc.

2

4.	Gums	These are the secretory products of plants. These are used pharmaceutically as suspending and emulsifying and binding agents e.g., agar etc.
5.	Resins	Resins are present in plants and are formed by oxidation and polymerization of volatile oils which are insoluble in water e.g., jalap, colocynth etc.
6.	Oleoresins	The mixture of volatile oils and resins forms oleoresins e.g., bark of pine tree etc.
7.	Tannins	Tannins are the chemical substances which are non-nitrogenous plant constituents e.g., tincture of catechu (plant acacia) etc.
8.	Antibacterials	These substances are obtained or derived from bacteria, mold and fungi e.g., penicillin, streptomycin etc.
9.	Toxins	Physiologically active toxins are obtained from many marine sources as well.

1.3   Briefing on important alkaloids

Alkaloids may be defined as chemical group having heterocyclic natural products containing heterocyclic Nitrogen. The alkaloids are considered to be alkaline in nature because they possess:

- Primary amine
- Secondary amine
- Tertiary amines

Some of the alkaloids are neutral in action and some of them possess phenolic activity which actually contributes the acidic nature of the molecule. The alkaloids display an exceptionally wide array of biological activities, being present in plants, fungi, bacteria, amphibia, insects, marine animals and humans. Alkaloids may also naturally exist as salts which are the product of a reaction of acid and base.

The alkaloids are classified based upon their chemical nucleus, as under:

1.	Pyridine
2.	Piperidine
3.	Pyrrolizidine
4.	Phenyl-alkyl amine
5.	Quinoline
6.	Isoquinoline
7.	Indole
8.	Tropane
9.	Xanthine
10.	Imidazole

Some important alkaloids are briefed below:

A. OPIUM

Opium is the sun-dried gummy exudate of the unripe capsule of the "opium poppy" (papaver somniferum) and contains 20 % of 30 different alkaloids. Opium contains isoquinoline type of alkaloids. It is cultivated in China, Persia, India, Pakistan, Afghanistan, Egypt, Southeren Eastern Europe and Golden Triangle. Some major alkaloids are mentioned below.

1.	Morphine	13 %
2.	Apomorphine	3%
3.	Codeine	0.3%
4.	Thebaine	0.4%
5.	Papaverine	0.8%
6.	Methadone	0.9%
7.	Norcotine	5%
8.	Noscopine And many others	0.7%

Apart from alkaloids, it also contains gums, sugars, organic acids, resins, proteins. It is used as supreme pain- relieving action, C.N.S. stimulant, smooth muscle relaxant, veterinary sedative, male impotence and cough depressant / expectorant.

B. RAUWOLFIA

The plant rauwolfia serpentina is also called as "snake root" (apocynaceace) and is cultivated in China, Indian sub-continent, South America, Middle East, Western African countries. In 1931, two Indian research brothers (Siddiqui and Siddiqui brothers) were awarded the **Noble Prize** for the isolation of very important alkaloid "AJMALINE' from rauwolfia serpentina. Major alkaloids are mentioned below.

1.	Reserpine	0.14%
2.	Yohimbine	---
3.	Ajmaline	---
4.	Ajmalicine	-
5.	Neo-ajmaline	-
6.	Serpentine	-
7.	Reserpinine	-
8.	Isoreserpinine And many others	-

It is used as super hypotensive, mental diseases also indicated in snake bite.

C. CANTHARANTHUS

Cantharanthus rosea is also known as "Vinca rosea" or "Madagascar periwinkle". It belongs to indole type of alkaloids (apocynaecace). It is cultivated all over but is indigenous to Madagascar. It is also called as garden plant in many countries. In different places, it has different flower colors. Some major alkaloids are mentioned below.

1.	Vincristine	0.0002%
2.	Vinblastine	0.0005%
3.	Vinrosidine	-
4.	Vinleurosine	-
5.	Vinglycinate	-
6.	Vindesine	-
7.	Vinorelbine And many others	-

Vincristine and vinblastine are the major alkaloids which are very important, potent and commonly used in cancer therapy.

D. STRYCHNOS NUX VOMICA

It is known as "Nux vomica" (looganiaceae). It is very highly poisonous and is evergreen tree. It belongs to South East Asian countries but cultivated widely in India and China. Some major alkaloids are mentioned below.

1.	Strychnine	1.5%
2.	Brucine	1.023%
3.	Vomine And many others	0.3%

It is used to increase the male sexual potency, rodenticide, analeptic, increases tone of the skeletal muscles followed by general anesthesia, respiratory stimulant in deep centrally depressant.

E. CINCHONA

Cinchona is a genus of 25 species with evergreen foliage (rubiaceae). It is also known as "Jesuit's bark' or "Peruvian bark". It is cultivated in entire South America and China. It contains quinoline type of alkaloids. Some major alkaloids are mentioned below.

1.	Quinine	16%
2.	Quinidine	-
3.	Cinchonine	-
4.	Cinchonidine	-
5.	Dihydroquinine	-
6.	Dihydroquinidine And many others	-

It is used since about 500 years in folk medicine. Used to treat malaria, kills bacteria / parasites / germs, hypothermia, regulating heartbeat, stimulates digestion, reduces spasm and decreases secretions.

F. ERGOT

Ergot is also known as "Claviceps purpurea" (clavicpitaceae). It has about 50 species known and is cultivated in Central Asian countries, South American countries of tropical regions. It belongs to the indole alkaloid family. Some major alkaloids are mentioned below.

1.	Ergometrine	21%
2.	Ergocrystine	-
3.	Ergonovive	-
4.	Ergocrystinine	-
5.	Ergotoxin	-
6.	Ergosine	-
7.	Ergokryptine And many others	-

It is used as antihypertensive, oxytocic, in migraine, depresses the vasomotor centers and causes hallucination.

G. HYOSCYAMUS NIGER

It is also known as "Black henbane" or "henbane" (Solanaceae). It belongs to the category of tropane alkaloids and is cultivated in Central Asia, Middle east, South America, China and Eastern European countries. Some major alkaloids are mentioned below.

1.	Hyoscymine	18%
2.	Scopolamine methyl bromide	-
3.	Scopolamine	-
4.	Hyoscine And many others	-

It is used as spasmolytic and anticholinergic.

H. BELLADONA

It is known as "Deadly nightshade" or "Atropa belladonna" (Solanaceae). It is cultivated in Europe, North Africa, Central and Western Asia. It is a type of tropane alkaloid. Belladona means beautiful lady. Some major alkaloids are mentioned below.

1.	Atropine	11%
2.	Homatropine	-
3.	Amprotropine	-
4.	Adephinine	-
5.	Dicyclomine	-
6.	Hyoscymine And many others	-

It is very powerful mydriatic, powerful cholinergic blocking agent, pre-anesthesia, motion sickness and antispasmodic.

I. PHYSOSTIGMA

It is also called as "Calabar bean" or "Physostigma venenosum" or "African vine" or "Ordeal bean" (fabaceae) and is cultivated in Tropical African countries. It is a indole type of alkaloid which contains 6 alkaloids. Some major alkaloids are mentioned below.

1.	Physostigmine	9%
2.	Neostigmine	-
3.	Pyridostigmine And others	-

It is used in glaucoma, Alzheimer's disease, myasthenia gravis, stimulation of peristalsis, miosis and stimulation of skeletal muscles.

J. IPECACUANHA

It is also known as "Psychotria ipecacuanha" or "Cepkaelis ipecacuanha" (rubiaceae) and cultivated in Brazil, Peru and Columbia. It belongs to the group of isoquinoline group of alkaloids. Some major alkaloids are mentioned below.

1.	Physostigmine	8%
2.	Neostigmine	-
3.	Pyridostigmine And others	-

It is used as an emetic, nauseant, expectorant, amebiasis induce seating, diarrhea, fever and bronchitis.

K. COCA

It is also called as "Erythroxylum coca" (erythroxylaceae) and is cultivated in Colombia, Peru and Bolivia. It is a tropane alkaloid. Traces of coca have been also found in mummies dating to about three thousand years back and it is a major drug of abuse as with heroin. Some major alkaloids of coca are mentioned below.

1.	Cocaine	1.5%
2.	Methylecgonine	-
3.	Benzylecgonine	-
4.	Hydroxytropacocaine	-

| 5. | Ecgonine | - |
| 6. | Hygrine and some others | - |

It is very highly stimulant, suppresses hunger thirst, sever pain, fatigue, local anesthetic, hallucinant and euphoric.

L. PILOCARPUS JABORANDI

It is known as "Pilocarpus jaborandi holms" with about 13 species (rutaceae) and is cultivated in South American countries. It is of an imidazole type of alkaloid. Most important alkaloid of this plant is:

Pilocarpine 1%

It is used as a sympathomimetic causing salivation and tachycardia, its main use is in miosis after atropine, as an antidote for scopolamine, atropine and hyoscyamine poisoning and to contract the pupil after the use of atropine.

M. EPHEDRA VULGARIS

It is also known as "ephedra distichal" or "Ephedra sinical" or "Ma Huang' (Ephedraceae) and is cultivated in Southern Europe, part of Central and Western Asia. It belongs to the group of phenylalkylamine group of alkaloids. Most important alkaloid of this plant are:

Ephedrine	2.5% (80 % ephedrine and pseudoephedrine)
Pseudoephedrine	As above
And many others	-

Main uses are in colds, (other bronchial conditions), C.N.S stimulant, vasoconstrictor and bronchodilator in severe asthma.

N. DATURA

It is also called as "Datura stramonium" or "Throne apple". It has also many other names, like; Jismon weed, Stink weed, Loco weed, Korean morning glory, Jamestown weed, Angel's trumpet, Devil's trumpet, Devil's snare, crazy tea, Zombie cucumber and Anushka (Solanaceae) and is cultivated in South and Central America and Central Asia. It is used in travel sickness, preparative medication and hallucinogenic.

O. ASHWAGANDHA

It is called by many of the following names:

- Winter cherry
- Withania somnifera
- Indian ginseng
- Agagandha
- Kanaje hindi
- Samm al ferakh

Family is Solanaceae and is cultivated in India, Nepal, Pakistan, Sri Lanka, North Africa, Middle east and Bangladesh. Most important alkaloid s / lactones of this plant are:

1.	Withanine	0.31%
2.	Somniferine	-
3.	Somnine	-
4.	Somniferinine	-
5.	Withananine	-
6.	Peeudowithanine	-
7.	Withanolide (steroidal lactone) And some others	-

It is used as analgesic, sedative, enhances fertility in both sexes, antioxidant, anti-inflammatory and anticancer as well.

P. VASAKA

Vasaka alkaloid is obtained from the plant "Justicia Adhotoda" (Acanthaceae) and is cultivated in Central Asia, China, Nepal and South America. It belongs to the quinazoline group of alkaloids. It is also the official provincial flower of "PUNJAB STATE "of Pakistan. It is also called by many other different names like:

- Adhatoda
- Adalodakam
- Malabar nut

Most important alkaloid of this plant are:

1.	Vasicine	-
2.	Vasicinone	-
3.	Deoxyvasicine	-
4.	Maiontone And many others	-

It is used in respiratory discomfort, cough / expectorant, cardiac tonic, skin diseases oxytocic and possess abortifacient activity.

Q. CAT'S CLAW

It is known as "Uncaria tomentosa" or "Vilcacora" Rubiaceae) and cultivated in Tropical jungles of South / Latin / Central America and Central Asia. I t belongs to the tetracyclic and pentacyclic oxinadole group of alkaloids. Most important alkaloid of this plant are:

Rhychophylline
Isorhychophylline
some others

It is used to reduce the speed and contraction of the heart, ataxia, sedative, treatment of cancer, for HIV infection, arthritis / rheumatism and diabetes.

R. TONGAT ALI

It is known as "Eurycoma longifolia" or "Pasak bumi" (Simaroubaceae) and is cultivated in Thailand, Indonesia and Malaysia. It is used as antimalarial, antipyretic, antiulcer, cytotoxic with aphrodisiac properties as well.

S. MURRAYA

It has 12 species (rutaceae) and belongs to the family of carbazole alkaloids. It is cultivated in India, China, Australia, South East Asia and Golden triangle. It is also called as:

Murraya alata (drake)
Murraya koneigi (curry tree or curry pata)
Murraya periculata (orange jasmine or Chinese box or lakeview jasmine)
Murraya ovatifoliolata (domin)
Murraya stenocarpa (swingle)

It is used as antidiabetic, antioxidant, antimicrobial, anti-inflammatory, hepatoprotective, analgesic and anti-hypercholesterolemia.

T. TOBACCO

Tobacco contains nicotine alkaloid approximately 0.6–3.0% (maximum 5%) of the dry weight of tobacco in the edible family solanaceae including potatoes, tomatoes, and eggplants, though sources disagree on whether this has any biological significance to human consumers. It functions as an antiherbivore chemical; consequently as an insecticide. Nicotine addiction is well known that its dependence causes distress. Nicotine also acts as a receptor agonist at most nicotinic acetylcholine receptors.

U. COFFEE BEAN

Caffeine is the source which is obtained from coffee bean It is a methylxanthine alkaloid and is chemically related to the adenine and guanine bases of deoxyribonucleic acid (DNA) and ribonucleic acid (RNA). It is cultivated in Africa, East Asia and South America. Evidence of a risk during pregnancy is equivocal. Coffee leaves contain 3.5% caffeine and coffee roots contain 2.2%.

1.4   Marine medicinal chemistry

Marine environment are potential sources for new bioactive compounds. First development was the discovery of "arabinose nucleosides" from marine invertebrate demonstration that sugar moietys other than ribose and deoxyribose can yield bioactive nucleoside structures. Later marine drug was approved from the snail toxin "ziconitide" to treat sever neuropathic pain. Several other marine derived compounds are in clinical use for different type of diseases. Another drug "bryostatin" is used against cancer therapy. Marine life forms the following forms from which the medicinal products are developed:

- Microscopic life
- Plants, coral and algae
- Marine invertebrates
- Fish
- Reptiles
- Seabirds
- Marine mammals (whales, sea cow, seals, sea lion, walrus, sea otter polar bear)

Marine drugs

The drugs obtained from marine sources are being used since a long from shark, cod-liver oil, sodium alginate, agar-agar. Many of the species contain very toxic agents. Important marind medicinal compounds are listed below:

No.	Pharmacological system	Chemical name of the medicinal compound
1.	Cardiovascular agents	Anthopleurins (hog fish) Eptatretin (hog fish) Laminine (algae) Octopamine (octopus) Saxitoximussel (mussel) Autonomium (fish) Halothurins (plants) Asterosaponins (plants) Spongosine (sponge) Eledosin (sponge)
2.	Cytotoxic agents	Cytosine arabinose (sponge) Crassin acetate (corals) Geranyl hydroquinone (corals) Aplysistatin (algae) Halitoxin (sponge) Majusculamine-C(algae) Acanthifolicin (sponge) And many others
3.	Anti -microbial agents	Halotoxin (sea cucumber) Tetrabromoheptanone (brown algae) Polythaloacetones (red algae) Aeoplysinin (sponge) Eunicin (corals)

4.	Antibiotic compounds	Tribromophenol-2yl-phenol (bacterium) Cycloeudesmol (algae) Variabillin (sponge) Dibromo-4-hydroxy benzine-acetamide (sponge)
5.	Anti-inflammatory and antispasmodic agents	Manoalide (sponge) Dendalone (sponge) Flexibillide (coral) Flustramine (coral) Tetradotoxin (puffer fish) And many others
6.	Toxin agents	Ciguatoxin (octopus) Palytoxin (fish) Red tide toxin (fish) Many others
7.	Anticonvulsant agent	Kainic acid (red algae)
8.	Ascaris / Pin worms	Domoic acid (red algae)
9.	Insecticide	Annelid (coral)
10.	Allergy	Didemnins (sponge)
11.	Antidepressant	Aplysinopsin (yellow sponge)
12.	Anticoagulant	Laminarin (plants)
13.	Prostaglandins	Gorgonian (coral)

1.5 Isolates of important plant extracts

1.5.1   Isolation of Cinchona alkaloids

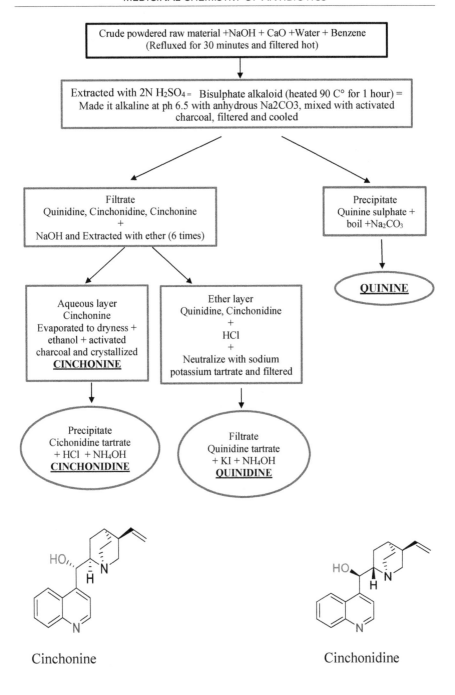

Crude powdered raw material +NaOH + CaO +Water + Benzene
(Refluxed for 30 minutes and filtered hot)

Extracted with 2N H_2SO_4 = Bisulphate alkaloid (heated 90 C° for 1 hour) =
Made it alkaline at ph 6.5 with anhydrous Na2CO3, mixed with activated
charcoal, filtered and cooled

Filtrate
Quinidine, Cinchonidine, Cinchonine
+
NaOH and Extracted with ether (6 times)

Precipitate
Quinine sulphate +
boil +Na_2CO_3

QUININE

Aqueous layer
Cinchonine
Evaporated to dryness +
ethanol + activated
charcoal and crystallized
CINCHONINE

Ether layer
Quinidine, Cinchonidine
+
HCl
+
Neutralize with sodium
potassium tartrate and filtered

Precipitate
Cichonidine tartrate
+ HCl + NH_4OH
CINCHONIDINE

Filtrate
Quinidine tartrate
+ KI + NH_4OH
QUINIDINE

Cinchonine

Cinchonidine

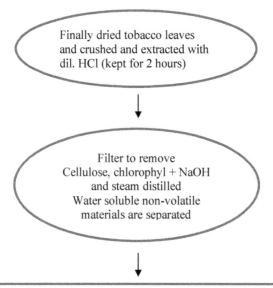

Quinine   Quinidine

1.5.2   Isolation of Nicotine alkaloid

Finally dried tobacco leaves
and crushed and extracted with
dil. HCl (kept for 2 hours)

Filter to remove
Cellulose, chlorophyl + NaOH
and steam distilled
Water soluble non-volatile
materials are separated

Again steam distilled and acidified with oxalic acid +
Heat to concentrate to thich mass and cooled
Crystalline Nicotine oxalate is formed.
Transfered to separating funnel with the addition of potassium
hydroxide in excess

Nicotine will be separated at the top of the
two layers in the separating funnel in brown
colour, separated upper layer and again
extracted with excess of ether solution
Evaporate
Crystals of nicotine are obtained
NICOTINE

Nicotine

1.5.3 Isolation of Cocaine alkaloid

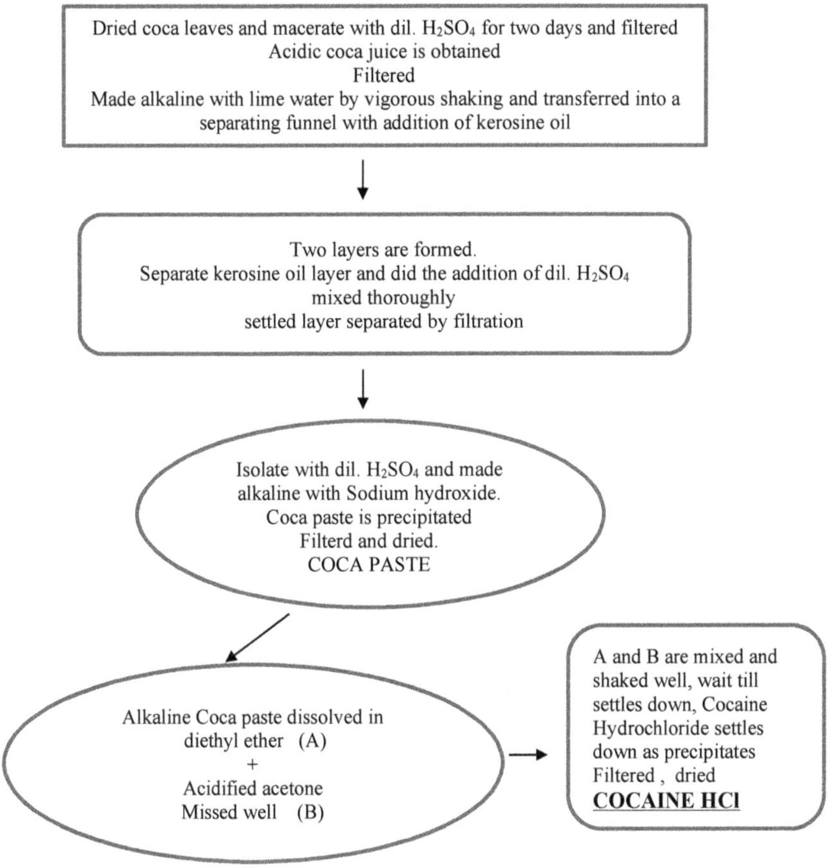

Dried coca leaves and macerate with dil. H_2SO_4 for two days and filtered
Acidic coca juice is obtained
Filtered
Made alkaline with lime water by vigorous shaking and transferred into a
separating funnel with addition of kerosine oil

Two layers are formed.
Separate kerosine oil layer and did the addition of dil. H_2SO_4
mixed thoroughly
settled layer separated by filtration

Isolate with dil. H_2SO_4 and made
alkaline with Sodium hydroxide.
Coca paste is precipitated
Filterd and dried.
COCA PASTE

Alkaline Coca paste dissolved in
diethyl ether (A)
+
Acidified acetone
Missed well   (B)

A and B are mixed and
shaked well, wait till
settles down, Cocaine
Hydrochloride settles
down as precipitates
Filtered , dried
COCAINE HCl

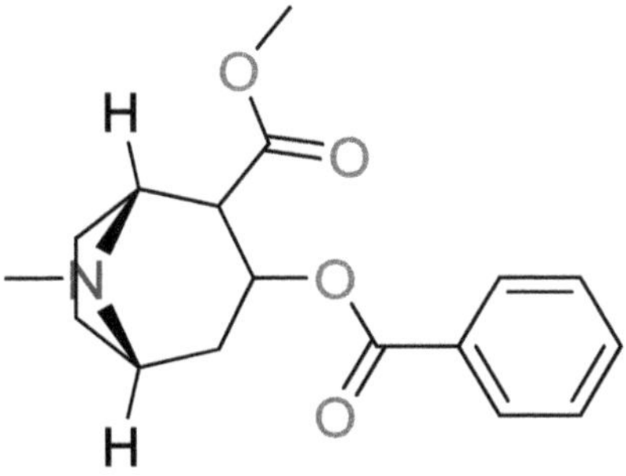

Cocaine

1.5.4 Isolation of Caffeine from xanthine alkaloids

Green tea leaves + hot water (hot extraction)
Tea extract solution (based upon purine nucleus) contains caffeine 2.5%,
theobromine 0.17%, theophylline 0.013%

After cooling in ice bath, transferred to separating
funnel already containing dichloromethane and
extracted 3 times

The lower layer is removed. Theobromine will remain in aqous layer
and the rest of extract separated and added with anhydrous sodium
sulphate. All rest of the impuriries will be separated.

Solution is filtered and evaporated to
dryness. Crystals of caffeine are
obtained.

Caffeine

1.5.5 Isolation of Morphine alkaloid from opium (method condensed)

The opium is cut into thin slices and treated with hot water until a paste is obtained. The opium is exhausted with cold water and the resultant liquor concentrated to a syrupy consistency and precipitated when hot with powdered sodium carbonate and heated as long as ammonia is given off; alkaline to phenolphthalein. After standing for twenty-four hours, the resultant precipitate is filtered and washed with cold water.

The precipitate is dissolved in alcohol at 85° and evaporated, to dryness and the residue is exhausted with dilute acetic acid as neutralization proceeds. The acetic acid solution is treated with decolorizing charcoal, then filtered and precipitated with ammonia, filtered the precipitated.

The precipitate is washed and purified by crystallization from alcohol; concentration of the alcoholic mother-liquor yields a further quantity of morphine.

1.5.6   Biosynthesis of Morphine

1.6   Nomenclature of various organic / inorganic groups

1.6.1   The nomenclature helps to define the stereo-chemical nature of the drug

ORGANIC GROUPS	NAMING DRUG
Acetamido	CH_3CONH-
Acetoxy	CH_3COO-
Acetyl	CH_3CO-
Acrylolyl	$CH_2=CHCO-$
Allyl	$CH_2=CH-CH_2-$
Allyloxy	CH_2CH-CH_2O-

Amidino	$H_2NC(=NH)-$
Amino	H_2N-
Anilino	C_6H_5NH-
Benzamido	C_6H_5CONH-
Benzhydryl	$(C_6H_5)_2CH-$
Benzhydryloxy	$(C_6H_5)_2CHO-$
Benzoyl	C_6H_5CO-
Benzoyloxy	C_6H_5COO-
Benzyl	$C_6H_5CH_2-$
Bis (2-chloroethylamino)	$(ClCH_2CH_2)_2N-$
Bromo	$Br-$
Butoxy	$CH_3(CH_2)_3O-$
n-Butyl-(butyl)	$(CH_2)_4-$
Sec-Butyl	$CH_3CH_2CH(CH_3)-$
Tertiary-Butyl	$(CH_3)_3C-$
Butylamino	$CH_3(CH_2)_3NH-$
Butyryl	$CH_3(CH_2)_2CO-$
Carbamoyl	H_2NCO-
Carbamoyloxy	H_2NCOO-
Carboxy	$HOOC-$
Chloro	$Cl-$
Cyano	$NC-$
Diethylamino	$(CH_3CH_2)_2N-$
2-Diethylamino ethyl	$(CH_3CH_2)_2NCH_2-CH_2-$
Diethylamino ethyl	$(CH_3CH_2)_2NCH_2-$
Diethylcarbamoyl	$(CH_3CH_2)_2NCO-$
Dimethyl amino	$(CH_3)_2N-$
2-Dimethylamino ethyl	$(CH_3)_2NCH_2CH_2-$
Dimethyl carbamoyloxy	$(CH_3)_2NCOO-$
Ethoxy	CH_3CH_2O-
Ethoxy carbonyl	CH_3CH_2OCO-
Ethyl	CH_3CH_2-
Ethynyl	$CH-C-$
Fluoro	$-F-$

Formyl	OHC-
Glycyl	H_2NCH_2CO-
Guanidino	$H_2NC(=NH) NH-$
Hydroxy	HO-
2-Hydroxy ethyl	$HOCH_2CH_2-$
Hydroxy mercuri	HOHg-
Iodo	I-
Isobutyl	$(CH_3)_2CHCH_2-$
Isopentyl	$(CH_3)_2CHCH_2CH_2-$
Isopropyl	$(CH_3)_2CH-$
Mercapto	HS-
Methoxy	CH_3O-
Methyl	CH_3-
Methyl amino	CH_3NH-
1-Methyl butyl	$CH_3(CH_2)_2CH(CH_3)-$
Methyl sulphonyl	CH_3SO_2-
Methyl thio	CH_3S-
Nitro	NO_2-
Nitroso	$-N=O$
Phenethyl	$C_6H_5CH_2CH_2-$
Phenoxy	C_6H_5O-
2-Phenoxy ethyl	$C_6H_5OCH_2CH_2-$
Phenoxy methyl	$C_6H_5OCH_2-$
Phenyl	C_6H_5-
Phenyl acetamido	$C_6H_5CH_2CONH-$
Propionyl	CH_3CH_2CO-
Propionyloxy	CH_3CH_2COO-
Propoxy	$CH_3CH_2CH_2O-$
n-Propyl	CH_3CH_2CH2-
Sulphamoyl	H_2NSO_2-
Sulphanil amido	$P-NH_2C_6H_4SO_2NH-$
Sulphonyl	$R-S(=O)_2-R'$
Trifluoro methyl	F_3C-
Vinyl	$CH_2=CH-$

1.7   Heterocyclic nuclei

A cyclic organic compound containing all carbon atoms in the ring formation is called as a "carbocyclic compound "and the branch of chemistry is known "carbocyclic or homocyclic chemistry". In case if at least one carbon atom in the ring formation is replaced by other atom, the compound is called as "heterocyclic compound" and thee branch is designated as "heterocyclic chemistry". Nitrogen, oxygen and sulphur are the common hetero atoms but some other atoms may also be replacing carbon in the system. Heterocyclic compounds may be classified into aliphatic and aromatic systems.

The aliphatic heterocyclics are the cyclic analogues of amines, ethers, thio-ethers and amides. Their properties are usually influenced by the presence of strain energy in the ring. These compounds generally consist of 3 or 4 membered and 5-9 membered.

The aromatic heterocyclic compounds are those which have a hetero atom in the ring and behave in a manner similar to benzene in some of their properties. Furthermore, these compounds also comply with the general rule proposed by Huckel. This rule states that aromaticity is obtained in cyclic conjugated and planar systems containing ($4n$ +2) electrons. The conjugated cyclic rings contain 6 electrons as in benzene and this forms a conjugated molecular orbital system which is thermodynamically more stable than the non-cyclically conjugated system.

A hetero ring may comprise of 3-9 (may be 3-10) (10th is under research trials) atoms which may be saturated or unsaturated. Although the ring may contain more than one hetero atom of similar or dissimilar type. The chemistry of heterocyclic compounds is as logical as that of aliphatic or aromatic compounds. Heterocyclic compounds occur widely in nature and in a variety of non-naturally occurring compounds.

A large number of heterocyclic compounds are essential to life. Various compounds like alkaloids, antibiotics, amino acids, vitamins, haemoglobin, hormones, chlorophyll, nucleic acids, bile pigments and many synthetic drugs, synthetic dyes and vast distribution of chemicals / medicines that contain heterocyclic compounds. A study of heterocyclic chemistry is very essential and important in biosynthesis and in the metabolism of drugs. For example, nucleic acids are basically important in biological processes of heredity changes. There are number of heterocyclic compounds with other important applications and many of them are involved as an intermediate in the synthesis of numerous compounds.

1.7.1   Nomenclature

International Union of Pure and Applied Chemistry (IUPAC) have systemized the nomenclature of heterocyclic compounds. According to this system, three to ten membered rings are named by combining the appropriate prefixes with the stems shown below.

Prefix to hetero atoms;

Hetero atom	Valence	Prefix
O	2	Oxa
N	3	Aza
S	2	Thia
Se	2	Selena
Te	2	Tellura
P	3	Phospha
As	3	Arsa
Si	4	Sila
Ge	4	Germa

1.7.2 Common name endings for heterocyclic compounds (3-9 membered)

Ring size	Suffixes for unsaturated compounds		Suffixes for unsaturated compounds	
	With Nitrogen	Without Nitrogen	With Nitrogen	Without Nitrogen
3	-irine	-irene	-iridine	-irane
4	-ete	-ete	-etidine	-etane
5	-ole	-ole	-olidine	-olane
6	-ine	-in	-------------------	-ane
7	-epine	-epin	-------------------	-epane
8	-ocine	----------	-ocin	-ocane
9	-azonine	----------	-azonane	-ocane

Some examples are given below:

Oxirane (ethylene oxide)	Oxerene	Aziridine	Pyridine

Numbering of the heterocyclic rings becomes essential when substituents are placed on the ring. Normally the hetero atom is designated at position 1 and the substituents are then counted around the ring giving the lowest possible numbers. In case the heterocyclic ring contains more than one hetero atom, the order of preference for numbering is Oxygen, Sulphur and Nitrogen. The position of a single hetero atom controls the numbering in a monocyclic compound.

Therefore, the study of heterocyclic chemistry focuses especially on unsaturated derivatives, and the preponderance of work and applications involves unstrained 5- and 6-membered rings. Included are pyridine, thiophene, pyrrole, and furan. Another large class of heterocycles refers to those fused to benzene rings. For example, the fused benzene analogs of pyridine, thiophene, pyrrole, and furan are quinoline, benzo-thiophene, indole, and benzofuran, respectively. The fusion of two benzene rings gives rise to a third large family of compounds. Analogs of the previously mentioned heterocycles for this third family of compounds are acridine, dibenzothiophene, carbazole, and dibenzofuran, respectively. The unsaturated rings can be classified according to the participation of the heteroatom in the conjugated pi system.

Pyridine is a heterocyclic compound and the Nitrogen atom replacing C in the ring is known as "hetero atom".

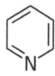

1.7.3   Classification of heterocyclic groups

1. Three membered Heterocyclic Compounds with One Hetero Atom.
2. Three membered Heterocyclic Compounds with Two Hetero Atoms.
3. Four membered Heterocyclic Compounds with One Hetero Atom.
4. Four membered Heterocyclic Compounds with Two Hetero Atom.
5. Five membered Heterocyclic Compounds with one Hetero Atom
6. Five membered Heterocyclic Compounds with Two Hetero Atoms
7. Six membered Heterocyclic Compounds with One Hetero Atom.

8. Six membered Heterocyclic Compounds with Two Hetero Atoms.
9. Six membered Heterocyclic Compounds with Three Hetero Atoms.
10. Six membered Heterocyclic Compounds with Four Hetero Atoms.
11. Six membered Heterocyclic Compounds with Five Hetero Atoms.
12. Seven membered Heterocyclic Compounds with One Hetero Atom.
13. Eight membered Heterocyclic Compounds with One Hetero Atom.
14. Nine membered Heterocyclic Compounds with One Hetero Atom.
15. Bicyclic ring systems derived from (5)
16. Bicyclic ring systems derived from (7)
17. Bicyclic ring systems derived from Pyridine (8)

1.7.4   Melting and boiling points of hetero atom compounds

MELTING AND BOILING POINTS OF HETERO ATOM COMPOUNDS							
Ring system with position of substituents	Substituents						
	H	CH$_3$	C$_2$H$_5$	COOH	COOC$_2$H$_5$	CONH$_2$	NH$_2$
Benzene	80	111	136	122	212	129	184
Pyridine (2)	115	129	148	137	243	107	57
Pyridine (3)	115	144	165	237	224	130	65
Pyridine (4)	115	145	168	315	219	156	158
Pyrrole (1)	130	113	129	95	178	166	175
Pyrrole (2)	130	148	164	208	39	174	285
Pyrrole (3)	130	143	179	148	40	152	---
Furan (2)	31	65	92	133	34	142	---
Furan (3)	31	66	92	122	175	168	---

Thiophene (2)	84	113	134	129	218	180	---
Thiophene (3)	84	115	186	138	208	178	146
Pyrazole (1)	68	127	136	102	213	141	---
Pyrazole (3)	68	204	209	214	158	159	38
Pyrazole (4)	68	206	247	275	78	---	81
Isoxazole (3)	95	118	138	149	---	134	---
Isoxazole (5)	95	122	138	146	---	174	---
Imidazole (1)	90	196	208	---	218	---	315
Imidazole (2)	90	144	80	164	178	312	---
Imidazole (4)	90	56	76	281	157	215	---
Pyrimidine (2)	124	138	152	197	64	166	127
Pyrimidine (4)	124	141	140	240	39	194	151
Pyrimidine (5)	124	153	175	270	38	212	170
Pyrazine (2)	55	137	155	225	50	189	118

Names in italics are retained by IUPAC

1.7.5. Basic Heterocyclic ring system nuclei with one Hetero atom

SATURATED			UNSATURATED		
THREE MEMBERED HETEROCYCLIC NUCLEI					
NITROGEN	**OXYGEN**	**SULPHUR**	**NITROGEN**	**OXYGEN**	**SULPHUR**
Azeridine	Oxirane	Thiirane	Azirene	Oxirene	Thiirene

FOUR MEMBERED HETEROCYCLIC NUCLEI					
NITROGEN	**OXYGEN**	**SULPHUR**	**NITROGEN**	**OXYGEN**	**SULPHUR**
Azitidine	Oxitane	Thietane	Azete	Oxete	Thiete

30

FIVE MEMBERED HETEROCYCLIC NUCLEI

NITROGEN	OXYGEN	SULPHUR		NITROGEN	OXYGEN	SULPHUR
Pyrrolidine	Oxolane	Thiolane		Pyrrole	Furan	Thiophene

SIX MEMBERED HETEROCYCLIC NUCLEI

NITROGEN	OXYGEN	SULPHUR		NITROGEN	OXYGEN	SULPHUR
Piperidine	Oxane	Thiane		Pyridine	Pyran	Thiopyran

SEVEN MEMBERED HETEROCYCLIC NUCLEI

NITROGEN	OXYGEN	SULPHUR		NITROGEN	OXYGEN	SULPHUR
Azepane	Oxepane	Thiepane		Azepine	Oxepine	Thiepine

EIGHT MEMBERED HETEROCYCLIC NUCLEI

NITROGEN	OXYGEN	SULPHUR		NITROGEN	OXYGEN	SULPHUR
Azocane	Oxocane	Thiocane		Azocine	Oxocine	Thiocine

NINE MEMBERED HETEROCYCLIC NUCLEI						
NITROGEN	OXYGEN	SULPHUR		NITROGEN	OXYGEN	SULPHUR
Azonane	Oxonane	Thionane		Azonine	Oxonine	Thionine

1.8 Nomenclature of various heterocyclic ring systems

Those containing one heteroatom are, in general, stable. Those with two heteroatoms are more likely to occur as reactive intermediates. The C-X-C bond angles (where X is a heteroatom) in oxiranes and aziridines are very close to 60° and the peripheral H-C-H bond angles are near to 180°.

1.8.1 Three-membered rings with one heteroatom

3-Atom Ring	Two Hetero Atoms		
		Diaziridine	HN−NH \/
		Oxaziridine	HN−CH$_2$ \ / O
		Diazirine	N=N \ / C R^1 R^2

Heteroatom	Saturated	Unsaturated
Boron	Borirane	Borirene
Nitrogen	Aziridine	Azirine
Oxygen	Oxirane	Oxirene
Phosphorus	Phosphirane	Phosphirene
Sulfur	Thiirane	Thiirene

Three membered with two hetero atoms

Heteroatom	Saturated	Unsaturated
Nitrogen	Diaziridine	Diazirine
Nitrogen/oxygen	Oxaziridine	NOT EXISTING
Oxygen	Dioxirane	NOT EXISTING

Some medicinally important three carbon membered monocyclic ring system name	Medicinal example	Chemical structure
Aziridine		
	Carboquone	

	Mitomycin	
Oxirane		
	Stramonin B	
	Fumagillin	
Thiirane		

Many others.........................

1.8.2 Four-membered rings with one heteroatom

Heteroatom	Saturated	Unsaturated
Nitrogen	Azetidine	Azete

34

Oxygen	Oxetane	oxete
Sulfur	Thietane	Thiete

Four-membered rings with two heteroatoms

Heteroatom	Saturated	Unsaturated
Nitrogen	Diazetidine	Diazete
Oxygen	Dioxetane	Dioxete
Sulfur	Dithietane	Dithiete

Some medicinally important four carbon membered monocyclic ring system name	Medicinal example	Chemical structure
β -lactam		
	Penicillin G	
	Ampicillin	

	Amoxicillin	
	Carbenicillin	
	Cephalosporin	
	Cephaloridine	
	Cephalexin	

Many thousands more...

1.8.3 Five-membered rings with one heteroatom

Heteroatom	Saturated	Unsaturated
Antimony	Stibolane	Stibole
Arsenic	Arsolane	Arsole
Bismuth	Bismolane	Bismole
Boron	Borolane	Borole
Nitrogen	Pyrrolidine	Pyrrole
Oxygen	Tetrahydrofuran	Furan
Phosphorus	Pholane	Phophole
Selenium	Selenolane	Selenophene
Silicon	Silacyclopentane	Silole
Sulphur	Tetrhydrothiophene	Thiophene
Tellutium	NOT EXISTING	Tellurophene
Tin	Stannolane	Stannole

Five-membered rings with two heteroatoms

The 5-membered ring compounds containing two heteroatoms, at least one of which is nitrogen, are collectively called:

* Azoles
* Thiazoles
* Isothiazoles

Heteroatom	Saturated	Unsaturated (and partially unsaturated)
Nitrogen/nitrogen	Imidazolidine	Imidazole
Nitrogen/oxygen	Oxazolidine	Oxazole
Nitrogen/sulfur	Thiazolidine	Thiazole
Oxygen/oxygen	Dioxolane	NOT EXISTING
Sulfur/sulfur	Dithiolane	NOT EXISTING

Five-membered rings with at least three heteroatoms

A large group of 5-membered ring compounds with *three* or more heteroatoms also exists. One example is the class of dithiazoles, which contain two sulphur atoms and one nitrogen atoms.

Heteroatom	Saturated	Unsaturated
3 Nitrogen	NOT EXISTING	Triazoles
2 Nitrogen 1 oxygen	NOT EXISTING	Oxadiazole
2 Nitrogen 1 sulfur	NOT EXISTING	Thiadiazole
1 Nitrogen 2 oxygen	NOT EXISTING	Dioxazole
1 Nitrogen 2 sulfur	NOT EXISTING	Dithiazole
4 Nitrogen	NOT EXISTING	Tetrazole
4 Nitrogen 1 Oxygen	NOT EXISTING	Oxatetrazole
4 Nitrogen 1 Sulfur	NOT EXISTING	Thiatetrazole
5 Nitrogen	NOT EXISTING	Pentazole

Some medicinally important five carbon membered monocyclic ring system name	Medicinal example	Chemical structure
Pyrrole / Azole		

	Viprynium	
Pyrrolidine		
	Pentolinium	
1-Pyrazoline		
2-Pyrazoline		
3-Pyrazoline		
	Phenazone	
Pyrazole		

	Sulphaphenazole	
Pyrazolidine		
	Phenylbutazone	
Imidazole		
	Metronidazole	
Imidazolidine		

	Clonidine	
2-Imidozoline		
	Naphazoline	
Triazole		
	Fluconazole	
Tetrazole		

	Pentetrazole	
4-Imidozoline		
	Carbimazole	
Furan		
	Frusemide	
Oxazole		
Oxazolidine		

	Furazolidine	
	Phenytoin	
Isoxazolidine		
	Cycloserine	
Isoxazole		

	Cloxacillin	
Thiazole		
	Thiobendazole	
1,3,4 Thiadiazole		
	Acetazolamide	

Many thousand others...

1.8.4   Six-membered rings with one heteroatom

Heteroatom	Saturated	Unsaturated	Ions
Antimony		Stibinin	
Arsenic	Arsinane	Arsinine	
Bismuth		Bismin	
Boron	Borinane	Borinine	Boratabenzene anion
Germanium	Germinane	Germine	
Nitrogen	Piperidine (Azinane is not used)	Pyridine (Azine is not used)	Pyridinum cation
Oxygen	Tetrahydropyran	Pyran (2H-Oxine is not used)	Pyrylium cation
Phosphorus	Phosphenane	Phosphinine	
Selenium			Selenopyrylium cation
Silicon	Silinane	Siline	
Sulfur	Thiane	Thiopyran (2H-Thiine is not used)	Thiopyrylium cation
Tin	Stanninane	Stannine	

Six-membered rings with two heteroatoms

Heteroatom	Saturated	Unsaturated
Nitrogen / nitrogen	Diazinane	Diazine
Oxygen / nitrogen	Morphuline	Oxazine
Sulfur / nitrogen	Thiomorpholine	Thiazine
Oxygen / oxygen	Dioxane	Dioxine
Sulfur / sulfur	Dithianane	Dithiin
Boron / nitrogen		1,2-dihydro-1,2-azaborine

Six-membered rings with three heteroatoms

45

Heteroatom	Saturated	Unsaturated
Nitrogen	Triazinane	Triazine
Oxygen	Trioxane	NOT EXISTING
Sulfur	Trithiane	NOT EXISTING

Six-membered rings with four heteroatoms

Heteroatom	**Saturated**	**Unsaturated**
Nitrogen	NOT EXISTING	Tetrazine

Carborazine is a six-membered ring with two nitrogen heteroatoms and two boron hetero-atom.

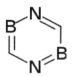

Six-membered rings with five heteroatoms

Heteroatom	Saturated	Unsaturated
Nitrogen	NOT EXISTING	Pentazine

Six-membered rings with six carbon monocyclic ring system

Some medicinally important six carbon membered monocyclic ring system name	Medicinal example	Chemical structure
Pyridine	I.N.H.	

Piperidine	Pethidine	
Pyridazine	Sulphamethoxy-pyridazine	
Pyrimidine	Pyrimethamine	
Pyrazine	Amiloride	
Piperazine	Diethylcarbamazine	
Barbituric acid	Amylobarbitone	
Morpholine	Morpholinium chloride	

Many thousand others.....................................

1.8.5 Seven-membered rings with one hetero-atoms

With 7-membered rings, the heteroatom must be able to provide an empty pi orbital (e.g., boron) for "normal" aromatic stabilization to be available; otherwise, homo-aromaticity may be possible. Compounds with one heteroatom include:

Heteroatom	Saturated	Unsaturated
Boron	NOT EXISTING	Borepine
Nitrogen	Azepane	Azepine
Oxygen	Oxepane	Oxipine
Sulfur	Thiepane	Thiepine

Seven-membered rings with two heteroatoms

Heteroatom	Saturated	Unsaturated
Nitrogen	Diazepane	Diazepine
Nitrogen/sulfur	NOT EXISTING	Thiazepine

Some medicinally important seven carbon membered monocyclic ring system name	Medicinal example	Chemical structure
Thiazepines		

Benzothiazepine	Diltiazem	
	Artesunate	
Tropone		
	Strychnine	

	Colchicine	
	Artemisinin	

1.8.6 Eight-membered rings with one hetero-atoms

Heteroatom	Saturated	Unsaturated
Nitrogen	Azocane	Azocine
Oxygen	Oxocane	Oxocine
Sulfur	Thiocane	Thiocine

Some medicinally important eight carbon membered monocyclic ring system name	Medicinal example	Chemical structure

Azocine		
	Sosegon	
Azocaine		
	Guanethidine	

1.8.7 Nine-membered rings with one hetero-atoms

Heteroatom	Saturated	Unsaturated
Nitrogen	Azonane	Azonine
Oxygen	Oxonane	Oxonine
Sulfur	Thionane	Thionine

Some medicinally important nine carbon membered monocyclic ring system name	Medicinal example	Chemical structure

Oxonine		
Thionine		

Many hundred others.................................

1.9 Nomenclature of various fused heterocyclic ring system

Some medicinally important fused ring systems	Medicinal example	Chemical structure
Indole	Indomethacin	
Indoline	Indocaine	
Isoindoline	Chlorthalidone	

Benzimidazole	Thiabendazole	
Xanthine	Caffeine, theobromine	
Purine	Mercaptopurine	
Quinoline	Quinine	
	Chloroquine	
Isoquinoline	Papaverine	

Pteridine	Folic acid, methotrexate, triamterene	
Tropane	Atropine	
	Hyoscine	
	Cocaine	
	Pethidine	
Phenothiazine	Chlorproma-zine	

	Promethazine	
Phenantherine		
	Cholesterol	

Many hundred others...

1.10 Diazanaphthalene

(medicinally important class of aromatic heterocyclic compounds
consisting of a naphthalene double ring)

Diaza-naphthalene are a class of aromatic heterocyclic chemical
compounds.

Consisting of a naphthalene double ring in which two of the carbon
atoms have been replaced with nitrogen atoms.

There are 10 potential isomers of naphthyridines which differ by the
location of the nitrogen atoms.

Examples are as follows:

Naphthalene

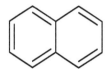

Quinoline

1,8-naphthyridine

NAME	CHEMICAL STRUCTURE
Cinnoline	
Quinazoline	
Phthalazine,	
Benzopyrazine / quinoxaline,	

Naphthyridine	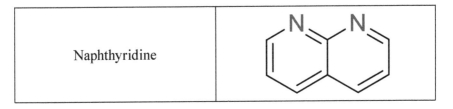

Many hundred others..

1.11 Medicinally important heterocyclic compounds

Acridine		
	Proflavine	
	Tetracycline	
	Doxycycline	

	Oxytetracycline	
	Chlortetracycline	
	Minocycline	
Quinoline		
Isoquinoline		

	Quinine	
	Quinidine	
	Chloroquine	
	Hydroxychloroquine	

Many hundred others...

1.12 Arrangement of heterocyclic ring systems

When one heterocyclic ring is present, it is considered as "parent compound".

In case of more than one heterocyclic ring is present, the preference of a ring containing nitrogen is preferred.

The fused heterocyclic compounds are named by giving the example of "purine" which has both the pyrimidine and imidazole heterocycles. Among the two hetero systems (purine), the pyrimidine is considered as the base component due to its large size but this explanation is not complete till the fusion is not described. The fusion of imidazole is from peripheral side. It is also evident that the "d" side of pyrimidine is involved in fusion with imidazole to form purine.

1.13 Functional groups

The functional groups are the atoms or group of atoms that replaces Hydrogen atom from the hydrocarbons. They may be -OH, -COOH, -CO, -CHO, -Cl, -COCl, -COOR etc. They are responsible for the characteristics of a molecule. The following is a list of common functional groups. In the formulas, the symbols R and R' denotes attached Hydrogen or a hydrocarbon side chain of any length or group of atoms.

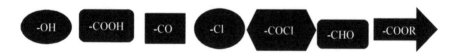

Chemical class	Group	Formula	Graphical Formula	Prefix	Suffix	Example
Alcohol	Hydroxyl	ROH		hydroxy-	-ol	 Methanol
Aldehyde	Aldehyde	RCHO		oxo-	-al	 Acetaldehyde
Alkane	Alkyl	RH		alkyl-	-ane	 Methane
Alkene	Alkenyl	$R_2C=CR_2$		alkenyl-	-ene	 Ethylene
Alkyne	Alkynyl	$RC\equiv CR'$		alkynyl-	-yne	$H-C\equiv C-H$ Acetylene
Amines	Primary amine	RNH_2		amino-	-amine	 Methylamine
	Secondary amine	R_2NH		amino-	-amine	 Dimethylamine
	Tertiary amine	R_3N		amino-	-amine	 Trimethylamine
Carboxylic acid	Carboxyl	RCOOH		carboxy-	-oic acid	 Methanoic acid
Ester	Ester	RCOOR'			-oate	 Methyl methanoate
Ketone	Ketone	RCOR'		keto-, oxo-	-one	 Butanone

1.14 Carbocyclic or homocyclic chemistry / carbocyclic or homocyclic compounds

(Homocyclic Chemistry / Homocyclic compounds)

A compound having 6 carbon atoms in the ring is called "carbocyclic or Homocyclic compound. The branch of chemistry is known as "homocyclic or carbocyclic chemistry".

OH

Followings are the examples of carbocyclic or homocyclic...........

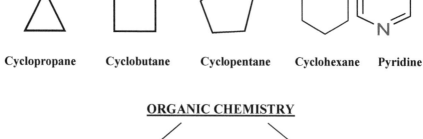

Cyclopropane   Cyclobutane   Cyclopentane   Cyclohexane   Pyridine

ORGANIC CHEMISTRY

Carbocyclic / homocyclic chemistry   Heterocyclic chemistry

Carbocyclic / homocyclic compound   Heterocyclic compound

- <u>Carbocyclic or homocyclic compound:</u>

Cyclic compound whose ring contains only one type of atom i.e., Carbon atoms based upon the ring system or a cyclic organic compound containing all corresponding Carbon atoms in the respective ring formation.

- <u>Heterocyclic compound:</u>

Cyclic compound whose ring contains more than one kind of atom apart from Carbon atom e.g., N, O, S, P (especially N atom). The compound to be designated as heterocyclic must have the removal of at least one carbon atom from the ring system.

Carbocyclic or homocyclic chemistry:

Toluene   Benzoic acid

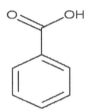

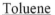
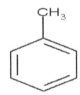

Heterocyclic chemistry: e.g. Pyridine
(basic unit to constitute D.N.A. / R.N.A

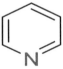
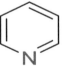

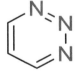   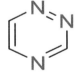   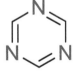

Triazines

Thiopyran   Furan

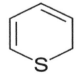   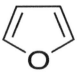

1.15 Classification of drugs

The medicinal compounds are broadly classified into the following groups:

1.15.1   By pharmacological or biological effects

Medicinal compounds are grouped based upon their biological actions e.g., analgesics, antipyretics, antibiotics, anti-hypertensives etc. In this category, the focus is placed on the pharmacological / biological activity of the compounds while these compounds may not be from the same chemical group. However, it should be emphasized that such grouping may contain large variety of drugs. This is because there is very less chance that the disease/s can be cured in a single way.

There are many biological systems by which the medicinal chemist can target to get the desired results. Moreover, another point is that most of the medicinal compounds may not fit into one category. For example, a sedative might act as anticonvulsant or certain antihistamines may act to reduce the gastric acid secretion. The antibacterial drugs are the realistic group of medicines that are classified according to their pharmacological / biological effects.

1.15.2   By chemical structure

Many medicinal compounds having same common skeleton are grouped together e.g., penicillin, barbiturates, opiates, steroids and catecholamines etc. However, it may be mistaken that all the medicinal compounds of certain chemical groups have the same pharmacological / biological action. It is also important to consider that most of the drugs may act at several sites of the body and have various pharmacological effects. The opiates, penicillin and cephalosporins are the groups of drugs with similar basic chemical skeleton.

1.15.3 By target system

The medicinal compounds falling under this category are classified according to their effect on certain target system in the body, usually involving chemical messenger for example, antihistamine, cholinergic etc. It is still a system with different stages for example, all the antihistamines to be the similar medicinal compounds since the system by which histamine is synthesized, released, interacts with its receptor and finally vanished, can be attacked at all these stages.

1.15.4 By site of action

These are the medicinal compounds which are grouped according to the enzyme or receptor with which they interact. For example, anticholinesterases are a group of medicinal compounds which act through inhibition of the enzyme acetylcholinesterase. Presently the pharmaceutical industries try their best to develop a new medicinal compound that targets the enzyme system only based upon the fact that no other physiological part of the body be affected by action of that particular drug.

1.16 Pharmacologically influential physicochemical properties of organic medicinal agents:

- ❑ Solubility
- ❑ Partition coefficient
- ❑ Ionization
- ❑ Hydrogen bonding
- ❑ Protein binding
- ❑ Chelation
- ❑ pKa value
- ❑ Redox potential
- ❑ Isomers

- ☐ Steric effect
- ☐ Surface activity
- ☐ Lipophilicity

Solubility	Spectroscopy	pKa	Partition coefficient
Melting point	Particle size	Shape	Crystal properties and Polymorphism
Surface area	Microscopy	Powder flow	
Stability studies	Excipient compatibility	Compression properties	

- ❖ **The solubility expression: in terms of its affinity/ lipophilicity or repulsion/phobicity for either an aqueous (hydro) or lipid (lipo-) solvent.**

- ☐ hydrophilic...................water-loving
- ☐ lipophobic....................lipid-hating
- ☐ lipophilic......................lipid-loving
- ☐ hydrophobic.................water-hating
- ☐ Examination of the structure of chloramphenicol (indicates the presence of both lipophilic (nonpolar) and hydrophilic (polar) groups and substituents. The presence of oxygen and nitrogen containing functional groups usually enhances water solubility. While lipid solubility is enhanced by non-ionizable hydrocarbon chains and ring systems.

66

1.16.1   Ionization

o   Ionization or ionisation, is the process by which an atom or a molecule acquires a negative or positive charge by gaining or losing electrons to form ions, often in conjunction with other chemical changes.

o   *Ionisation = protonation or deprotonation resulting in charged molecules.*

o   Ionization can result from the loss of an electron after collisions with subatomic particles, collisions with other atoms, molecules and ions, or through the interaction with electromagnetic radiation.

o   Heterolytic bond cleavage and heterolytic substitution reactions can result in the formation of ion pairs.

o   Ionization can occur through radioactive decay by the internal conversion process, in which an excited nucleus transfers its energy to one of the inner cell electrons causing it to be ejected.

o   *(sodium chloride, Hydrochloic acid, Carbonic acid, Nitric acid etc.,)*

Factors affecting ionization are;

❖   pH of the medium
❖   pKa (acid dissociation constant) of the drug
❖   Acidic drug tend to ionize in more basic medium
❖   pH – pKa = log (ionized / nonionzized)
❖   Basic drug tend to ionize in more acidic medium
❖   pH – pKa = log (nonionized / ionized)

1.16.2   Factors effecting physical degradation of medicinal compounds:

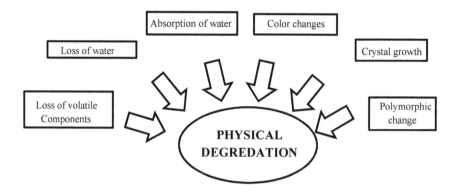

1.16.3 Importance of pH level in the body

☐ The pH level of water measures how acidic it is (pH stands for potential hydrogen, referring to how much hydrogen is mixed with the water.) 7 is a balanced pH for water. Anything below 7 indicates the water is acidic, and if it is above 7 it is alkaline. ... This is important because the human body has a natural pH of 7.4.

☐ The body's pH level influences its health. The acid-base balance of your blood is significant for normal daily function, healing and digestion.

☐ The acidity or alkalinity level of your body is determined by a pH, potential of hydrogen, scale.

☐ The scale ranges from zero, which indicates high acidity 0-5.9 and highly alkaline from 7-16, which indicates high alkalinity. Optimal acid-base balance is a pH of 7.35 to 7.45, which indicates the body is alkaline. In the event of acidosis or alkalosis, neutralizing pH is necessary.

FLUID	pH
Aqueous humor	7.2
Blood	7.4
Colon	5.8
Duodenum (fasting)	4.4-6.6

Saliva	6.4
Small intestine	6.5
Stomach (fasting)	1.4-2.1
Stomach (random)	3-7
Sweat	5.4
Urine	5.5-7.0

1.16.4 Chelation

Chelation is the process by which a molecule encircles and binds to the metal and removes it from tissue.

❏ Complex formation involving a metal ion and polar groupings of a single molecule.
❏ In haem, the Fe^{2+} ions chelated by the porphyrin ring.
❏ Chelation can be used to remove an ion from participation in biological reactions,
❏ as: (the chelation of Ca^{2+} of blood by EDTA, which thus acts as an anticoagulant.)

1.17 Principles of drug design

Metabolism

Metabolism is a term that is used to describe all chemical/bio-chemical reactions involved in maintaining the living state of the cells and organism.

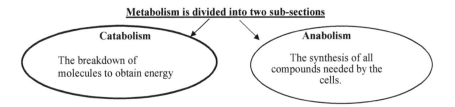

Metabolism is divided into two sub-sections

Catabolism
The breakdown of molecules to obtain energy

Anabolism
The synthesis of all compounds needed by the cells.

- Metabolism plays a central role in the elimination of drugs, after brake down in many fragments, and other foreign compounds (xenobiotics) from the body.
- Drug metabolism reactions are called as "detoxification" or "de-toxication".

Drug metabolism reactions have been divided in two phases.

Phase I (functionalization)	**Phase II** (conjugation)

(oxidative, reduction and hydrolytic biotransformation)	The purpose of these reactions on the other hand is to attach small, polar and ionizable endogenous compounds as glucuronic acid, sulphate, glycine to form water soluble conjugated products.
• The purpose of these reactions is to introduce a polar functional group into the xenobiotic molecule by direct introduction or by modification.	
	Conjugation takes place by the activity of enzymes.
• Phase I reactions tend to provide a functional group in the molecule that can undergo subsequent phase II reactions.	**Polar**: water soluble **Metabolite:**
	During or after the metabolism, the parent compound is converted to a newer active or inactive compound that is called "metabolite".

Phase I (functionalization)	**Phase II** (conjugation)
Phase I reactions not always produce hydrophilic or pharmacologically inactive metabolites.	Conjugated metabolites are excreted in urine and are generally devoid of any pharmacological activity or toxicity.

Oxidative reactions	
✓ Oxidation of aromatic compounds ✓ Oxidation of olefins ✓ Oxidation of C atoms (aliphatic and aromatic) ✓ Oxidation of C-N systems ✓ Oxidation of C-S systems ✓ Oxidation of alcohols and aldehydes ✓ Oxidation of C-Heteroatom system	✓ Glucuronic acid conjugation ✓ Sulphate conjugation ✓ Amino acids conjugation ✓ Glutathione/Mercapturic acid conjugation (protects the body) ✓ Acetylation (no biological activity) ✓ Methylation (no biological activity)

1.17.1 Site of drug biotransformation

❖ Although biotransformation reactions may take place in many tissues, but the liver is, by far, the most important organ in drug metabolism.

❖ Liver is rich in almost all the drug metabolizing enzymes.

❖ The liver is well perfused organ and plays a major role in detoxification and metabolism of endogenous and exogenous compounds present in the blood stream.

❖ Orally administered drugs that are absorbed through G.I.T., must pass through liver. Therefore, they are susceptible to

"hepatic metabolism "before reaching the systemic circulation. "Hepatic metabolism" is called as: *first pass effect ".*

Metabolites may also be pharmacologically active, sometime more than the parent drug.

• Chemical inactivation of a drug by converting it into a more water-soluble compound or metabolite, that can be excreted from the body. LIVER is the primary site of metabolism of drugs.

- The chemical reactions of metabolism are organized into metabolic pathways.
- These pathways allow the basic chemicals from nutrition / food or drugs to be transformed through a series of steps into another chemical, by a sequence of enzymes.
- Enzymes are crucial to metabolism because they allow organisms to drive desirable reactions that require energy.
- As enzymes acts as a catalyst, they allow these reactions to proceed quickly and efficiently.
- Enzymes also allow the regulation of metabolic pathways in response to changes in the cell's environment or signals from other cells.

1.17.2   Development of new medicinal compound

- In general, the medicinal chemist is developing drugs with four objectives in mind:
    - To increase activity.
    - To reduce side effects.
    - To provide easy and efficient administration to the patient.
    - To ease synthesis. This is a substantial part of the medicinal chemistry.

There are many chemicals to whome is called the drugs and are taken every day and they have biological effect.

- Morphine ---------- acts to bring pain relief,
- Snake venom----- causes death,
- Strychnine---------- in male dysfunction but may cause death,
- LSD----------------- acts to produce hallucination,
- Coffee-------------- acts to wake up,
- Penicillin------------ reacts with bacterial cell to kill them,
- Sugar---------------- reacts with the tongue to produce a sense of taste,

- Tea, coffee and cocoa (containing caffeine) Caffeine is a stimulant drug,
- Nicotine.................. in the cigarette causes cancer,
- Alcohol.................. the most unsatisfactory drug.

- ❖ A) choose a disease.
- ❖ B) choose a drug target.
- ❖ C) identify a bioassay.
- ❖ D) find "LEAD COMPOUND" (the active principle isolated).
- ❖ E) isolate and purify the lead compound.
- ❖ F) determine the structure of a lead compound.
- ❖ G) identify structure – activity relationship (SAR).
- ❖ H) identify the pharmacophore.
- ❖ I) improve pharmacokinetic properties
- ❖ J) study drug metabolism and test for toxicity
- ❖ K) design a manufacturing process
- ❖ L) carry out clinical trials
- ❖ M) patent the drug market the drug and make profits.
- ❖ *The discovery and development of a new basic drug may take 5 to 10 years before it is marketed.*

1.18 Antibiotics

Antibiotic are the chemical compounds or substances obtained from various kinds of microorganisms which destroy or inhibits the growth of other kinds of microorganisms at low concentration. The term antibiotic was first employed by Waksman that antibiotics are substances which are produced by microorganisms and are antagonistic to refer to the substances produced by growth of other microbes. Later it was suggested broadening the definition to include inhibitory substances of plant or animal origin. Afterwards, an antibiotic be defined as "a compound possessing inhibitory, i.e., static, degenerative, killing activities for vegetable, or animal microorganisms such as viruses, rickettsia, bacteria, actinomycetes, fungi, algae or protozoa.

It is a well-defined reproducible substance formed originally by living cells and first isolated from such cells or their metabolic products by chemical manipulation or by a biosynthetic process." In a wider, though not accepted globally definition, antibiotics are sb-ubstances of biological origin which, without possessing enzyme character, in low concentrations inhibit cell growth process.

The development of the antibiotic drugs is unquestionably one of the major advances in chemotherapy in recent years. Not only has the practice of medicine been basically influenced by the introduction of these substances, but certain of the antibiotic drugs have attained exclusively important applications in nutrition, agriculture and the food processing industry. Before 1935, the search of chemical agents active against bacterial infections in the blood serum was unproductive till the "sulphonamide drugs" were introduced. With the advent of the antibiotics, the use of sulphonamide drugs began to decline.

Uptill now, thousands and thousand antibiotics have been isolated from microbial origin and more than 50,000 are produced syntheticall or by semi-synthetic processes. These antibiotics are among the most efficient compounds to treat the infectious diseases. Antibiotics are also used in veterinary medicine, as plant protection agents, animal feed and food preservatives.

1.18.1   Chemotherapeutic agents and development of chemotherapy

To combat pathogenic microorganisms such as viruses, bacteria, fungi, protozoa and also more highly organized parasites such as worms, which are responsible of numerous diseases, medicines today made use of large variety of *antibiotics* and *chemotherapeutic agents*. The treatment of infectious and cancer diseases by means of these *chemical agents* is given the general term *chemotherapy*. The aim of chemotherapy is to achieve a selective toxic action, for example in the system drug-host-parasite, the drug must be more toxic for the parasite (virus, bacterium, worm, cancer cell etc.) than for the host. In the ideal case, the drug should be highly toxic for the parasite and completely a toxic for the host.

Antibiotics and chemotherapeutic agents fundamentally differ from each other in how they are produced and not in their action and use. Antibiotics are substances which are metabolically produced by *microorganisms*, whereas chemotherapeutic agents are synthetically prepared compounds which do not occur in nature. There is, however, no sharp distinction between these two classes of compounds. Active compounds which have been prepared by modification of the structure of an antibiotic, for example semi-synthetically, such as certain penicillin, cephalosporins, kanamycin, sisomicin, tetracyclines, rifamycin, lincomycin, bleomycin or compounds which had originally been detected and isolated as metabolic products of micro-organisms but which are today prepared by total synthesis, such as chloramphenicol, tetracycline group, penicillin etc. are also classified as antibiotics. Even the chloramphenicol analogues, thiamphenicol and azidamfenicol, which do not occur in nature and are obtained by total synthesis, are classed as antibiotics.

The chemotherapeutic agents are used to combat the most varied types of pathogenic parasites (viruses, fungi, bacteria, protozoa, worms) as well as cancer, but majority of antibiotics are practically confined to the treatment of infections caused by *bacteria and virus*. A relatively small number of antibiotics are therapeutically used in mycoses (griseofulvin and polyene antibiotics), against trichomonads (hachimycin), against amoebae (erythromycin, paromycin, thiamphenicol, tetracyclines), against nematodes (avermactins) as well as cancer (mitomycin C, bleomycin, peplomycin, streptozocin, dactinomycin, daunorubicin, doxorubicin, mitramycin, aclarubicin). The great development of chemotherapy in the last few decades has led to a marked decrease in the rate of deaths caused by infectious diseases.

1.18.2 Historical data outlining the development of chemotherapy:

YEAR	DESCRIPTION	STRUCTURE
1632	First importation of cinchona bark from Peru to Europe to treat malaria.	
1683	Discovery of bacteria by A. van Leuwenhoek, the founder of microbiology.	
1820	P. J. Pelletier and J. B. Caventou isolated the alkaloid *quinine* from the cinchona bark, the active constituent against malaria.	
1844	Preparation of cis-dichloro-diammine-platinum(II) by M. Peyrone. The cytotoxic properties of this square platinum complex were discovered by B. Rosenberg et al. in 1969. Today, cisplatinum is successfully employed in the treatment of cancer (e.g. testicular carcinoma).	
1871	Isolation of *emetine*, the alkaloid active component obtained from ipecac which was known in Brazil for curative effect against amoebic dysentery.	

1876	Robet Koch showed for the first time with the *anthrax bacillus* that a living microorganism was the specific cause of an infectious disease. This was the beginning of medical bacteriology.	
1877	L. Pasteur and J. F. Joubert observed that two different microorganisms did not grow equally well in the same culture medium and that one microorganism was apparently damaged by the other one.	
1882	Robert Koch discovered the tuberculosis pathogen (*mycobacterium tuberculosis*).	
1889	Principle of the concept *"antibiosis"* was defined by P. Vuillemin and from which the term *"antibiotic "*is derived.	
1892	Discovery of the anti-infective properties of the synthetically prepared 8-hydroxyquinoline derivative *chiniofon*. About 30 years later, this compound was successfully used in the treatment of amoebic dysentery.	

1896	B. Gosio discovered that microorganisms can form substances active against bacteria. He observed that *"mycophenolic acid"* isolated from *Penicillium brevicompactum* inhibit the growth of *Bacillus anthracis* (anthrax bacillus). Mycophenolic acid shows also antifungal, anti-viral and antitumor properties.	
1899	R. Emmerich and O. Low isolated" pyocyanase" from cultures of *Pseudomonas aeruginosa*, found to be effective against various bacteria and at first wrongly referred to as an enzyme mixture.	
1907	Paul Ehrlich and S. Hata discovered by systematic research "salvarsan", a synthetic arsenic compound which is very effective against trypanosomes and the spirochete *treponema palladium* (syphilis pathogen).	

1910	Salvarsan was introduced into clinical medicine and thus constituted the beginning of modern chemotherapy.	
1917	R. Greig-Smith observed that various actinomycetes produce substances with antibacterial activity.	
1920	The pharmaceutical company, Bayer Leverkusen, Germany introduced the synthetically prepared "suramin" as a medicament against the African sleeping sickness caused by *trypanosomes*. Suramin has also been found to possess ant filarial activity.	
1928	The first industrially produced and therapeutically applied antibiotic "pyocyanase" to control anthrax.	

1929	Alexander Fleming discovered penicillin (beginning of the antibiotic era). He observed that a staphylococcal culture was inhibited in its growth on an agar plate by the metabolic product of a contaminating mould colony (*penicillium notatum*). This metabolic product was called "penicillin ". Shortly after the beginning of the world war II, H. W. Florey and E. Chain succeeded in isolating the first small amount of impure but clinically effective penicillin. Due to various difficulties (instability of penicillin, lack of efficient production methods, etc.), this valuable antibiotic became available as a therapeutic only at the end of the war, as a result of gigantic Anglo-American research and development programme.	
1932	The synthetic azo dye stuff "prontosil" was discovered by G. Domagk.	

1934	Discovery of the synthetic antimalarial agent "chloroquine" by H. Andersag. The high activity and therapeutic value of this 4-aminoquinoline derivative was rediscovered in the United States during the course of an antimalarial development program in World war II. Chloroquine was introduced into practical medicine in 1947.	
1934	The "prontosil" became the first representative of the "sulphonamide" group to be introduced in therapy (beginning of the sulphonamide era). In the same year, J. Trefouel detected that the *in vivo* activity of "prontosil" was attributed to its metabolite (sulphanilamide) *p-aminobenzenesulphonamide*. Practically all the present day valuable sulphonamides are derived from "sulphanilamide", mainly by substitution at the N1 position by heterocyclic groups.	
1938	Discovery of the Sulphacetamide	

	Sulphapyridine	
	Sulphathiazole (imino + amino tautomers)	
1938	R. J. Dubos isolated "tyrocidine" and "gramicidin" from *Bacillus brevis*.	

1940	S. A. Waksman and H. B. Woodruff isolated "actinomycin D" from *"sreptomyces antibioticus "*, which 12 years later, proved to be the first cytostatically active antibiotic in man.	
1942	Discovery of the cytostatic action of "mechlorethamine" (nitrogen mustard). This synthetic, classical representative of the group of alkylating agents is particularly active against lymphomas.	
1942	G. F. Gause and M. G. Brazhnikova discovered and isolated "gramicidin S "from a strain of *bacillus brevis*.	
1944	Discovery of the pyrimidine sulphonamides Sulphadiazine (structure) Sulphamethazine (structure) Sulphamerazine (structure)	

	Sulphisoxazole (sulphifurazole) (structure)	
1944	Discovery of the antibacterially active a synthetic derivative "nitrofurantoin".	
1944	S. A. Waksman et al. discovered the antibiotic "streptomycin". It was isolated from "*streptomyces griseus* "and proved to be particularly active against tuberculosis bacteria, *(mycobacterium tuberculosis)*.	

| 1945 | B. A. Johnson et al. isolated "bacitracin" from" *Bacillus licheniformis* "and in the same year, Giuseppe Brotzu discovered (in cagliari Sardinia) the broad- spectrum antibiotic activity of "penicillin N and cephalosporin C "in the culture filtrate of "*Cephalosporium acremonium*". Isolation and structure elucidation of these antibiotics were later accomplished by E.P. Abraham and G. G. F. Newton in 195 and 1959 respectively. Cephalosporin C is the parent substance from which the clinically important cephalosporins are derived. | |

Many thousand others..

1.18.3   Discovery of important antibiotics since 1945

YEAR	NAME	YEAR	NAME
1947	Chloramphenicol	1963	Gentamycin
	Polymyxin		Daunorubicin
1948	Chlortetracycline	1964	Cephaloridine
1949	Neomycin		Dicloxacillin
1950	Oxytetracycline		Amoxacillin
1951	Fumagillin	1965	Carbencillin
	Nystatin		Ticarcillin
	Viomycin	1966	Rifampin
1952	Thiamphenicol		Clindamycin
	Erythromycin		Bleomycin

	Carbomycin	1967	Tobramycin
	Puromycin		Doxorubicin
1953	Tetracycline		Cephalexin
	Penicillin V	1969	Fosfomycin
	Leucomycin		Flucloxacillin
	Mithramycin	1970	Cefazolin
1954	Oleandomycin		Furbucillin
	Spiramycin	1971	Cefuroxime
1955	Cycloserine		Cephamendole
	Novobiocin		Cefoxitin
1956	Amphoteracin B	1972	Cefadroxil
	Vancomycin		Amikacin
1957	Kanamycin		Rosaramicin
	Demeclocycline	1974	Cefotiam
1958	Mitomycin C		Cefmetazole
1959	Streptozocin		Clavulanic acid
1960	Methicillin (Methacycline)		Furazlpcillin
		1975	Netilmicin
	Doxycycline		Aclarubicin
1961	Oxacillin	1976	Cefotoxime
	Cloxacillin		Nocardicin
	Ampicillin		Ceftizoxime
	Minocycline	1977	Salbactam
	Rifamycin		Peplomycin
	Spectinomycin	1978	Ceftazidime
1962	Cephalothin		Ceftriaxone
	Lincomycin	1979	Sulfazecin
	Capreomycin	1980	Azthreonam
	Fusidic acid		

1.18.4 Discovery of important chemotherapeutic agents since 1945

Year	Name	Chemical structure
1946	Thioacetazone (thiosemicarbazones)	
1946	p-Aminosalicylic acid (p-aminobenzoic acid antagonists	
1946	Primaquin (8-aminoquinolines)	
1947	Diethylcarbamazine (piprazines)	H_3C-N $N \cdot CON(C_2H_5)_2$
1948	Methotrexate (folic acid antagonists)	

1951	Pyrimethamine (folic acid antagonists)	
1952	Isoniazid (isonicotinic acid) (4-pyridinecarboxylic acid)	
	Isonicotinic acid hydrazide	
1952	Thiotepa (alkylating agent)	
1953	Busulfan (alkylating agent)	
1953	Chlorambucil (alkylating agent)	

1953	6-Mercaptopurine (purine antagonists)	
1956	Ethionamide (thioisonicotinic acid amide)	
1956	Cyclophosphamide (alkylating agent)	
1957	5-Fluorouracil (pyrimidine antagonists)	
1957	5-Fluorocytosine (pyrimidine antagonists)	
1957	Trimethoprim (folic acid antagonists)	

1959	Sulfamethoxazol (p-aminobenzoic acid antagonists)	
1959	Sulfadimethoxine (p-aminobenzoic acid antagonists)	
1959	Metronidazole (nitroimidazole)	
1959	Cytarabine (nucleoside antagonists)	
1959	Idoxuridine (nucleoside antagonists)	

1960	Sulfadoxine (p-aminobenzoic acid antagonists)	
1960	Niclosamide (salicylanilides)	
1961	Ethambutol (ethylinediamines)	
1961	Thiabendazole, (benzimidazoles)	
1962	Nalidixic acid (pyridone carboxylic acids)	
1962	Carmustine (alkylating agents)	

1963	Procarbazine (methylhydrazine compounds)	
1964	Ornidazole (nitroimidazoles)	
1964	Niridazole (nitrothiazole)	
1965	Benznidazole (nitroimidazoles)	
1967	Clotrimazole (imidazole)	

1969	Micanazole (imidazole)	
1971	Mefloquine (quinine analogues)	
1973	Pimpidic acid (pyridone carboxylic acids)	
1973	Alafosfalin (phosphonopeptides)	$$\overset{L}{H_2N-CH-CO-NH-\overset{L}{CH}-PO_3H_2}$$ $$\underset{CH_3}{\mid}\qquad\qquad\underset{CH_3}{\mid}$$
1973	Fludalanine (D-Alanine antagonists)	$$F-CH_2-\overset{D}{\underset{\underset{NH_3^+}{\backslash}}{C}}-COO^-$$

1975	Praziquantel (piperazines)	
1976	Doxifluridine (nucleoside antagonists)	
1976	Ketoconazole (imidazole)	
1977	Acyclovir (nucleoside antagonists)	

Many thousand others...

The great discoveries achieved by S. A. Waksman and G. Brotzu caused a further acceleration in the already intensive investigation on the metabolic products of actinomycetes and fungi isolated from soil samples. The total research on antibiotics has undergone tremendous development since 1945, which in a relatively short period, has led to the discovery of many antibiotics still therapeutically used today.

A very important advance was the discovery of the mutual potentiation of sulphonamides, specially sulphamethoxazole (SMZ) and the 2,4-diaminopyrimidine derivative trimethoprim (TMP). This leads to the practical application of the combination SMZ + TMP in 5:1 ratio as broad-spectrum antibacterial agent exhibiting the same therapeutic effect as that of penicillins, cephalosporins, tetracyclines and chloramphenicol.

1.19 Natural occurrence of antibiotics

Over 5,000 antibiotics known to date, which have been isolated from biological sources, originate from bacteria or fungi. With regard to the number of antibiotics produced, the bacterial order of "*actinomycetales*", occupies the first position, followed by fungi (mainly fungi) and the bacterial order of "*Eubacteriales*". The antibiotics dealt with and the microorganisms from which they stem are briefly described as under:

Antibiotic	Microorganism

<u>**Bacteria**</u>

<u>**(Eubacteriales)**</u>

Bacitracins	*Bacillus (B) licheniformis*
Gramicidins	*B. brevis*
Polymyxins	*B. polymyxa, B. circulans*
B. polymyxa, B. circulans	
Sulfazecin	*Pseudomonas acidophila*
Pseudomonas acidophila	
Tyrocidins	*B. brevis*

(Actinomycetales)

Aclarubicin	*Streptomyces (S) galilaeus*
Amphomycin	*S. canus*
Amphotericin B	*S. nodosus*
Avermectins	*S. avermitilis*
L-Azaserine	*S. fragilis*
Bleomycins	*S. verticillus*
Candicidin	*S. griseus*
Capromycin	*S. capreolus*
Carbomycin	*S. halstedii*
Cephalosporin C	*S. spp.*
Cephamycin C	*S. clavuligerus*
Chloramphenicol	*S. venezuelae*
Chlortetracycline	*S. aureofaciens, S. sayamaensis*
	S. Lusitanus, S. omiyaensis
Clavulanic acid	*S. clavuligerus*
D- Cycloserine	*S. lavendulae*
Dactinomycin	*S. antibioticus*
Daunorubicin	*S. peucetius,*
	S. coeruleorubidus
Deacetoxycephalosporin C	*S. spp.*
Deacetylcephalosporin C	*S. spp.*
Demeclocycline	*S. aureofaciens*
6-Diazo-5-oxo-L-norlucine	*S. sp.*
Doxorubicin	*S. peucetius var. caesius*
Erythromycin	*S. erythreus*

Fosfomycin	*S. fradiae*
Fusidic acid	*Fusidium coccineum*
Gentamycins	*Micromonospora purpurea, M. Echinospora, M. sagamiensis*
Hachimycin	*S. hachijonsis, S. abikoensis*
Kanamycins	*S. kanamyceticus*
Leucomycins	*S. kitasatoensis*
Lincomycin	*S. lincolnensis*
Mikamycins A and B	*S. mitakaensis*
Mithramycin	*S. sp.*
Mitomycin C	*S. caespitosus*
Natamycin	*S. natalensis*
Neomycins	*S. fradiae*
Nocardicins	*Nocardia uniformis*
Novobiocin	*S. speroided, S. viveus*
Nystatin	*S. noursei*
Oleandomycin	*S. antibioticus*
Oxytetracycline	*S. rimosus, S. alboflavus, S. Aureofaciens, armillatus*
Paromomycins	*S. rimosus forma paromomycinus*
Penicillin N	*S. spp.*
Puromycin	*S. albo-niger*
Rifamycins	*Nocardia mediterranea*
Ristocetins	*Nocardia lurida*
Rosaramicin	*Micromonospora Rosaria*
Sarkomycin	*S. erythrochromogensis*
Sisomicin	*Micromonospora inyoensis*
Spectinomycin	*S. spectabilis*
Spiramycins	*S. ambofaciens*
Streptomycins	*S. griseus*
Streptonigrin	*S. flocculus*
Streotozocin	*S. achromogenes*
Tetracycline	*S. aureofaciens, S. sayamaensis,*
Thienamycin	*S. cattleya*

Tobramycin	*S. tenebrarius*
Vancomycin	*S. orientalis*
Viomycin	*S. flor*

Fungi

Cephalosporin C	*Cephaloporium spp.*
	Cephalosporium spp.
Deacetylcephalosporin C	*Cephalosporium spp.*
Fumagillin	*Aspergillus fumigatus*
Griseofulvin	*Penicillium janczewskil, P. Griseofulvum, P. nigricans*
Pecilocin	*Paecilomyces varioti Bainier var. antibioticus*
Penicillins	*Penicillium notatum, P. chrysogenum*

CHAPTER 2

BASIC PRINCIPLES AND TECHNIQUES OF MEDICINAL CHEMISTRY FOR ANTIBIOTICS / ANTIBACTERIALS

2.1 The bacterial / human cell

The antibacterial agent is considered as a selective only when the bacterial cell is affected by that particular agent rather than the animal cell. The bacterial and animal cells are quite different in their structure and in the biosynthetic pathways which processes inside them. The following is the difference described between the two:

BACTERIAL CELL	ANIMAL CELL
Has a cell wall and cell membrane.	has only a cell membrane.
Does not have a defined nucleus and the cell is relatively simple.	does have a defined nucleus contains a variety of structures called "organelles", mitochondria etc.
Biochemistry differs significantly as the bacteria may have to synthesize essential vitamins and must have the enzymes to catalyze these reactions.	vitamins are acquired from food since the reactions are not required.

The cell wall is crucial for the bacterial cell to survive. Apart from the bacteria have to survive a wide range of environments and osmotic pressures, but not the animal cells.

2.1.1   Detection of antibiotic activity

The detection process of an antibiotic action may be demonstrated in two ways:

1. It may be necessary to demonstrate that a particular microorganism produces an antibiotic or that an isolated substance has an antibiotic action. These points usually arise during the search of new antibiotics.
2. On the other side, the sensitivity of a specific microorganism (e.g. Clinically isolated pathogen) to an antibiotic or chemotherapeutic agent has to be determined. Such problems are to be dealt with in clinical-bacteriological laboratories.

The choice of method depends on the problem to be solved. Independent of the method chosen, one differentiates between a "bacteriostatic" and a "bactericidal" action. In bacteriostasis the inhibition of the growth takes place which disappears on the withdrawal of the antibiotic. A bactericidal action is the name given to irreversible damage that leads to the death of the cell. Often the same antibiotic can show both effects according to the experimental conditions and to the bacteria involved.

2.1.2   Minimal inhibitory concentration (MIC) of some basic antibiotics for different bacteria in µg/ml

GRAM- POSITIVE BACTERIA					
	Penicillin G	Amoxicillin	Cefamandole	Doxycycline	Gentamycin	Erythromycin
SA	0.006-0.3->100	0.05-0.1->100	0.25-1- 4	0.04-1.6->100	0.03-0.1-3->25	0.005-2->200
SPA	0.004-0.03	0.01-0.3	0.01-0.1	0.09-1.6-25	0.01-0.5-12->25	0.007-0.6
SF	0.15-1.5-3-6	0.4-1.6-3	16-64	1.6-50->100	0.1-1-25->100	0.1-1-5
SN	0.006-0.06	0.006-0.012	0.01-0.06	0.04-0.4	0.1-3-12->25	0.003-0.4

Staphylococcus aureus = (SA), Streptococcus pyogenes A = (SPA), Streptococcus faecalis = *(SF), Streptococcus pneumoniae = (SN)*

GRAM- NEGATIVE BACTERIA						
	Penicillin G	Amoxicillin	Cefamendole	Doxycycline	Gentamycin	Erythromycin
NG	0.006-0.06->5	0.01-0.2->5	0.01-2-16	0.09-0.4->4	0.8-1.5-3-6	0.004-6.25
PA	>100	>100	>100	25->100	0.1-0.5-12->100	>100
ST	3->100	0.4-1.5-3	0.2-1	0.5-2-10	0.2-1-4-8	>100
EC	>30	0.8-12.5->100	0.2-8->100	1.6-12.5->100	0.1-0.5-8->50	>100
KP	>100	50->100	0.1-4-64	6.3-50->100	0.1-0.4-8-50	>100
PM	30->100	1.5-12.5->100	0.2-8-64	4-50->100	0.4-1.5-16-50	>100
HI	0.3-3->100	0.1-0.5->100	0.1-1	1.6-6.3	0.4-1.5-3-8	0.1-1-5-20

Neisseria gonorrhoeae = *(NG), Pseudomonas aeruginosa* = *(PA), Salmonella typhi* = *(ST), Escherrichia coli* =*(EC), Klebsiella pneumoniae* = *(KP), Proteus mirabillis* = *(PM), Haemophilus infleunzae* = *(HI).*

The action of an antibiotic depends upon various following factors:

1. concentration of the antibiotic.
2. nature of the growth medium.
3. density of the population.
4. phase and rate of growth of the organism.
5. rate at which resistant mutants arises.

The general standard methods for detecting and determining an *in vitro* antibiotic activity includes:

1. serial dilution test (broth dilution test and agar dilution test)
2. plate diffusion test
3. streak test

2.1.3   Serial dilution test

In this test, the growth of the test organism is investigated in a liquid culture medium with decreasing concentrations of the antibiotic. After incubation (e.g.at 37 C), the lowest still inhibitory (bacteriostatic) concentration of the antibiotic, so called minimal inhibitory concentration (MIC) is given in mg/ml. In order to determine the minimal bacteriocidal concentration (MBC), it is necessary to expose the bacteria to a number of different concentrations of the antibiotic and after a shorter or longer period of time to transfer them to an antibiotic-free nutrient medium (subculture) to test if they again grow, or in other words if they are still capable of reproducing or not.

The agar dilution test is similar to the broth dilution test, but it does not allow the determination of the MBC because no subcultures can be made.

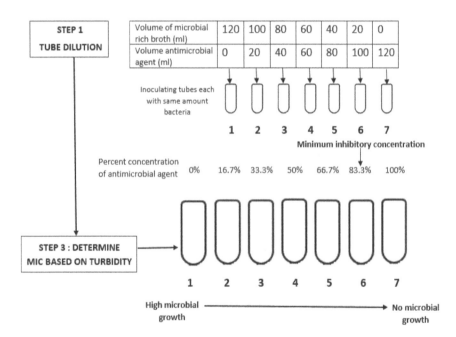

Minimum Inhibitory Concentration: Tube Dilution Assay is performed by constantly increasing the percent concentration of antimicrobial agent to microbial rich broth in a series of tubes. It is used to measure the Minimum Inhibitory Concentration [MIC] of an antimicrobial agent, which is the lowest concentration of antimicrobial agent which will inhibit the growth of microbes. The turbidity of the tubes indicates the amount of microbe growth, with the least turbid, or clear, tubes (tubes 6 and 7) correlating with the absence of microbes. The tube with no antimicrobial agent (tube 1) presents as opaque and most turbid because the microbes are able to flourish. As antimicrobial concentration increases, the turbidity decreases until the MIC is reached and microbes can no longer survive. Antimicrobials with low MICs are more effective than those with high MICs, as only a low dosage is necessary to eradicate microbes.

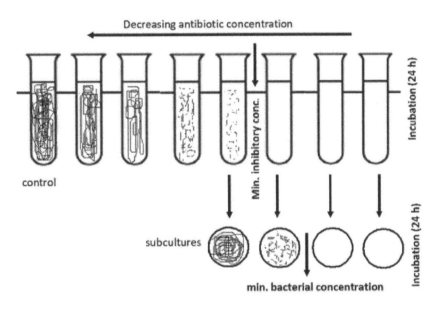

2.1.4   Plate diffusion test

In this test, the surface of an agar nutrient medium contained in a Petri dish is uniformly inoculated with a measured amount of the test bacterial culture. The test solutions are added to such a plate by pipetting them either into circular holes cut into the agar or into previously applied glass or metal cylinders or they are absorbed on to filter paper discs which are put on the surface of the agar **(disc test).**

The test substances diffuse into the agar with deceasing concentration towards the periphery. In the case of a positive reaction, an inhibitory zone can be observed after incubation (e.g. at 37 C) for several hours. The diameter of the inhibitory zone is proportional to the logarithm of the concentration of the antibiotic under constant experimental conditions:

- culture medium composition,
- thickness of agar,
- inoculum size,
- incubation time
- temperature etc.

2.1.5   Kirby-Bauer antibiotic testing

Kirby-Bauer is a test using antibiotic-impregnated paper disk to test whether particular bacteria are susceptible to specific antibiotics. A known quantity of bacteria is grown on agar plates in the presence of thin filter paper discs containing relevant antibiotics. If the bacteria are susceptible to a particular antibiotic, an area of clearing surrounds the wafer where bacteria are not capable of growing, it is called a zone of inhibition.

When comparing different antibiotics at known concentrations, the inhibitory zone diameter is taken as a measure of the antibiotic activity. Owing to its simplicity, the disc test is the most widely used method. An example is given below where the determination of the sensitivity to different antibiotics of a *Proteus strain,* isolated from the urine is shown. The amount of active drug in the disc is so adjusted that an inhibitory zone in the laboratory test indicates that an antibiotic effect can also be expected in the patient.

The formation of inhibitory zones round the disc with gentamycin (Gent), ampicillin (Amp), cephalothin (Ceph), streptomycin (strep) and nalidixic acid (NaI) is evidence for the activity of these compounds in contrast to penicillin G (Pen), tetracycline (Tetr), chloramphenicol (Chlor) and polymyxin B (Pol) which do not cause the formation of an inhibitory zone.

The picture obtained is called "antibiogram". On the basis of such antibiograms, the physician selects the antibiotic or chemotherapeutic agent which is most suitable for the therapy of the infection concerned.

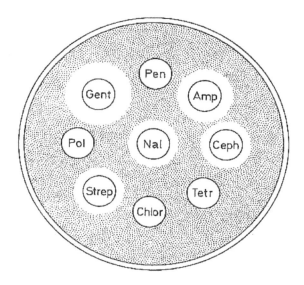

2.1.6   Streak test

This test permits the determination of the antibiotic effect of the test compound on several microorganisms simultaneously and is hence suitable for the determination of the *spectrum of activity.*

A filter paper disc impregnated with 10 mg of the antibiotic to be examined (penicillin G, tetracycline and griseofulvin) is placed in the middle of a Petri dish containing nutrient agar. The suspensions of the test organisms, as listed below, are streaked on the plate with a platinum loop.

1. *Staphylococcus aureus*
2. *Streptococcus*
3. *Escherichia coli*
4. *Pseudomonas aeruginosa*
5. *Candida albicans*
6. *Tricophyton*

❖ This method is used for testing individual isolates, specially actinomycetes which may be obtained from soil without any previous knowledge.

❖ The organism may come from one of the two methods.

❖ The purified isolate is streaked across upper third of plate containing medium which supports its growth as well as the test organism.

❖ A variety of media may be used for streaking the antibiotic.

❖ It is followed to grow for up to 7 days, in which time any antibiotic produced would have diffused a considerable distance from the streak.

❖ Test organisms are streaked at right angle to the original isolates and the extent of the inhibition of the various test organisms observed.

After incubation it is established that some of the test organisms have been inhibited in their growth in the diffusion area to different extents. The streak test is also particularly useful in testing for the formation of antibiotics by certain microorganisms, these being inoculated in the center of the agar plate and the indicator strains streaked on radially.

2.2 Screening, isolation, development and production of antibiotics

2.2.1 Screening

As microorganisms are very small, occur abundantly, and are thus readily dispersed, they are to be found everywhere although their most common habitat is in soil and ponds. One gram of soil sample contains millions of bacteria, fungi, protozoa and other microorganisms. Microorganisms grow in their natural environment in competition with one another, but without producing measurable quantities of antibiotics. Only when they are grown in the laboratory on an artificial culture medium, certain microorganisms are capable of producing antibiotics in large quantities as secondary metabolic products.

The fact that practically only bacteria and fungi are capable of producing substances which display a marked and selective toxic effect on (other) bacteria and fungi.

Most antibiotics have been discovered during screening programs. The various stages of such a program are from the dilution of the soil sample containing the microorganisms to the animal tests. The antibiotic produced by the microorganism is excreted into the culture solution.

Steps involved in antibiotic screening programme.

1. Preparation of dilution from soil samples or from other sources,
2. Preparation of agar plate by incubation with special nutrient medium,
3. Spraying of the test organism on the agar plate,
4. Evaluation of the sprayed plate to check inhibitory zone,
5. Streak test determination for the antibacterial spectrum,
6. Suitability test for submerged culture by keeping at 24 C for 7 days,
7. Fermenting culture in the fermenter culture,
8. Detection of chemotherapeutic activity,
9. Determination of chemical stability, structure activity relationship, chemical and instrumental analysis and rest of all chemical and physical work,
10. Determination of spectrum activity,
11. Determination of toxicity in animal,
12. Determination of therapeutic activity, tolerance, side effects *in vivo* (animal test).

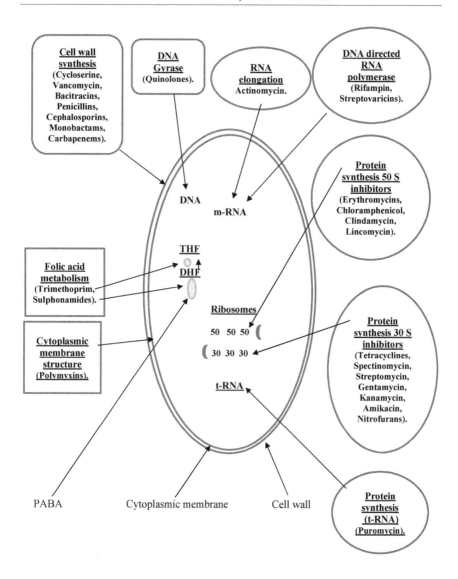

THF: Tetra-hydrofolic acid; DHF: Di-hydrofolic acid; DNA: Deoxyribonucleic acid t-RNA: Transfer Ribonucleic acid; m-RNA: Messenger Ribonucleic acid

2.2.2   Isolation

Complicated adsorption, precipitation or liquid-liquid extraction processes are frequently required to isolate the pure antibiotic.

Thus, for example:

Streptomycin is isolated from the filtered culture solution by adsorption on a cation exchanger.

Tetracyclines are obtained by precipitation of the calcium or magnesium complexes.

Benzylpenicillin

is extracted as the acid with butyl acetate, amyl acetate or chloroform from the cooled culture filtrate which is acidified to pH 2.0-2.5. for purification and concentration, benzyl-penicillin is re-extracted from the organic layer as an alkali metal salt by means of phosphate buffer (pH 7) and again extracted with butyl acetate as the acid after acidification. By the addition of salts soluble in organic solvents, benzyl-penicillin is precipitated or crystallized as the corresponding salt.

When an antibiotic isolated in the pure form has proved successful *in vivo* (animal test) with respect to its activity (ED_{50} in mg/kg, in the experimentally infected mouse) *, its tolerance is ascertained by determining the acute toxicity (LD_{50} in mg/kg) ** and the chronic toxicity during 6 months.

If there is a great enough safety margin between the active dose and the toxic dose, the antibiotic will be tested clinically in human after the formulation of suitable pharmaceutical preparations and the performance of stability tests.

If the clinical test is favorable, a development program is set up to find mutants of the microorganism which will give higher yields of antibiotic. This is usually accomplished by treating the microorganism with UV, X-rays or mutagenic substances.

* ED_{50} = effective dose 50% (dose at which 50% of the infected animals survive: when given per oral or subcutaneous).

** LD_{50} = lethal dose 50% (dose at which 50% of the animals die: when given intravenous).

2.2.3   Acute toxicity of various basic antibiotics in the mouse.

Antibiotic	LD50 (mg/kg)	Administration mode
Amikacin (sulphate)	300	i.v.
Amphotericin B	6	i.v.
Amphotericin B (methyl ester)	85	i.v.
Ampicillin	>10000	oral
Ampicillin (sodium salt)	6000	i.v.
Azlicillin (sodium salt)	4870	i.v.
Cefamandole	4000	i.v.
Cefazolin (sodium salt)	5000	i.v.
Cefoxitin	7950	i.v.
Cephalexin	1600-4500	oral
Cephalothin (sodium salt)	5000	i.v.
Chloramphenicol	2640	oral
Chloramphenicol	245	i.v.
Dibekacin (sulphate)	71	i.v.
Doxycycline (hydrochloride)	1650	oral
Doxycycline (hydrochloride)	244	i.v.
Erythromycin (estolate)	6450	oral
Fusidic acid (sodium salt)	975	oral
Gentamycin (sulphate)	77	i.v.
Kanamycin (sulphate)	280	i.v.
Neomycin (sulphate)	2880	oral
Neomycin (sulphate)	24	i.v.
Novobiocin	362	oral
Oxytetracycline (hydrochloride)	6696-7200	oral
Oxytetracycline (hydrochloride)	178	i.v.

Paromomycin (sulphate)	2275	oral
Paromomycin (sulphate)	160	i.v.
Penicillin G	3090	i.v.
Penicillin V	3940	oral
Polymyxin B (sulphate)	1187	oral
Polymyxin B (sulphate)	6.1	i.v.
Rifampin	858	oral
Streptomycin (sulphate)	9000	oral
Streptomycin (sulphate)	200	i.v.
Thiamphenicol	>5000	oral
Tobramycin (sulphate)	79	i.v.
Vancomycin (hydrochloride)	400	i.v.

2.2.4   Acute toxicity of various basic anti-tumor antibiotics in the mouse

Antibiotic	LD_{50} (mg/kg)	Administration mode
Aclarubicin	33.7	i.v.
Bleomycin (sulphate)	210	i.v.
Dactinomycin	0.7	i.v.
Daunorubicin (hydrochloride)	26	i.v.
Doxorubicin (hydrochloride)	20.8	i.v.
Mithramycin	0.35	i.v.
Mitomycin C	5	i.v

2.3   Mechanisms of biological activity of antibiotics

Owing to their inhibitory action on the cell metabolic reactions, antibiotics have proved to be of outstanding value in fundamental molecular biological research. The inhibitory action on a particular biosynthetic reaction by an antibiotic takes place by specific covalent or non-covalent binding which results in the inactivation of the substrate, enzyme or factor. This inhibition leads to the information of growth or death of the affected cell. To achieve, very often only very low concentrations of the antibiotic are required; it only requires a few molecules per cell of the most active antibiotic to inhibit the most sensitive microorganisms.

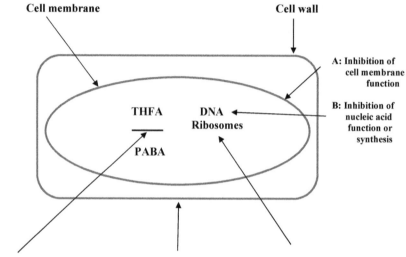

C: metabolism inhibition, D: cell wall synthesis inhibition, E: inhibition of protein synthesis.

A= Inhibition of membrane function: I.N.H and Amphotericin B.

B= Fluoroquinolones and Rifampin.

C= Sulphonamides and Trimethoprim.

D= β-lactams (Penicillin, Cephalosporins and Vancomycin.

E= Tetracyclines, Aminoglycosides, Macrolides, Chloramphenicol, Clindamycin.

2.3.1 Mechanism of antibacterial agent, site attack

2.3.1.1 Inhibition of cell metabolism

Antibacterial agents which inhibit cell metabolism are called "antimetabolites".

These compounds inhibit the metabolism of a microorganism but not metabolism of the host.

They do this by inhibiting an enzyme-catalyzed reaction which is present in the bacterial cell but not in animal cells. The examples of antibacterial agents acting in this way are the 'sulphonamide'.

2.3.1.2   Inhibition of bacterial cell wall synthesis

Inhibition of cell wall synthesis leads to bacterial cell lysis (bursting) and death. Agents operating in this way include "penicillin" and "cephalosporins". Since animal cells do not have a cell wall, they are unaffected by such agents.

2.3.1.   Interaction with the plasma membrane

Some antibiotics interact with the plasma membrane of bacterial cells to affect the membrane permeability. This has fatal results for the cell. Polymyxins and tyrothricin acts in this manner.

2.3.1.4   Disruption of protein synthesis

It means that essential enzymes are required for the survival of the cell. Agents of this type of activity are the "rifamycin, aminoglycosides, tetracyclines and chloramphenicol".

2.3.1.5   Inhibition of nucleic acid transcription and replication

Inhibition of nucleic acid function prevents cell division and / or the synthesis of essential enzymes. Agents acting in this way is "nalidixic acid ".

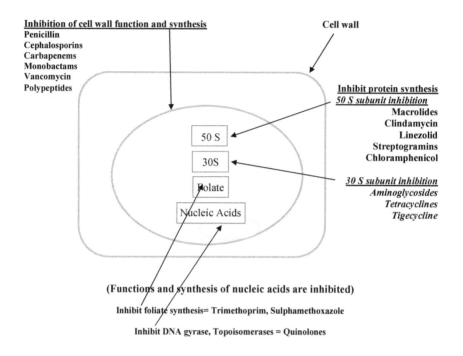

Inhibition of cell wall function and synthesis
Penicillin
Cephalosporins
Carbapenems
Monobactams
Vancomycin
Polypeptides

Cell wall

50 S

30S

folate

Nucleic Acids

Inhibit protein synthesis
50 S subunit inhibition
Macrolides
Clindamycin
Linezolid
Streptogramins
Chloramphenicol

30 S subunit inhibition
Aminoglycosides
Tetracyclines
Tigecycline

(Functions and synthesis of nucleic acids are inhibited)

Inhibit foliate synthesis= Trimethoprim, Sulphamethoxazole

Inhibit DNA gyrase, Topoisomerases = Quinolones

2.4   Combination and resistance of antibiotics

(Bactericidal and bacteriostatic antibiotics)

An infection should, if possible, be treated with a single antibiotic agent. Combination therapy is, however, administered when a synergistic effect can be achieved, e.g.,

sulphametthoxazole + trimethoprim	in infections due to *gram-negative* and gram positive pathogens,
sulphadoxime + pyrimethamine	in malaria,
clavulanic acid (salbactam) + amoxicillin	against b-lactamases *enterobacteria* and *staphylococci.*

azlocillin + tobramycin   in severe *pseudomonas* infections,

cefamandole + gentamycin   in severe infections due to *Enterobacteriaceae.*

flucytosine + amphotericin B   in disseminated *mycosis.*

Furthermore, drug combinations are used when a broader antibacterial spectrum is required, e.g.

cefamandole + gentamycin   in severe infections due to unknown pathogens and in severe mixed infections,

rifampin + isoniazid + ethambutol   in tuberculosis,

rifampin + trimethoprim   in infections due to gram positive and gram negative pathogens,

penicillin G (or ampicillin) + gentamycin   in *enterococcal endocarditis* increase the bacterial efficacy.

The activity of an antibiotic combination can markedly differ depending on the individual concerned. Indifference occurs when the activity of the combination is equal to that of the more active component. Addition takes place when the activity of the combination is equal to the sum of activities of the individual components. **Potentiation** (synergism) is observed when the activity of the combination is significantly higher than the sum of activities of the individual components. Antagonism takes place when the activity of the combination is lower than that of the more active component. The activity of combination is largely dependent on the bactericidal or bacteriostatic properties of the individual components.

2.4.1   Antibiotics classified into four groups

GROUP 1	GROUP 2	GROUP 3	GROUP 4
Bactericidal	**Bactericidal**	**Bacteriostatic**	**Bacteriostatic**
Tyrocidins	Penicillins	Chloramphenicol	D-Cycloserine
Gramicidins	Cephalosporins	Thiamphenicol	Capreomycin
Polymycins	Thienamycin	Azidamfenicol	Viomycin
Streptomycin	Bacitracin	Tetracycline	Lomefloxacin
Neomycins	Vancomycin	Fusidic acid	Rufloxacin
Paromomycins	Ristocetins	Erythromycin	
Kanamycins	Fosfomycin	Oleoandomycin	
Gentamycins	Rifamycins	Cabomycin	
Tobramycin		Rosaramycin	
Dibekacin		Lincomycin	
Amikacin		Clindamycin	
Pentisomicin		Novobiocin	
Ciprofloxacin		Nalidixic acid	
Norfloxacin		Chlortetracycline	
Ofloxaci		Oxytetracycline	
Levofloxacin		Minocycline	
Enoxacin		Methacycline	
Moxifloxacin			
Dihydrostreptomycin			

GROUP 1 = partially also on resting microorganisms
GROUP 2 = only on proliferating microorganisms
GROUP 3 = in high concentrations also bactericidal
GROUP 4 = exclusively bacteriostatic

In combinations made up of antibiotics from the above four groups, the following modes of action can generally be expected:

- The combination of antibiotics within the group 1, 2 and 4 usually does not show any antagonism.
- The combination of an antibiotic of group 1 with one of the groups 2, 3 or 4 only rarely give rise to antagonism. In general, the bactericidal agent predominates.
- The combination of an antibiotic of group 2 with one of the group3 frequently leads to a dominance of action of the bacteriostatic agent, the activity of the combination corresponds to the activity of the agent of group.
- Antagonism is thus possible.
- The combination of an antibiotic of group 2 with one of the group4 usually exhibits the dominant action of the bactericidal action.
- The combination of an antibiotic of group 3 with one of the group4 rarely shows any antagonism.

2.4.2 Bacterial persistence

Under the influence of a bactericidal antibiotic, a small number of microorganisms may persist *in vitro* in spite an unchanged susceptibility to the antibiotic. A similar persistence phenomenon can also be observed *in vivo,* despite optimal antibiotic concentration at the site of infection, pathogens may persist and lead to relapses or to carrier states after termination of the therapy.

Thus, even with bactericidal antibiotics a single massive dose is not recommended, but always a prolonged therapy, whereby the body's own defense mechanism plays an important role in the final elimination of the pathogens.

2.4.3 Bacterial resistance

The phenomenon of bacterial resistance was detected and described by P. Ehrlich at the beginning of the chemotherapy era in 1909. When the microorganisms continue to proliferate at a therapeutically achievable antibiotic concentration, when the minimal inhibitory concentration (MIC) is higher *in vitro* than the *in vivo* attainable serum or tissue concentration, bacterial resistance is present. This is caused by the lack of penetration of the antibiotic into the bacterial cell (permeability barrier), by modification in the cell so that it is insensitive to the antibiotic, or very importantly, by inactivation of the antibiotic due to the action of a bacterial enzyme.

Methicillin-resistant *Staphylococcus aureus* (MRSA) refers to a group of Gram-positive bacteria. Scanning electron micrograph of a human neutrophil ingesting MRSA.

The examples of enzymatic in-activation:

(A) Penicillin G and ampicillin are inactivated by the enzyme "penicillinase" of certain staphylococcal and gram -ive strains (including Neisseria gonorrhoeae and haemophilus influenzae) by hydrolytic cleavage of b-lactam ring to afford the corresponding "penicilloic acid ".

Cephalosporins (certain) and analogous of penicillin and ampicillin is inactivated by the action of b-lactamases from gram-negative bacteria. (Enterobacteriaceae and Pseudomonas aeruginosa) by cleavage of the b- lactam ring.

A great effort has been made in the search for b-lactamase-stable penicillin and cephalosporins and the several valuable compounds have been found to be effective.

(B)   Chloramphenicol is another example of enzymatic inactivation
      of antibiotic by the mechanism of acetylation by certain R-
      factor carrying bacteria (resistance factor) which produce a
      specific "acetyl-transferase "(e.g. Salmonellae) in typhoid fever.

Chloraphenicol → 3-O-acetylchloramphenicol
(Acetyltransferase, Acetyl CoA, CoA)

1-O-acetylchloramphenicol → 1,3-O,O-diacetylchloramphenicol
(Acetyltransferase, Acetyl CoA, CoA)

(C)   Kanamycin, an aminoglycoside antibiotic is also inactivated by the
      mechanism of O-phosphorylation. The "O-phosphotransferase",
      an enzyme, of many strains (Pseudomonas aeruginosa) are
      responsible for this inactivation. But some other antibiotics of
      the same group, for example "amikacin" is not attacked by the
      most of the O-phosphotransferases and by other inactivating
      enzymes.

Kanamycin B → Kanamycin B 3'-phosphate
(3'-O-Phosphotransferease, ATP, ADP)

Not only the various species of bacteria but also the bacterial strains of a species differ with respect to their antibiotic susceptibility. Even within a bacterial population there are variants with different susceptibility. Resistant microorganisms can readily be distinguished by means of a disc test the antibiotic concentration normally attainable in the blood of the patient being regarded as the susceptibility limit.

2.4.4   Types of resistance

Natural resistance

This type of resistance is due to a permanent genetically determined insensitivity to a bacterial species towards certain antibiotic, e.g., all Pseudomonas aeruginosa strains are resistant to "penicillin G ".

Primary resistance

It is a type of resistance in which some of the existing strains of a bacterial species are resistant, while others are susceptible, for example 30-60% of all E. coli strains are resistant to "tetracycline".

Secondary resistance

This is due to mutation or transfer of resistance in the case of individual organisms of an antibiotic-susceptible population. Secondary resistance may develop at different rates. A distinction is made between a rapid increase of resistance (one- step mutation) e.g., "streptomycin" and a slow increase (multi-step mutation) for example "penicillin".

Transfer resistance

This type of resistance is due to the transfer of genetic material, of either "chromosomal" or "extrachromosomal" origin from one bacterial cell to another.

Three types of genetic transfer mechanisms have been found:

1. transformation, involving transfer of naked DNA,
2. transduction, in which the DNA from the donor is carried to the recipient inside a phage,
3. conjugation, which requires contact of donor and recipient cells and in which the genetic material is transferred through a channel between mating cells.

The genes for drug resistance are carried on by "chromosomal" and "extra chromosomal" elements or "plasmids". These "plasmids "are also called as "R factors". Plasmid-carried resistance genes for several commonly used antibiotics have been found in "pathogenic staphylococci". These include genes conferring resistance to "penicillin, erythromycin, chloramphenicol, tetracycline and kanamycin.

2.5   Biogenesis of some basic antibiotics

Biogenesis is a study of biosynthesized a natural product. I case of the antibiotics, this being the pathway from the constituents of the culture medium to the complete antibiotic. The antibiotics are secondary metabolites of microorganisms, the biogenesis of which follows for a considerable way the synthetic route of the primary metabolites.

The formation of a secondary metabolite which comprises the uptake of a substrate and its conversion by the usual reaction mechanism into an inter mediatory product of general metabolism followed by the combination of such intermediary metabolic products in an abnormal way, where again the same general metabolic synthesis of secondary metabolites. Once a microorganism possesses the ability of making a secondary metabolite, it will produce not one such compound but a whole series.

The building units of antibiotics, whose biogenesis could be elucidated or for which plausible hypothesis exist, derive mainly from the amino acids, sugars and fatty acids (acetate and propionate) metabolism. Antibiotics may be classified on basis of their biogenetic origin.

The biosynthesis of peptide antibiotics, which are frequently built up of unusual D-amino acids, does not proceed according to the mechanism of normal protein synthesis in ribosomes, where only the usual protein amino acids of the L-series are linked together. The biogenesis of the following compounds are the examples;

❐ **Penicillins and cephalosporins**

❐ **7-Chlortetracycline**

❖ Penicillin G produced by *Penicillium chrysogenum (PC)* was formed from L-cysteine, L-valine and phenylacetic acid. Then 6-aminopenicillanic acid was isolated from the fermentation broth of *PC* where no precursor added and it was not established that it is a by-product of the penicillin G biosynthesis.

❖ The isolation of penicillin N from the fermentation broth of *Cephalosporium acremonium (CA)* was followed by further important discoveries and.

❖ First the tripeptide L-α-cysteinyl–D- valine was found in the mycelium of both PC and CA. Further it was found that PC and mycelium cultures contains small amounts of isopenicillin N and L- α - amino-adipyl side chain were present. Then enzyme system involved in the cyclization of the tripeptide was studied.

❖ Penicillin G is formed from iso-penicillin N by side chain exchange catalyzed by an acyl transferase. Experiments with labeled amino acids and acetates has revealed that cephalosporin C is actual formed from L-α-amino-adepic acid, L-cystein, L-valine and acetate. So, the penicillin N is a precursor of cephalosporin C.

❖ The enzymatic rearrangement of penicillin N to de-acetoxy-cephalosporin C was demonstrated by experiments with a cell-free system from protoplasts of *CA*. The skeleton of penicillin can also be converted into cephalosporins by means of sulphoxide rearrangement.

L-alpha-aminoadipic acid   L-Cysteine   L-Valine

2-ammonio-6-((1-((1-carboxy-2-methylpropyl)amino)-3-mercapto-1-oxopropan-2-yl)amino)-6-oxohexanoate

Isopenicillin N

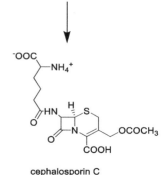

deoxycetoxycephalosporin C

deacetylcephalosporin C

cephalosporin C

General scheme of Penicillin and Cephalosporins Biogenesis.

❖ The hydro-naphthacenic carbon skeleton of the tetracyclines is built up of 9 acetate units with the participation of CO_2, biotin, co-enzyme A and some other necessary enzymes.

❖ The two N-methyl groups and the methyl group at C-6 originates from methionine. The linkage of C-atoms at different positions is still not known.

❖ The hypothetical presentation of the biogenesis of 7-chlorotetracycline is supported by numerous experiments.

❖ Accordingly, malonamoyl CoA acts as initiator for the enzymatic polymerization of 8 malonyl CoA units.

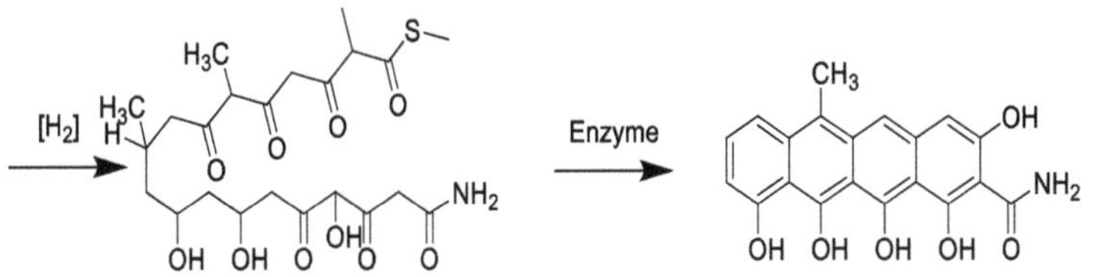

Reduced polypeptide amide

1,3,10,11,12-pentahydroxy-6-methyltetracene-2-carboxamide

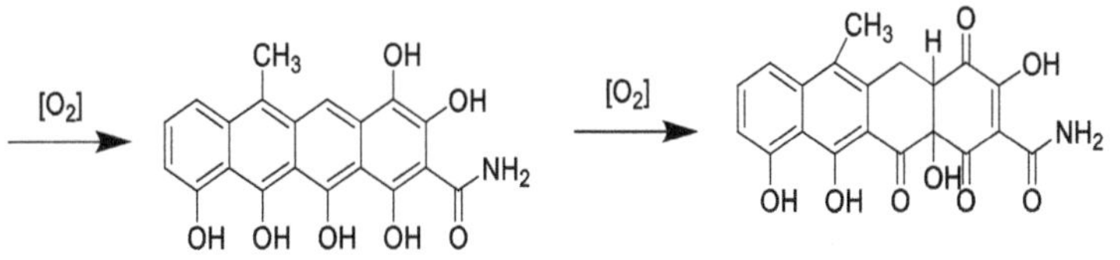

1,3,4,10,11,12-hexahydroxy-6-methyltetracene-2-carboxamide

3,10,11,12a-tetrahydroxy-6-methyl-1,4,12-trioxo-1,4,4a,5,12,12a-hexahydrotetracene-2-carboxamide

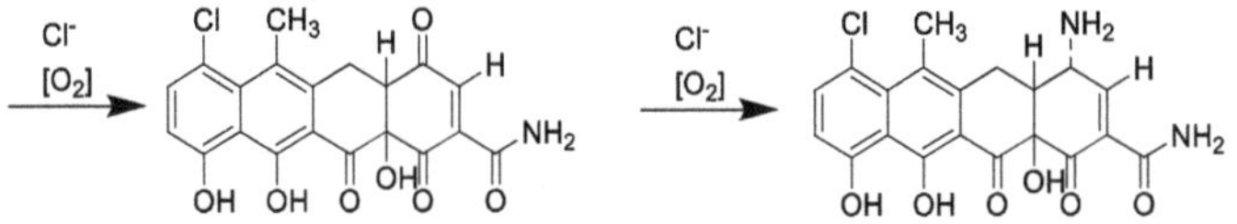

7-chloro-10,11,12-trihydroxy-6-methyl-1,4,12-trioxo-1,4,4a,5,12,12a-hexahydrotetracene-2-carboxamide

(4R)-4-amino-7-chloro-10,11,12a-trihydroxy-6-methyl-1,12-dioxo-1,4,4a,5,12,12a-hexahydrotetracene-2-carboxamide

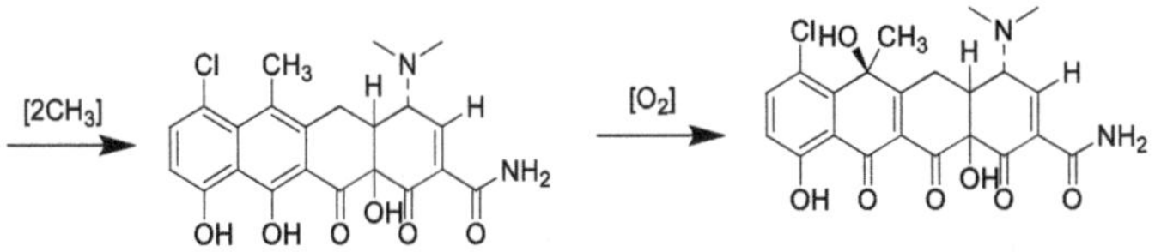

(4R)-7-chloro-4-(dimethylamino)-10,11,12a-trihydroxy-6-methyl-1,12-dioxo-1,4,4a,5,12,12a-hexahydrotetracene-2-carboxamide

(4R,6S)-7-chloro-4-(dimethylamino)-6,10,12a-trihydroxy-6-methyl-1,11,12-trioxo-1,4,4a,5,6,11,12,12a-octahydrotetracene-2-carboxamide

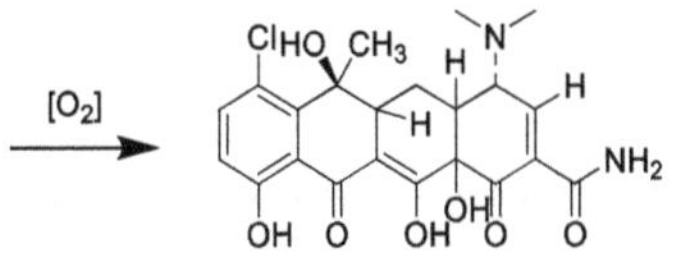

7-chlorotetracycline

CHAPTER 3

CHEMOTHERAPEUTIC PROPERTIES OF ANTIBIOTICS

3.1 Clinical uses and antibacterial spectrum

The best prerequisite for the correct choice of antibiotic, which, at the same time, will be fully active and well tolerated, is an exact clinical and bacteriological diagnosis. With serious infections the risk of a certain degree of toxicity must be accepted, when one antibiotic is clearly superior to others in its antibacterial action. For certain infectious diseases, the "antibiotic of choice" is known to which the pathogen is nearly always susceptible.

In case of pneumonia, pyelonephritis and other diseases which may be caused by several different pathogens with varying antibiotic susceptibilities, the choice of the most suitable antibiotic should be made by means of the antibiogram.

In the use of bacteriostatic antibiotic, the endogenous defensive mechanisms play a decisive role in the final destruction of the pathogens. Bactericidal antibiotics are more effective in some serious infections such as endocarditis, meningitis, septicemia; they are, above all. Indicated in infections where the bactericidal effect is the deciding factor, owing to the failure of the body's defense mechanism.

1. Typical diseases with known pathogens, e.g.

    syphilis antibiotic of choice = **penicillin G,** typhus abdominalis: therapeutic agents of choice = **co-trimoxazole, thiamphenicol**

2. Infectious diseases with various pathogens, e.g.

Pneumonia, urinary tract infections; specific treatment according to bacteriological data and antibiogram. When a bacteriological examination is not possible, the treatment must be carried out on the basis of the empirically most frequently occurring pathogen.

If the treatment with the first antibiotic administered is unsuccessful, one turns to another agent which has usually proved to be successful with this disease.

3. Ill-defined bacterial disease which cannot be localized and the state of the patient remains critical:

Begin the treatment by using a super broad-spectrum "**cephalosporin**" or a combination of two highly effective antibiotics which supplement each other in spectrum of activity, such as "**cephamandole**" and "**gentamycin**". The antibacterial spectrum and the clinical application of important antibiotics and chemotherapeutic agents have already been discussed.

3.2 Frequently occurring pathogens, typical diseases caused and their therapy with basic antibiotics / chemotherapeutic agents commonly used

Name	Normal occurrence	Typical diseases caused	Suitable antibiotics and chemotherapeutic agents
Streptococcus pyogenes (A)	Pharynx.	Erysipelas, scarlet fever, tonsillo-pharyngitis, rheumatic fever, puerperal fever, septicemia.	Peroral penicillins, penicillin G, cephalosporins, erythromycin, doxycycline, co-trimoxazole.

Staphylococcus aureus	Skin, upper respiratory tract.	Furuncle, wound infection, mastitis, septicemia, pneumonic abscesses, post-antibiotic enterocolitis, food poisoning, foreign body infections, osteomyelitis.	With non-penicillinase producing Staphylococcus. peroral penicillin, penicillin G. With penicillinase-producing Staphylococcus: flucloxacillin, dicloxacillin, cephalosporins, erythromycin, clindamycin, vancomycin, fusidic acid, co-trimoxazole.
Streptococcus faecalis	Intestinal tract, urinary tract.	Urinary tract infections, septicemia, endocarditis.	Amoxicillin, ampicillin, mezlocillin, erythromycin, doxycycline, co-trimoxazole, nitrofurantoin.
Streptococcus pneumoniae	Upper respiratory tract.	Lobar pneumonia, bronchitis, sinusitis, ulcus corneae, meningitis, pleural empyema, septicemia, otitis media.	Peroral penicillin, penicillin G, cephalosporins, erythromycin, doxycycline, co-trimoxazole.
Pseudomonas aeruginosa	Normally not on the skin or mucous membranes, frequently in the water and dirt.	Wound infections, particularly burns, chronic otitis, urinary tract infections, septicemia, chronic bronchitis, ecthyma gangraenosum, enteritis, umbilical infections.	Amikacin, tobramycin, gentamycin, azlocillin, piperacillin, superbroad- spectrum cephalosporins, cefsulodin, ticarcillin, carbencillin, polymyxin B, colistin, pipemidic acid.

Escherichia coli	Intestinal tract.	Urinary tract infections, enteritis, infant meningitis, wound infections, septicemia.	Cephalosporins, co-trimoxazole, mezlocillin, piperacillin, amoxicillin, ampicillin, doxycycline, amikacin, gentamycin, pipemidic acid, nalidixic acid, sulphonamides, nitrofurantoin.
Kiebsiella spp., Enterobacter spp.	Intestinal tract, respiratory tract.	Urinary tract infections, enteritis, infant meningitis, wound infections, septicemia.	Superbroad- spectrum cephalosporins, co-trimoxazole, cephamendole, cefoxitin, cephazolin, mezlocillin, piperacillin, amikacin, gentamycin, pipemidic acid, nalidixic acid, nitrofurantoin, sulphonamides.
Proteus mirabilis, Proteus Vulgaris, Proteus morganil, Proteus rettgeri.	Intestinal tract.	Urinary tract infections, less frequently in burns, wound infections, chronic otitis.	Superbroad- spectrum cephalosporins, co-trimoxazole, cephamendole, cefoxitin, mezlocillin, piperacillin, amikacin, amoxicillin, ampicillin, gentamycin, kanamycin, pipemidic acid, nalidixic acid, sulphonamides.
Haemophilus influenzae.	Respiratory tract.	Chronic bronchitis, broncho-pneumonia, middle ear infections, sinusitis, conjunctivitis, meningitis, septicemia.	Superbroad- spectrum cephalosporins, cephamendole, amoxicillin, ampicillin, thiamphenicol, co-trimoxazole, doxycycline, erythromycin.

Bacteroides spp. (gram-negative anaerobes)	Intestinal tract, mouth.	Mixed infections from intestine or mouth, dental infections, appendicitis, pneumonic abscesses, genital infections, septicemia, tonsillar abscesses, biliary infections, abscesses with fetid pus.	Clindamycin, ornidazole, metronidazole, moxalactam, cefoxitin, doxycycline, thiamphenicol, erythromycin, mezlocillin, azlocillin, piperacillin.
Candida albicans.	Skin, mouth, intestine.	Stomatitis, vaginitis, balanitis, esophagitis, septicemia, intertrigo and nail mucosa.	Amphotericin B, candicidin, nystatin, co-trimoxazole, miconazole, ketoconazole.
Halicobacter pylori	Intestinal tract, stomach acid.	Acid producing bacteria in the gastric region.	Combination therapy is given to eradicate Helicobacter pylori. 1.0 gm of Amoxicillin two times a day FOR SEVEN DAYS + 1.0 gm of Clarithracin two times a day FOR SEVEN DAYS + 20 mg of Esomeprazole magnesium trihydrate (Nexium) two times a day FOR SEVEN DAYS **and then** Followed by 20 mg of esomeprazole two times a day for 4-6 weeks.

3.3 Route of administration and major indications of important basic antibiotics / chemotherapeutic agents.

Drug	Administration	Major indication
Amikacin	i.v., i.m., infusion.	Severe infections with *Pseudomonas* and *Enterobacteriaceae,* particularly when tobramycin-, gentamycin, dibekasin-, sisomicin- and netilmicin – resistant.
Amoxicillin, ampicillin.	per oral, i.v., i.m.	Infections due to *E. coli, H. influenzae, P. mirabilis, S. faecalis,* particularly urogenital and respiratory infections.
Azlocillin.	i.v.	*Pseudomonas* infections.
Benzathine penicillin G (long acting)	i.m.	Prophylaxis of rheumatic fever and syphilis.
Carbencillin.	i.v.	*Pseudomonas* infections.
Cephalosporins. (cephalexin, cefaclor)	per oral.	Urinary and respiratory infections.
Cephalosporins. superbroad-specrtum (cefoperazone, moxalactam, ceftizoxime, cefataxime, ceftriaxone, ceftazidime, cephamandole, cefoxitin)	i.v., i.m.	Septicemia with unknown pathogens and other severe infections.
Clindamycin	per oral, i.v., i.m., infusion.	Severe infections due to anaerobes (esp. *Bacteroides*), staphylococcal infections with penicillin allergy or oxacillin resistance.
Co-trimoxazole	per oral, i.v., infusion.	Urinary tract infections, chronic bronchitis, typhoid, paratyphoid fever.
Doxycycline	per oral.	Infections due to *E. coli, H. Influenzae, Bacteroides, Brucella, Rickettsia, Mycoplasma, Chlamydia.*

Doxycycline	i.v.	Initial therapy of several infections Which have to be treated with tetracyclines.
Erythromycin	per oral, i.v., infusion.	Coccal infections (esp. with penicillin allergy or penicillin resistance), infections due to *Mycoplasma* and *Chlamydia*.
Flucloxacillin. (penicillinase- resistant)	per oral, i.v., i.m., infusion.	Staphylococcal infections.
Fusidic acid	per oral, i.v., infusion.	Staphylococcal infections (with penicillin allergy or oxacillin resistance).
Gentamycin	i.v., i.m., infusion.	Severe infections due to infusion *Pseudomonas* and *Enterobacteriaceae*.
Meslocillin.	i.v.	Infections caused by *Enterobacteriaceae, H. Influenzae, S. faecalis.*
Metronidazole	per oral.	Infections due to anaerobic bacteria, trichomoniasis, amoebiasis, lambliasis.
Nalidixic acid	per oral.	Uncomplicated urinary tract infections due to *Proteus, E. coli, Klebsiella, Enterobacter.*
Nitrofurantoin	per oral, i.v., infusion.	Urinary tract infections (esp. after treatment), prophylaxis after urological operations.
Ornidazole	per oral.	Infections due to anaerobic bacteria, trichomoniasis, amoebiasis, lambliasis.
Penicillin G (sodium)	i.v., i.m.	Sever streptococcal, pneumococcal and meningococcal infections.
Penicillin V	per oral	Mild to moderate infections due to penicillin- sensitive bacteria e.g., scarlet fever, tonsillo-pharyngitis, erysipelas" prophylaxis of rheumatic fever.

Piperacillin.	i.v.	*Pseudomonas* infections, Infections caused by *Enterobacteriaceae, H. Influenzae, S. faecalis.*
Procain penicillin G. (depot)	i.m.	Gonorrhea and syphilis.
Rifampin	per oral.	Tuberculosis (in combination e.g., with isoniazide and ethambutol
Streptomycin	i.m.	Tuberculosis, brucellosis, plague.
Sulphonamides	per oral, i.v.	Uncomplicated urinary tract infections.
Thiamphenicol	per oral, i.v., i.m.	Typhoid and paratyphoid fever, respiratory tract and urogenital infections (esp. gonorrhea), meningitis, (due to *H. influenazae),* peritonitis.
Ticarcillin.	i.v.	*Pseudomonas* infections.
Tobramycin	i.v., i.m., infusion.	Severe infections due to *Pseudomonas* and *Enterobacteriaceae.*
Vancomycin	i.v., infusion	Severe staphylococcal infections (with penicillin allergy or oxacillin resistance).

3.4   Pharmacokinetics of antibiotics in general

In the preparation of a therapy plan (choice of antibiotic, route of administration and dosage), the pharmacokinetics of the antibiotic must be taken into consideration.

1. Absorption and blood levels, tissue diffusion and distribution, protein binding, metabolism and excretion differ for each antibiotic.

2. Even with the same drug there can be considerable differences pharmacokinetically, according to illness, functional capability of the internal organs and the age of the patient.

3. Also the nature of the galenical formulation which may vary from preparation to preparation, can play an important role.

3.4.1   Absorption and blood levels

The extent rate of absorption following per oral administration affect the blood levels and are favorable for a number of antibiotics whereas with others absorption is insufficient so that the agents have to be administered parentally. Also i.m. administered antibiotics are absorbed at different rates,

e.g. penicillin G sodium salt and procaine penicillin G.

The height and duration of blood and tissue levels are relevant for the desired bactericidal activity of the antibiotic. With predominantly bacteriostatically acting antibiotics, nearly constant average levels are necessary, which should at least reach or even exceed the minimal inhibitory concentration for the pathogen.

3.4.2   Tissue diffusion and distribution

The tissue diffusion of antibiotics is of great importance for therapy. Determination of tissue concentration is practically, however, difficult and with many antibiotics is still too little investigated. In general, there tends to be an equilibrium between concentrations in blood and tissue. In the kidneys, glomerular filtration, tubular secretion and reabsorption from the renal tubules affect the blood and tissue levels. Antibiotics with good diffusion capacity (**thiamphenicol**) is to be distinguished from those exhibiting poor tissue distribution (**polymyxins**). Moreover, diffusion capacity is different in the various organs, as shown by the high concentrations of antibiotic always found in the lungs and liver compared with those in the eye or bones.

The antibiotic levels in the body fluids (liquor, bile, urine etc.) are important for the therapy of certain diseases (meningitis, cholangitis and urinary tract infections). However, it has to be taken into consideration that an antibiotic can have considerably different pharmacokinetics when given to an ill or to a healthy individual. Thus, penicillin diffuses better into the liquor of persons with meningitis than in healthy ones: conversely, the antibiotic concentration in the bile can be reduced by obstructive jaundice.

3.4.3   Protein binding

The binding of an antibiotic to serum proteins is important in as much as only the free, non-bonded portion is anti-bacterially effective. The degree of protein binding varies with the antibiotic, in addition it,

- ❐ depends upon the concentrations
- ❐ pH value
- ❐ presence of other drugs
- ❐ and other factors

Bound and unbound portions of the antibiotic in the plasma and tissue are at a concentration-dependent equilibrium which is determined by the absorption isotherm. Therefore, the protein-bound portion of an antibiotic is not lost for the therapy.

3.4.4   Serum protein binding of some basic antibiotics

Antibiotic	Protein binding (%)
Amikacin	4-10
Amoxicillin	17
Ampicillin	18
Azlocillin	About 30
Carbencillin	50
Cefamandole	67-80
Cefazolin	70-85

Cefoxitin	50-60
Cefuroxime	33
Cephalexin	10-15
Cephaloridine	22-31
Cephalothin	62-65
Chloramphenicol	About 50
Clindamycin	84
Demeclocycline	70
Dicloxacillin	97
Doxycycline	96
Erythromycin	60
Flucloxacillin	95
Fosfomycin	No binding
Fusidic acid	90-97
Gentamycin	No binding
Kanamycin	No binding
Lincomycin	20-30
Mezlocillin	About 30
Oxacillin	93
Oxytetracycline	40
Penicillin V	60
Penicillin G	About 50
Propicillin	80-85
Rifampin	75-80
Streptomycin	30
Thiamphenicol	10-20
Tobramycin	No binding

3.4.5   Metabolism

Metabolism occurs in all antibiotics, but, to different degrees. The metabolites formed by oxidation, reduction, hydrolysis or conjugation may be antibacterially inactive and appear in this form in the blood, urine, bile and feces.

The inactivation is frequently accompanied by a detoxification of the antibiotics as e.g.in the case of "chloramphenicol", by coupling with D-glucuronic acid (metabolized in liver).

Chloramphenicol   Chloramphenicol glucuronide

3.4.6 Excretion and half-life

Most antibiotics are eliminated predominantly via the kidneys by glomerular filtration, partly by tubular secretion. In a very few cases, as with "**erythromycin, rifampin** and **fusidic acid** ", the antibiotic is mainly excreted into the bile and feces. This elimination may be accompanied by a re-absorption in the intestine which may be useful for therapy.

Renal insufficiency causes accumulation of particularly those antibiotics which are largely excreted through the kidneys so that toxic side effects may be induced. In case of a reduction of the kidney function, best characterized by the creatinine clearance, a prolongation of the dosing interval is therefore required for several antibiotics.

3.4.7 Half - life of some basic antibiotics and dosing interval in renal impairment

Antibiotic	Half-life (hours)		Dosing interval (hours) with creatinine clearance (ml/min.)			
	normal	Severe renal insufficiency	> 80	80-85	50-10	<10
Amikacin	2.3	72-96	8	24	24-72	72-96
Ampicillin	1.0	8.5	6	8	12	24

Azlocillin	1.25	8-10	6	8	8	12-24
Carbencillin	1.0	15	6	8	12	24
Cefazolin	1.5	5-20	6	8	12	24-48
Cefoxitin	0.75	5-10	6	8	12	24
Cefuroxime	1.2	5-20	6	8	12	24-48
Cephalexin	1.0	30	6	6	8	24-48
Cephalothin	0.65	3-18	4-6	6	6	8
Chloramphenicol	3.0	3-4	8	8	8	8
Clindamycin	3.0	3-5	6	6	8	12
Colistin	2.0	24-36	8	24	36-60	60-92
Doxycycline	15.0	15-24	24	24	24	24
Erythromycin	2.0	5-8	6	6	6	6
Flucloxacillin	0.75	8	6	8	8	12
Gentamycin	2.0	60	8	12	18-24	48
Kanamycin	2-3	72-96	8	24	24-72	72-96
Lincomycin	5.0	10-13	8	8	12	12
Mezlocillin	0.8	6-14	6	8	8	12-24
Oxacillin	0.4	2	4-6	6	6	8
Penicillin G	0.65	7-10	6	8	8	12
Tetracycline	8-9	30-128	6	12	48	72-96
Thiamphenicol	3.0	30	8	12	12-48	72
Vancomycin	6.0	216	12	72	240	240

3.4.8 Administration and dosage

The route of administration:
Per oral
Parenteral (i.m., i.v.), local
depends upon the followings factors;

- ❖ nature of the illness
- ❖ condition of the patient
- ❖ external circumstances

Some antibiotics, such as "**penicillin V** and **propicillin** ", can only be given per orally whereas others, such as "**gentamycin or**

cephamandole", are administered parenterally, as practically no absorption from the intestine occurs. Certain antibiotics, such as "

neomycin, paromomycin and nystatin", are suitable for systemic use owing to their toxicity, and hence can only be applied locally. Number of antibiotics can be given per orally and parenterally.

Better absorption usually occurs after parenteral administration than after per oral administration. Therefore, with serious infections, treatment is recommended with i.v. antibiotics, in order to rapidly reach high and possibly bactericidal effective blood and tissue levels.

3.4.9 Dosage of important basic antibiotics commonly used in adults.

Drug	Daily dose	Number of single doses daily	Administration
Amikacin	1 g	2-3	i.m., i.v. infusion
Amoxicillin	1-1.5(-3) g	3-4	Per oral, iv., i.m.
Ampicillin, parenteral	1.5-2(-10-20) g	3-4	i.m., i.v.
Ampicillin, peroral	2-3-4 g	3-4	Per oral
Azlocillin	6-15 g	3	i.v.
Carbenicillin	12-30-40 g	4-6	i.v.
Cefaclor	2-4 g	3-4	Per oral
Cefamandole	1.5-3-6(-12) g	3-6	i.v., i.m.
Cefazolin	3-4(-6) g	3-4	i.v., i.m.
Cefoxitin	3-6(-12) g	3-4	i.v., i.m.
Cefuroxime	2.25-4-8 g	3-4	i.v., i.m.
Cephalexin	3-4 g	3-4	Per oral
Cephalothin	3-4-6-8 g	3-4-6	i.v.
Chloramphenicol	1.5-2-3 g	3-4	Per oral, i.v., i.m.
Clindamycin	0.6-1.2 g	3-4	Per oral., i.m., i.v. infusion
Co- trimxazole	(0.96-)1.92(-2.88) g	2	Per oral, i.v. infusion

Demeclocycline	0.6(-1.2) g	2	Per oral
Dicloxacillin	2-4(-6-10) g	4-6	Per oral
Doxycycline	0.1-0.2 g	1	Per oral, i.v.
Erythromycin	1-2 g	2-3	Per oral, i.v. infusion
Fluclacillin	2-4(-6-10) g	4-6	Per oral, i.m., i.v. infusion
Fusidic acid	1.5(-3) g	3	Per oral, i.v. infusion
Kanamycin	1 g	2	i.m.
Mezlocillin	6-15 g	3	i.v.
Minocycline	0.2 g	1-2	Per oral, i.v. infusion
Oxytetracycline	1-1.5(-2) g	2-4	Per oral
Penicillin G	0.6-1.2-3(-12-24-60) g	4 -6	i.v ., i.m.
Per oral, penicillin	0.9(-2.5-5) g	3	Per oral
Piperacillin	2-16 g	3	i.v.
Pivampicillin	1.4-2.8 g	3-4	Per oral
Rifampin	0.6-0.75 g	1-2	Per oral
Streptomycin	(0.7-) 1 (-1.5) g	1-3	i.m.
Thiamphenicol	1.5(-3) g	3	Per oral, i.v., i.m.
Tobramycin; Gentamycin	0.16-0.24(-0.32) g	2-3	i.m., i.v. infusion
Vancomycin	1-2 g	2-4	i.v. infusion

A desired depot effect may be obtained by the i.m. injection of sparingly soluble antibiotics such as **"penicillin G "**. With per oral administration, there are often marked differences in the degree of absorption between antibiotics. Whereas, e.g., **amoxicillin, pivampicillin, cephalexin, doxycycline** and **thiamphenicol** are completely absorbed. While **penicillin V, ampicillin** and **oxytetracycline** is incompletely absorbed.

Tolerance to an antibiotic can be different in peroral and parenteral administration. A rapid i.v. injection, e.g., of **oxytetracycline,** may

140

readily cause vascular irritation and undesired general reactions whereas with per oral **oxytetracycline** treatment, intestinal disturbances are more frequently observed. For local use, antibiotics are preferred which are not or rarely used per orally or parenterally, as the danger of sensitization is considerably greater in local administration. Above all **penicillin** and **streptomycin** should be avoided.

It has to be noted that the dosage of an antibiotic must provide a concentration at the site of infection sufficient for bacterial inhibition. The establishing of the does to be given must be determined by the special conditions of each individual case. For this the following must be taken into consideration:

❖ the susceptibility of the pathogen
❖ the pharmacokinetics
❖ tolerance at a particular age
❖ site of action in particular diseases

3.4.10   Side effects

❖ As for other drugs, antibiotics may also cause undesirable side effects. But there is is a difference among toxic, allergic, biological side effects and between acute and chronic toxicity. Acute toxic reaction ca be observed after high polymyxin doses and chronic toxic effects may occur after administration of chloramphenicol.

❖ As a measure of acute toxicity, the LD_{50} values (mg / kg) are determined in animal tests. These values usually give the information on the possible toxicity in humans.

❖ Antibiotics with low toxicity such cephalosporin / penicillin / erythromycin stand in contrast to potentially toxic antibiotics such as aminoglycosides antibiotics, polymyxins, chloramphenicol, novobiocin and amphotericin B which may cause partially reversible and irreversible damage.

❖ On account of their toxicity, the followings are: (neomycin, paromomycin, bacitracin, gramicidin and nystatin) are totally unsuitable for systemic use and are therefore only applied in local treatment.

❖ Allergic side effects can be observed in therapy with penicillin which may occur any time during the treatment. The most dangerous is anaphylactic shock that may be fatal.

❖ Biological side effects due to growth inhibition of the normal bacterial flora on the skin or mucous membranes, are frequently encountered in treatment with broad spectrum antibiotics as; tetracyclines. Super infections, such as stomatitis, glossitis, esophagitis and enterocolitis can be caused by an overgrowth of the fungus *Candida albicans* or resistant bacteria as *Pseudomonas aeuginosa and Klebsiella pneumoniae.*

❖ Furthermore, it has been shown that clindamycin associated pseudomembranous colitis is due to overgrowth of resistant, toxin producing clostridia *(Clostridium difficile).*

General scheme of antibiotics contraindicated during pregnancy.

Chloramphenicol	Gray Baby Syndrome
Metronidazole	Teeth discoloration and hepatic failure
Aminoglycosides	Ototoxicity
Tetracyclines	Liver failure

3.4.11   Average serum concentrations after a single administration of various basic antibiotics

Drug	Dose / g	Route of administration	Average serum concentration µg/ml at 1-4 hours after administration 1 2 3 4			
Amikacin (sulphate)	0.5	i.m.	21			2.1 (after 10 hours)

Amoxicillin	0.5	peroral	3.5	4.0	2.5	1.4
Ampicillin	0.5	peroral	1.5	1.6	0.7	0.3
Ampicillin (sodium salt)	0.5	i.m.	10.0	5.0	2.0	0.9
Azlocillin (sodium salt)	1.0	i.v.	23	9	4	1
Carbencillin (disodium salt)	1.0	i.v.	25	12		
Cefaclor	0.25	peroral	5.0	1.9	0.9	0.3
Cefoxtin (sodium salt)	0.5	i.m.	7.4	3.5	1.0	
Cefuroxime (sodium salt)	0.5	i.m.	21.6	11.9	7.2	4.0
Cephalexin	0.25	peroral	7.3	3.7	1.5	0.7
Cephaloridine	0.5	i.m.	15.9	11.2		3.8
Cephalothin (sodium salt)	0.5	i.m.	7.3	2.7		0.3
Cephamendole	0.5	i.m.	13.5	6.0	4.7	2.0
Cephazolin (sodium salt)	0.5	i.m.	31.5	25.4		12.5
Chloramphenicol	0.5	peroral	2-3		3-4	
Clindamycin (hydrochloride)	0.15	peroral	2-4	1.4-2.4	1-1.8	0.7-1.4
Co-trimoxazole	0.96	peroral	1-2 (after 3 hours)			40-60 (after 3 hours)
Dicloxacillin (sodium salt)	0.5	peroral	3	6.5	5	2
Doxycycline (hydrochloride)	0.2	peroral	0.2-0.6	2-4	2-4	0.7-1.1 (after 24 hours)
Doxycycline (hydrochloride)	0.2	i.v.	3.5-5	3-4	3-4	0.7-1.4 (after 24 hours)
Erythromycin (ethylsuccinate)	0.5	peroral	1.5	1.5	0.7	0.4
Fucidic acid (sodium salt)	0.5	peroral	17	28		11 (after 8 hours)
Gentamycin (sulphate)	0.08	i.m.	5.1	4.5	3.1	2.0
Kanamycin (sulphate)	0.5	i.m.	15-20			4.8 (after 5-7 hours)
Mezlocillin (sodium salt)	1.0	i.v.	7.8	2.9	1.5	0.9

Penicillin G (sodium salt)	0.3	i.m.	4.8	2.4	1.2	
Piperacillin (sodium salt)	1.0	i.v.	10	3	1	
Pivampicillin (hydrochloride)	0.7	peroral	7.0	5.5	2.8	1.0
Procaine penicillin G	0.6	i.m	1.0	1.0		0.9 (after 6 hours)
Propicillin (potassium salt)	0.28	peroral	3.1	2.3	1.4	0.7
Rifampin	0.6	peroral		7-14		2 (after 12 hours)
Streptomycin (sulphate)	1.0	i.m.	40	37	32	10 (after 10 hours)
Thiamphenicol	0.5	peroral	2.8	4.7	3.6	2.5
Vancomycin (hydrochloride)	1.0	i.v.	25-40		10	

3.4.12 pK_a values for some of the basic antibiotics

pK_a values				pK_a values		
Antibiotic name	HA	HB+		Antibiotic name	HA	HB+
Adriamycin		8.2		Erythromycin		8.8
Amoxicillin	2.4	7.4, 9.6		Erythromycin estolate	10.7	
6-Amino-penicillanic acid	2.3	4.9		Flucloxacillin	2.7	
Amphotericin B	5.5	10.0		Fusidic acid	5.4	
Ampicillin	2.5	7.2		Gentamycin		8.2
Azlocillin	2.8			Kanamycin		7.2
Bacampicillin		6.8		Lincomycin		7.5
Carbencillin	2.7			Methacycline	3.5, 7.6	9.5
Cefaclor	1.5	7.2		Methicillin	3.0	
Cafamandole	2.7			Minocycline	2.8, 5.0, 7.8	9.5
Cefazolin	2.1			Mitomycin		10.9
Cefotaxime	3.4			Nafcillin	2.7	
Cefoxitin	2.2			Nalidixic acid	6.0	

144

Ceftzidime	1.8, 2.7	4.1		Natamycin	4.6	8.4
Ceftriaone	3.2, 4.1	3.2		Novobiocin	4.3, 9.1	
Cephalexin	3.2			Nystatin	8.9	5.1
Cephaloridine	3.4			Oxacillin	2.7	
Cephalothin	2.5			Oxytetracycline	3.3, 7.3	9.1
Cephradine	2.6	7.3		Penicilloic acid	5.2	
Chlortetracycline	3.3, 7.4	9.3		Penicillin G	2.8	
Ciprofloxacin	6.0	8.8		Penicillin V	2.7	
Clindamycin		7.5		Pivampicillin		7.0
Cloxacillin	2.8			Polymyxin		8.9
Cyclacillin	2.7	7.5		Rifampin	1.7	7.9
Demeclocycline	3.2	7.2, 9.3		Rolitetracycline	7.4	
Daunorubicin		8.4		Tetracycline	3.3, 7.7	9.7
Demeclocycline	3.3, 7.2	9.4		Ticarcillin	2.6, 3.4	
Dihydrostreptomycin		7.8		Tobramycin		6.7, 8.3, 9.9
Doxorubicin		8.2, 10.2		Trimethoprim		7.2
Doxycycline	3.4, 7.7	9.5		Viomycin	8.2, 10.3, 12.0	

3.4.13   pH values for tissue fluids

Fluid	Type	pH
Aqueous humor		7.2
Blood		
	Arterial	7.4
	Venous	7.4
	Maternal umbilical	7.3
Cerebrospinal (SPF)		7.4
Colon		
	Fasting	5-8
	Fed	5-8
Duodenum		

	Fasting	4.4-6.6
	Fed	5.2-6.2
Faces		7.1 (4.6-8.8)
Ileum		
	Fasting	6.8-8.6
	Fed	6.8-8.0
Intestine		
	Micro-surface	5.3
Lacrimal (LF)	Tears	7.4
Milk	Breast	7.0
Muscle	Skeletal	6.0
Nasal secretions		6.0
Prostatic (PF)		6.5
Saliva		6.4
Semen		7.2
Stomach		
	Fasting	1.4-2.1
	Fed	3.0-7.0
Sweat		5.4
Urine		5.8 (5.5-7.0)
Vaginal secretions		
	Pre-menopause	4.5
	Post-menopause	7.0

3.4.14   Acute toxicity of various basic antibiotics in the mouse.

Antibiotic	LD_{50} (mg/kg)	Mode of administration
Aclarubicin	33.7	i.v.
Amikacin (sulfate)	300	i.v.
Amphotericin B	6	i.v.
Amphotericin B methylate	85	i.v.
Ampicillin	>10000	oral
Ampicillin (Na salt)	6000	i.v.

Azlocillin (Na salt)	4870	i.v.
Bleomycin (sulfate)	210	i.v.
Cefazolin (Na salt)	~5000	i.v.
Cefamandole (sulfate)	7950	i.v.
Cefoxitin (Na salt)	1600-4500	oral
Cephalexin	6696-7200	oral
Cephalothin (Na salt)	~5000	i.v.
Chloramphenicol	245	i.v.
Chloramphenicol	>5000	oral
Dactinomycin	0.7	i.v.
Daunorubicin (hydrochloride)	26	i.v.
Dibekacin (sulfate)	71	i.v.
Doxorubicin (hydrochloride)	20.8	i.v.
Doxycycline (hydrochloride)	244	i.v.
Doxycycline (hydrochloride)	2640	oral
Erythromycin (estolate)	6450	oral
Fucidic acid (Na salt)	975	oral
Gentamycin (sulfate)	77	i.v.
Kanamycin (sulfate)	160	i.v.
Kanamycin (sulfate)	280	i.v.
Mithramycin	0.35	i.v.
Mitomycin C	5	i.v.
Neomycin (sulfate)	2880	oral
Neomycin (sulfate)	24	i.v.
Novobiocin	362	oral
Oxytetracycline (hydrochloride)	178	i.v.
Oxytetracycline (hydrochloride)	1650	oral
Paromomycin (sulfate)	2275	oral
Penicillin G (Na salt)	3090	i.v.
Penicillin V	3940	oral
Polymyxin B (sulfate)	1187	oral
Polymyxin B (sulfate)	6.1	i.v.
Rifampin	858	oral
Streptomycin (sulfate)	200	i.v.

Thiamphenicol	9000	oral
Tobramycin (sulfate)	79	i.v.
Vancomycin (hydrochloride)	400	i.v.

3.4.15 Possible side effects of different basic antibiotics and chemotherapeutic agents.

Antibiotic or chemotherapeutic agents	Side effects					Contra-indications (expect vital indication)		
	Allergic	Heamatotoxic	Nephrotoxic	Hepatotoxic	Neurotoxic	Gravid, M.1-111	Neonates	Severe renal insufficiency
Amikamycin	+		+		++	×		×
Amoxicillin, ampicillin	++				s			
Amphotericine B	s	s	++	s	s	×	×	×
Azlo- mezlo-, piperacillin	++				s			
Capreomycin	+	s	s		++	×	×	×
Cephalosporins (except cephaloridine)	+	s						
Cephradine	+	s	++					×
Chloramphenicol	s	+ 2			s	×	×	
Clindomycin[4]	s			s				
Co-trimazole	++	s				×	×	×
d- Cycloserine	s				++		×	×
Erythromycin	s							
Ethambutol	s			s	++			
Flu- dicloxacillin	++				s			
Flucytocine		+		+		×	×	×
Fusidic acid	s							
Gentamycin, tobramycin	s		+		++	×		×
Griseofulvin	+	s	s	s	s	×		
Isoniazid	s	s		+	++			
Ketoconazole	+					×		

148

Nalidixic acid	s	s			+		×	×
Nitrofurantoin	++	s		s	++	×	×	×
Ornidazole	s				s	×		
Penicillin G	++				+			
Polymyxin B, colistin	+		+		++			×
Rifampin	+	+	+	++	+	×	×	
Streptomycin	++	s	s		++	×		×
Sulfonamides	++	s		s			×	×
Tetracyclines	s	s		s		×	×	×
Thiamphenicol	s	$+^3$				×		×
Ticarcillin, carbenicillin								
Vancomycin	++		s		+	×	×	×

CHAPTER 4

CLINICALLY IMPORTANT ANTIBIOTICS

4.1 Pharmaceutical And Medicinal Chemistry Of Clinically Important Antibiotics / Structure Determination

4.1.1 Structure determination

When a new antibiotic with promising chemotherapeutic activity has been discovered and isolated in the pure state, attempts have been made to determine its chemical structure. Firstly, the new compound is characterized by certain physical properties such as:

1. melting point
2. chromatographic or electrophoretic properties (rf values)
3. optical activity
4. solubility in different solvents

For further characterization and for determination of the structure, the following methods, usually in conjunction, are used:

1. **Physical analytical methods:**
   a) Infrared (IR)
   b) Ultraviolet / visible (UV/V)
   c) Nuclear magnetic resonance (NMR)
   d) Mass spectroscopy (MS)
   e) X-ray diffraction
   f) Optical rotatory dispersion (ORD)
   g) Circular dichroism (CD)

h) Molecular weight determination

2. Chemical analytical methods
a) Elemental analysis
b) Establish the empirical formula based upon the molecular weight
c) Microanalysis for the determination of functional groups
d) Potentiometric microtitration (for the determination of pKa values, the isoelectric point and equivalent weight)

3. Chemical degradation

Identification and separation of the degradation products by analysis and if required, by synthesis and chromatographic techniques respectively. Prior to the development of spectroscopic techniques, x-ray differential analysis, NMR and analysis, the chemical degradation and the partial / total synthesis played a crucial role in the structure determination of the antibiotics and other natural products. The X-ray diffraction analysis was the most reliable method for structure determination: it affords information on the spatial position of the atoms in the molecule (relative and, under certain conditions, the absolute configuration). A prerequisite of this method is, however, that the substance concern forms clearly defined crystals of sufficient size. In the search for new antibiotics in screening programs, very often already known antibiotics are found. To determine whether an antibiotic, possibly only in a crude state is really a new, mostly combination of chemical, physical, instrumental and microbiological methods for analysis is used.

4.2 Classification of antibiotics

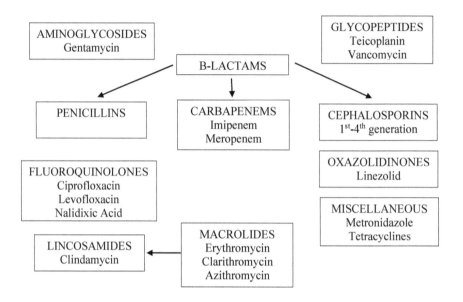

Gram +ive		Gram -ive		Gram +ive and Gram -ive	
Penicillin	Amoxacillin	**Aminoglycosides**	Streptomycin Tobramycin Gentamycin	**Tetracyclines**	Tetracycline Doxycycline
Macrolides	Azithromycin Clarithramycin Erythromycin			**Cephalosporins**	Kaliflex Cefol Cefeprime
Lincosamides	Clindamycin			**Flouroquinolones**	Ciprofloxacin Moxifloxacin Levofloxacin
				Carbapenams	Meropenam
				Metronidazole	Flagyl
				Sulphonamides	Trimethoprim + Sulphamethox-azole

4.2.1 Classification of penicillin

Chemical structure of Penicillin G. The sulfur and nitrogen of the five membered thiazolidine ring. The image shows that the thiazolidine ring and fused four-membered β-lactam are not in the same plane.

4.2.2   Antibiotics derived from one amino acid

This group includes the reserve D-cycloserine, Chloramphenicol, Thiamphenicol, Azidamphenicol, as well anti cancer antibiotics L-azaserine and 6-diazo-5-oxo-L-norleucine. A few of the structural diagrams are described below:

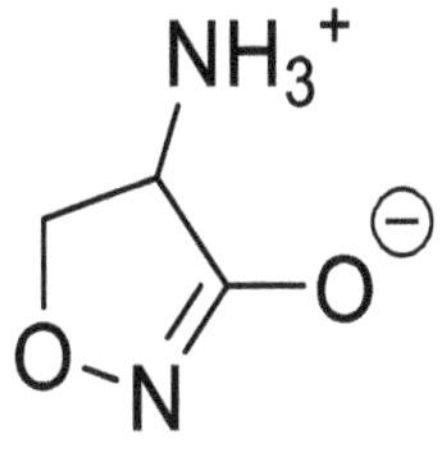

D-cycloserine

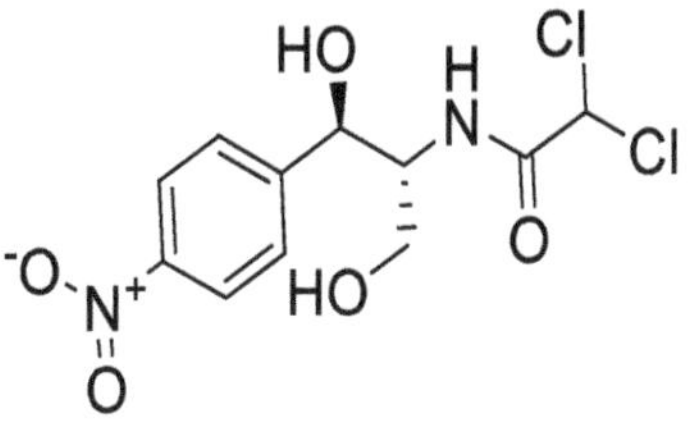

Chloramphenicol

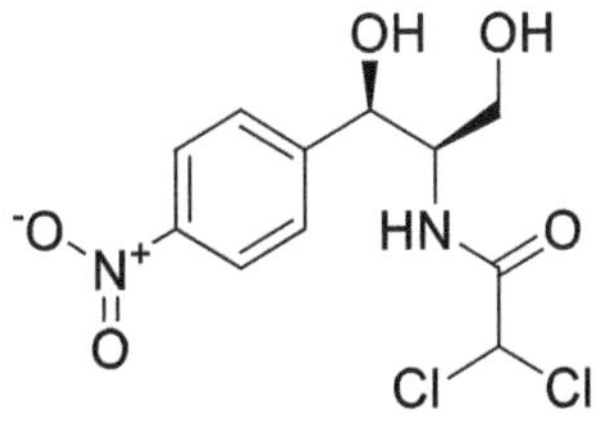

Thiamphenicol

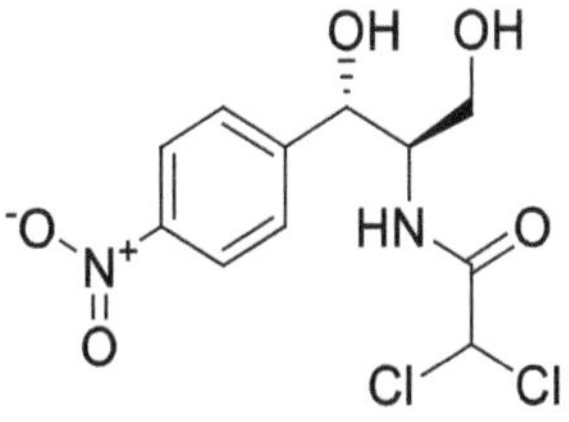

Azidamphenicol

Thiamphenicon has proved to be a suitable substitute for chloramphenicol since it does not cause irreversible haematological side effects. Azidamphenicol shows good results regarding water solubility and local tolerance especially for opthalmic use.

AMPHENICOLS

Amphenicols are a class of antibiotics with **"phenylpropanoid structure"**. They function by blocking the enzyme **"peptidyl transferase"** on the 50 S ribosome subunit of bacteria. The examples of amphenicols are:

153

- Chloramphenicol
- Thiamphenicol
- Azidamphenicol
- Florfenicol

4.2.3 Antibiotics derived from two amino acids

This group is composed of β-lactam antibiotics, such as Penicillin and Cephalosporins. Several representatives of this group belong to the most potent and valuable agents used in antibacterial therapy.

4.2.3.1 Penicillins

Penicillins are N-acyl derivatives of 6-aminopenicillanic acid. The latter is produced by chemical or enzymatic cleavage of the side chain of penicillin G or V. Acid stability and peroral activity of certain penicillins is due to the presence of an electron-attracting group at the alpha position of the side chain amide carbony, preventing the penillic acid rearrangement from taking place. Further better improvement is achieved by esterification as in pivampicillin and some others. These esters are prodrugs of ampicillin, being easily hydrolysed to ampicillin by esterases present in blodd and tissues.

Example:

6-aminopenicillanic acid   Penicillin

4.2.3.2 Cephalosporins

The cephalosporins a class of β-lactam originally derived from the fungus acremonium, which was previously known as "cephalosporium". Formally regarded as derivatives of 7-aminocephar Losporonic acid which is prepared by chemical cleavage of the side chain of cephalosporin C.

Together with cephamycin, they constitute a subgroup of β-lactam antibiotics called cephems. Cephalosporins were discovered in 1945.

Cefacetril	CH_3COOCH_2-	$-CH_2CN$
Cefadin	CH_3-	

Cefroxadin	CH_3O-	
Cefaloglycin	CH_3COOCH_2-	
Cefaclor	$-Cl$	
Cefalexin	CH_3-	
Cefadroxil	CH_3-	
Cefadroxil	CH_3-	

Cefetrizin		
Cefazedon		
Cefapirin	CH_3COOCH_2-	
Ceftezol		
Cefazolin		
Zefazaflur		
Cefalutin	CH_3COOCH_2-	

| **Cefaloridin** | 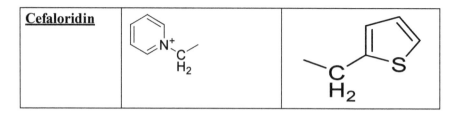 |

The novel β-lactam antibiotics with very interesting biological properties and structures considerably differing from those of penicillin and cephalosporins have been discovered. For example, "Clavulanic acid "(an irreversibly β-lactamase-inhibiting compound with low intrinsic antibacterial activity.

4.2.3.3   Clavulanic acid

4.2.4   Polypeptide antibiotics

This group includes "tyrocidin, gramicidin, bacitracin, capreomycin, viomycin, amphomycin, mikamycin, vernamycin, straphlomycin and viginiamycin which are predominantly active against gram-positive bacteria and are only suitable for local application. Polymixins are active against gram-negative bacteria. Anti-tumor antibiotics: bleomycin, peplomycin and dactinomycin are also belonging to this group.

Example: Bleomycin

4.2.5 Antibiotics derived from sugars

This group includes "streptomycin and dihydrostreptomycin which are effective against tuberculosis and plague. Neomycin used locally for skin infections. Paromomycin is used for G.I.T. problems.

Kanamycin, gentamycin, tobramycin, are effective in severe infections. Spectinomycin is active against penicillin-resistant gonorrhea.

Example: Gentamycin

4.2.6 Antibiotics derived from acetates / propionates

(a)   Antibiotics containing condensed ring systems.

This group includes broad-spectrum "Tetracyclines ".
Griseofulvin is active against fungal infections.
Fusidic acid used in penicillin allergy or oxacillin resistance.

Rest all are described in section (Chlortetracycline, Oxytetracycline, Tetracycline, Minocycline, Doxycycline and Methicillin).

Example: Methicillin.

(b)   Macrolide antibiotics

These antibiotics are so designated because of the presence of a macrocyclic lactone ring.

These antibiotics are predominantly active against gram-positive bacteria. The examples are "erythromycin, oleandomycin, carbomycin and spiramycin". Rosaramycin active against gram-negative. Avermectin is effective against nematodes.

Example: Erythromycin.

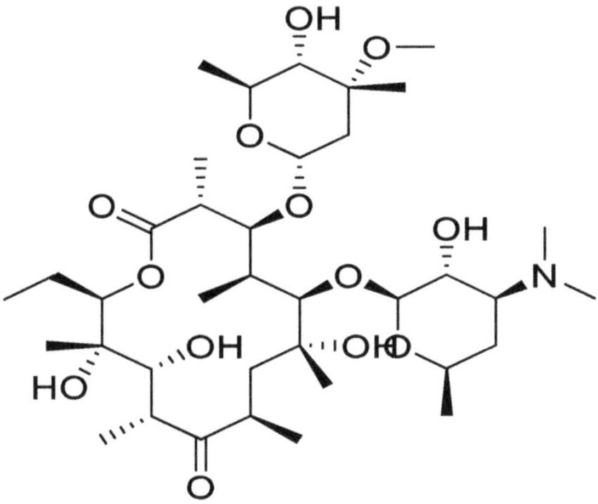

(c) Polyene antibiotics

These antibiotics chiefly owe their name to the presence of several conjugated double bonds. Classical representatives of this class are "natamycin, trichomycin, amphotericin B and fumagillin".

Example: Fumagillin

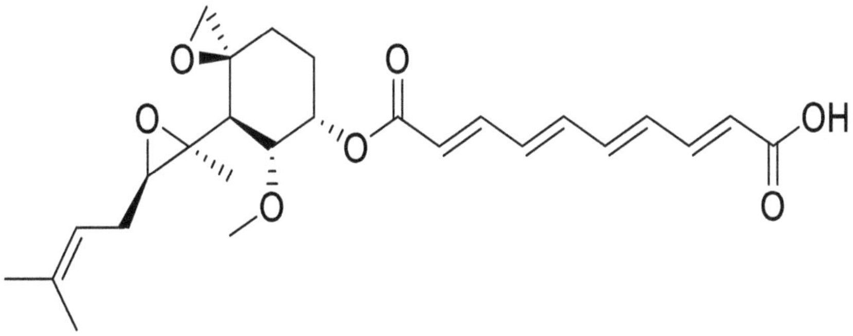

(d) Rifamycin antibiotics

Rifamycin comprise a group of macrocyclic antibiotics which are redominantly effective against gram-negative organisms. Rifamycin

B is produced by fermentation. Rifamycin SV and Rifamide are administered parentally.

Example: Rifamycin

4.2.7 Antibiotics derived from various structures

This group include vancomycin and ristocetin in infections to penicillin allergy or oxacillin resistance. Lincomycin and Clindamycin are highly effective against gram-negative and others.

Fosfomycin, Novobiocin and Puromycin are also effective but are more toxic.

Example: Lincomycin.

4.2.8   Anti-tumor antibiotics

This chemically heterogeneous group of antibiotics includes:

Sarkomycin, L-azaserine, 6-diazo-5-oxo-L-norleucine, Mitomycin C,
Streptogramin, Bleomycin, Peplomycin, Streptozocin, Dactinomycin
(Actinomycin A), Daunorubicin (Daunomycin), Doxorubicin
(Adriamycin), Aclarubicin A and Mithramycin (Aeraulic acid).

Example: Mithramycin

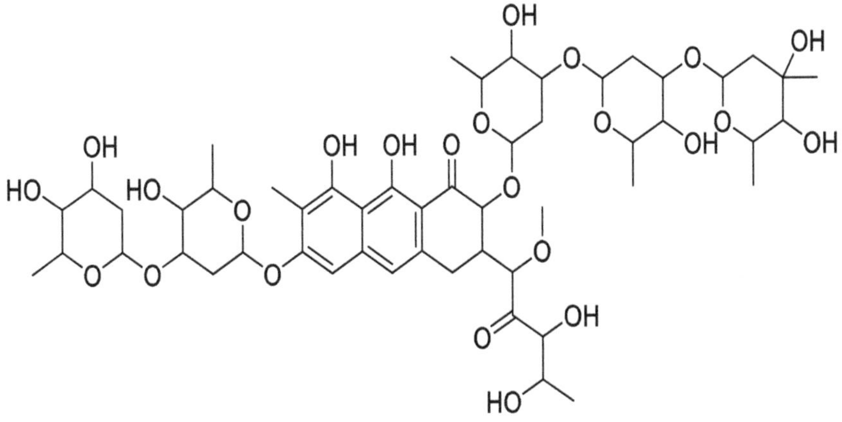

4.2.9   Quinolone antibiotics

(synthetic anti-bacterial)

A quinolone antibiotic is a member of a large group of broad-
spectrum bactericidal that share a bicyclic core structure related
to the substance quinoline. They are used in human and veterinary
medicine to treat bacterial infections, as well as in animal husbandry.
Nearly all quinolone antibiotics in use are fluoroquinolones, which
contain a fluorine atom in their chemical structure and are effective
against both gram negative and gram-positive bacteria. One example
is ciprofloxacin, one of the most widely used antibiotics worldwide.

Example: The second-generation fluoroquinolone, ciprofloxacin. The two ringed nitrogen containing system with a ketone is called a quinolone.

CHAPTER 5

STRUCTURAL FORMULAE, CHEMISTRY, CHEMICAL CLASSIFICATION AND STRUCTURE ACTIVITY RELATIONSHIP (SAR) OF ANTIBIOTICS

5.1 List of chemical groups of antibiotics

i.   Antibiotics derived from two amino acids.
  • β- lactam penicillin
  • β-lactam cephalosporin

ii.   Antibiotics derived from one amino acid.

iii. Antibiotics from polypeptide group.

iv.   Antibiotics derived from sugars (Aminoglycosides).

v.   Antibiotics derived from acetates and propionate groups.

vi.   Antibiotics from macrolide group.

vii. Antibiotics derived from polyene group.

viii. Antibiotics derived from rifamycin group.

ix.   Antibiotics with various structures.

x.   Anti-tumor antibiotics.

xi.   Quinolone antibiotics.

xii. Tetracycline group of antibiotics.

xiii. Streptomycin (aminoglycoside, derived from sugars)

xiv. Dihydrostreptomycin (aminoglycoside, derived from sugars)

xv.   Neomycin (aminoglycoside, derived from sugars)

xvi. Kanamycin (aminoglycoside, derived from sugars)

xvii. Gentamycin (aminoglycoside, derived from sugars)

xviii. Tobramycin (aminoglycoside, derived from sugars)

xix. Erythromycin (macrolide group)
xx. Nystatin (polyene group)
xxi. Vancomycin (from various structures)
xxii. Azithromycin (derived from erythromycin)
xxiii.Rifamycin B (rifamycin group)
xxiv. Mitomycin (anti-tumor)
xxv. Fusidic acid derived from acetates)
xxvi.Lincomycin (miscellaneous group)
xxvii. Ciprofloxacin (quinolone group)

5.2 Antibiotics derived from respective chemical groups

SERIAL NO.	NAME OF ANTIBIOTICS DERIVED FROM RESPECTIVE CHEMICAL GROUP
A	ANTIBIOTIC DERIVED FROM ONE AMINO ACID. FIRST GENERATION (Penicillin) (β-lactamase sensitive) (*narrow spectrum*)
	ANTIBIOTIC DERIVED FROM TWO AMINO ACID. **PENICILLINS**
B	ANTIBIOTIC DERIVED FROM TWO AMINO ACID. **PENEMS**
C	ANTIBIOTIC DERIVED FROM TWO AMINO ACID. SECOND GENERATION (β-lactamase resistant) (*narrow spectrum*)
D	ANTIBIOTIC DERIVED FROM TWO AMINO ACID. THIRD GENERATION (Aminopenicillins) (*extended spectrum*)
E	ANTIBIOTIC DERIVED FROM TWO AMINO ACID. FOURTH GENERATION (Carboxypenicillin) (*extended spectrum*)

F	ANTIBIOTIC DERIVED FROM TWO AMINO ACID. FOURTH GENERATION (Ureidopenicillins) (*extended spectrum*)
G	ANTIBIOTIC DERIVED FROM TWO AMINO ACID. FOURTH GENERATION (Miscellaneous) (*extended spectrum*)
H	ANTIBIOTIC DERIVED FROM TWO AMINO ACID. **PENEMS** FIRST GENERATION (Penicillin) (*narrow spectrum*)
I	ANTIBIOTIC DERIVED FROM TWO AMINO ACID. Carbapenems (Penicillin)
	ANTIBIOTIC DERIVED FROM TWO AMINO ACID. **CEPHALOSPORINS**
J	ANTIBIOTIC DERIVED FROM TWO AMINO ACID. FIRST GENERATION (*moderate spectrum*)
K	ANTIBIOTICS DERIVED FROM TWO AMINO ACIDS SECOND GENERATION (*moderate spectrum*)
L	ANTIBIOTICS DERIVED FROM TWO AMINO ACIDS THIRD GENERATION (*broad spectrum*)
M	ANTIBIOTICS DERIVED FROM TWO AMINO ACIDS FOURTH GENERATION (*broad spectrum*)
N	ANTIBIOTICS DERIVED FROM TWO AMINO ACIDS FIFTH GENERATION (*broad spectrum*)
O	**TETRACYCLINE GROUP OF ANTIBIOTICS** (*broad spectrum*) Chlortetracycline, Oxytetracycline, Tetracycline, Doxycycline, Minocycline Metacycline (metacycline), Demeclocycline (declomycin)
P	**POLYPEPTIDE ANTIBIOTICS**

Q	ANTI-TUBERCLOSTATICS
R	ANTIBIOTICS DERIVED FROM SUGARS
S	ANTIBIOTICS DERIVED FROM ACETATES / PROPIONATES
T	MACROLIDE ANTIBIOTICS
U	POLYENE ANTIBIOTICS
V	MACROCYCLIC ANTIBIOTICS
W	ANTIBIOTICS WITH VARIOUS STRUCTURES
X	QUINOLONE GROUP OF ANTIBIOTICS (MACROCYCLIC)
Y	ANTITUMOUR ANTIBIOTICS WITH VARIOUS STRUCTURES

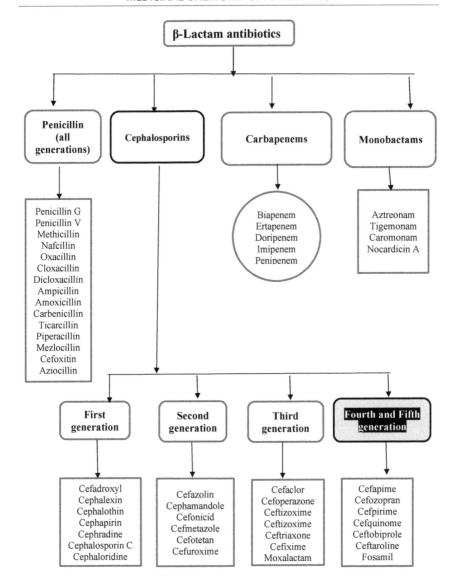

5.3 Chemistry of β-lactam

BETA–LACTAMS (β-lactam)

2-Azetidinone is the simplest β-lactam ring and it forms the central core structure of the several β-lactam antibiotic families, the principal ones being the;

A. **PENICILLIN** *(Penams).*
B. **PENICILLIN** *(Panems).*
C. **CARBAPENEMS.**
D. **CEPHALOSPORINS.**
E. **MONOBACTAMS.**

Nearly all of above β-lactam antibiotic families work by inhibiting bacterial cell wall biosynthesis and has lethal effect on bacteria. Other lactams are not active biologically or less active than β-lactam.

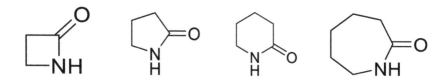

From left to right, general structures of a β-lactam, a γ-lactam, a δ-lactam, and an ε-lactam. The specific structures are β-propiolactam, γ-butyrolactam, δ-valerolactam, and ε-caprolactam.

"Cyclobutane" is the base for the formation of β-lactam antibiotics. It is also called as "four membered heterocyclic ring system". The β -lactam antibiotics are derived from two amino acids.

$$H_2C \text{ ------ } CH_2$$
$$| \qquad\qquad |$$
$$H_2C \text{ ------ } CH_2$$

Cyclobutene is a cycloalkane and organic compound. Commercially it is available as a liquefied. Cyclobutene itself is of no biological significance, but more complex derivatives are important in biology and biotechnology. When Nitrogen atom is added in the cyclobutene, it is converted to a compound which is called as "Azete".

Azete is a heterocyclic chemical compound consisting of an unsaturated four-membered ring with three carbon atoms and one hetero nitrogen atom.

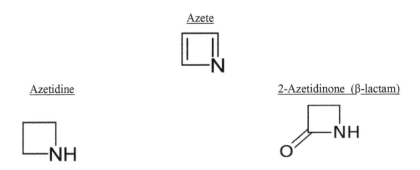

Azete

Azetidine

2-Azetidinone (β-lactam)

The antibiotic which basically contain β-lactam ring is known as β-lactam antibiotic. Azetidine is a saturated heterocyclic organic compound containing three carbon atoms and one NITROGEN atom. It is a liquid at room temperature with a strong odor of ammonia and is strongly basic compared.

- Azetidines do not occur as frequently in nature.
- Azetidinone ring is called as β-lactam because the functional CO group is present in azetidine ring at the beta position.
- Azetidine ring is incorporated with CO group and this ring system is called as β-lactam or "2-Azitidinone".
- 2-Azetidinone is the simplest β-lactam ring and it forms the central core structure of the β-lactam.
- β-lactam ring is formed by the internal cyclization when alpha (α) and gamma (Υ) amino acids are heated together.
- A β-lactam ring is a four-membered lactam (a lactam is a cyclic amide.) It is named as such because the nitrogen atom (N) is attached to the β-carbon atom relative to the carbonyl group (CO).
- A new study has suggested that β-lactams can undergo ring-opening polymerization to form amide bond.

Structure activity relationship (SAR)

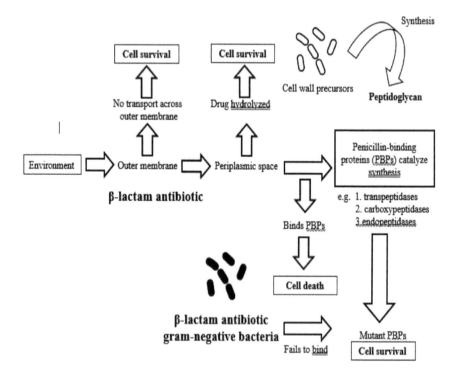

o β-Lactam ring and R should be cyclic, aromatic or heterocyclic for the minimal activity.
o Substitution on α-position of benzyl penicillin have resistance to acid hydrolysis.
o Increase in stability is due to electron withdrawing group on amide carbonyl group.
o α-carbon atom of an acyl group could be part of an aromatic or heterocyclic ring.

BETA-LACTIM RING (β – lactim)

The amide tautomer is referred to as the lactam structure, while the imidic acid tautomer is referred to as the lactim structure. These tautomeric forms are predominant at pH 7.

The concept of tautomerization is called tautomerism. The reaction interconverting the two is called tautomerization. In β–lactim ring, the H of NH group in beta lactam ring is shifted on carbonyl group, the comparison is shown below. This reaction commonly results in the relocation of a proton. Tautomerism is relevant to the behavior of amino acids and nucleic acids, two of the fundamental building blocks of life. The concept of tautomerizations is called tautomerism.

The β – lactims has no antibacterial activ ity.
(comparison of β–lactims and β-lactams)

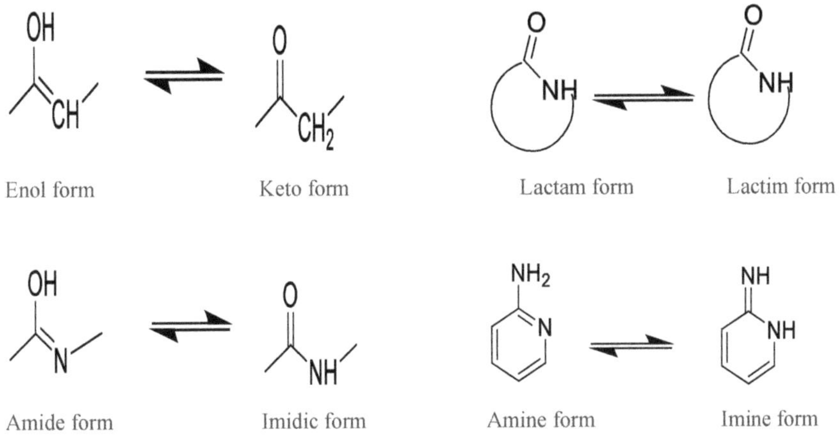

| Enol form | Keto form | Lactam form | Lactim form |

| Amide form | Imidic form | Amine form | Imine form |

A lactim is a cyclic carboximidic acid compound characterized by an endocyclic carbon-nitrogen double bond. They are formed when lactams undergo tautomerization as shown below:

173

Lactam   Lactim

5.3.1   Nomenclature of β-lactams

By convention, the bicyclic β-lactams are numbered starting with the position occupied by sulfur in the penams and cephems, regardless of which atom it is in a given class. That is, position 1 is always adjacent to the β-carbon of β-lactam ring. The numbering continues clockwise from position one until the β-carbon of β-lactam is reached, at which point numbering continues counterclockwise around the lactam ring to numb.

β-Lactams fused to saturated five-membered rings:
β-Lactams containing thiazolidine rings are named penams.
β-Lactams containing pyrrolidine rings are named carbapenams.
β-Lactams fused to oxazolidine rings are named oxapenams.
β-Lactams fused to unsaturated five-membered rings:
β-Lactams containing 2,3-dihydrothiazole rings are named penems.
β-Lactams containing 2,3-dihydro-1H-pyrrole rings are named carbapenems.
β-Lactams fused to unsaturated six-membered rings:
β-Lactams containing 3,6-dihydro-2H-1,3-thiazine rings are named cephems.
β-Lactams containing 1,2,3,4-tetrahydropyridine rings are named carbacephems.
β-Lactams containing 3,6-dihydro-2H-1,3-oxazine rings are named oxacephams.
β-Lactams not fused to any other ring are named monobactams.

β-lactams are classified according to their core ring structures.

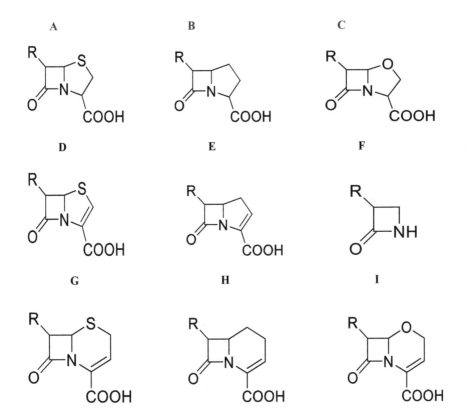

The β-lactam core structures. (A) A penam. (B) A carbapenam. (C) An oxapenam. (D) A penem. (E) A carbapenem. (F) A monobactam. (G) A cephem. (H)A carbacephem. (I) An oxacephem.

Greek prefixes in alphabetical order indicate ring size:

> α-Lactam (3 ring atoms)
> β-lactam (4 ring atoms)
> γ-Lactam (5 ring atoms)
> δ-Lactam (6 ring atoms)
> ε-Lactam (7 ring atoms)

This ring-size nomenclature stems from the fact that a hydrolyzed α-Lactam leads to an α-amino acid and a β-Lactam to a β-amino acid.

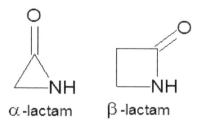

α-lactam   β-lactam

5.4   Penicillin and its derivatives

Classification of natural penicillin

Benzyl penicillin	Penicillin G
Pentyl penicillin	Penicillin F
3-Pentyl penicillin	Penicillin K
Phenoxymethyl penicillin	Penicillin V

PENEMS

Natural penicillin β-lactamase sensitive	Penicillin G (Benzylpenicillin) Benzathine penicillin G (Benzathine benzylpenicillin) Penicillin K (Bezyl penicillin potassium) Penicillin N (isopenicillin) Penicillin O (Almicillin) Penicillin V or VK (Phenoxymethylpenicillin) Procaine penicillin G (Procaine bezylypenicillin)	FIRST GENERATION
β-lactamase inhibitors	Clavulanic acid Salbactam Tozabactam	SECOND GENERATION

176

β-lactamase-resistant	Methicillin Nafcillin Oxacillin Cloxacillin Dicloxacillin Flucloxacillin	SECOND GENERATION
Aminopenicillins	Ampicillin Amoxicillin Pivampicillin Hetacillin Bacampicillin Metampicillin Talampicillin Epicillin	THIRD GENERATION
Carboxypenicillins	Carbencillin Ticarcillin Temocillin Carindacillin	FOURTH GENERATION
Ureidopenicillins	Mezlocillin Pipercillin Azlocillin	FOURTH GENERATION
Micellaneous	Mecillinam Pivmecillinam Salbenicillin	

PENEMS

- Faropenem
- Ritipenem

CARBAPENEMS

- Ertapenem
- Doripenem (antipeudomonal)
- Imipenem (antipeudomonal)
- Meropenem (antipeudomonal)
- Biapenem
- Panipenem

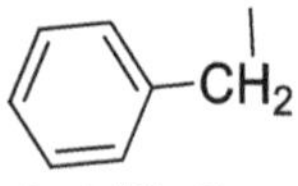

Penicillin G

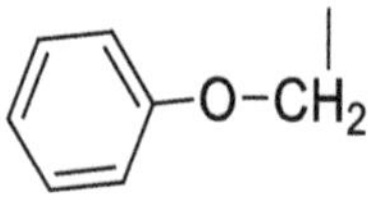

Penicillin V

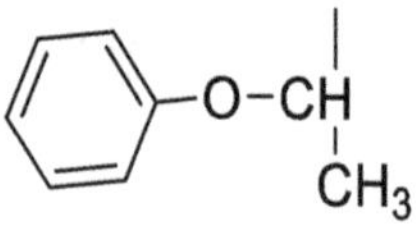

Phenethicillin

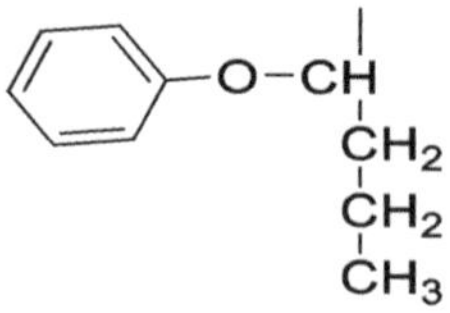

Propacillin

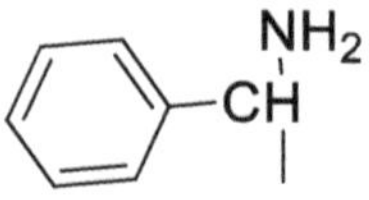

Ampicillin

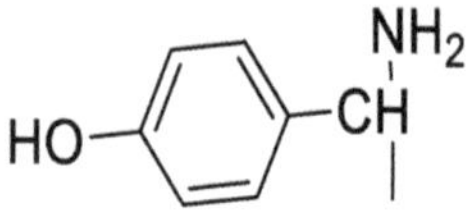

Amoxicillin

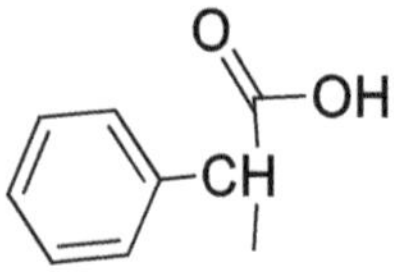

Carbenecillin

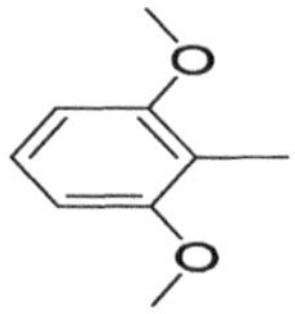

Methicillin

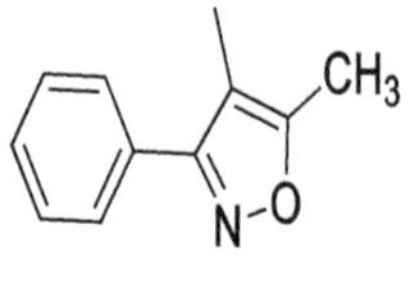

Oxacillin

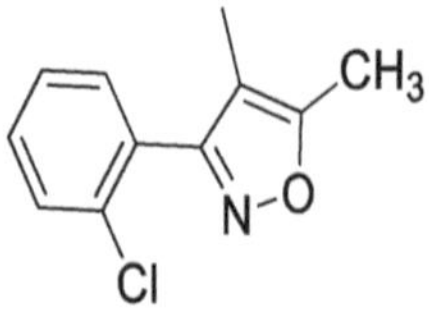

Cloxacillin

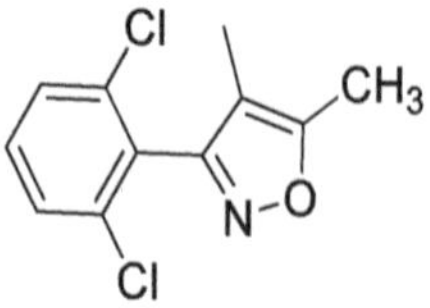

Docloxacillin

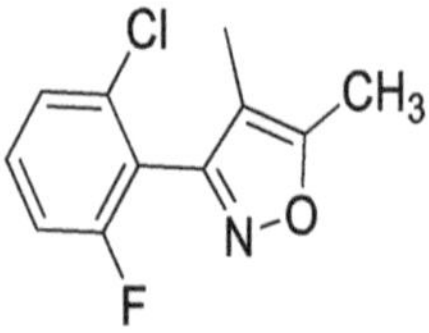

Flucloxacillin

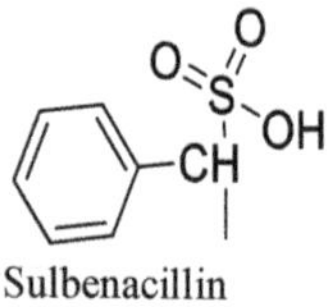

Sulbenacillin

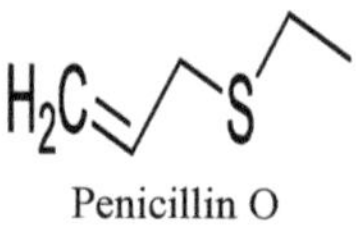

Penicillin O

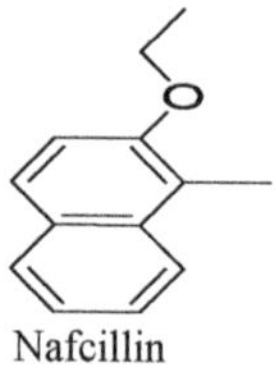

Nafcillin

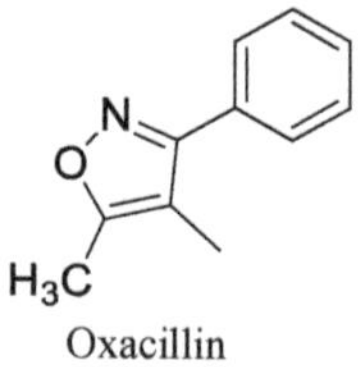

Oxacillin

This group is composed of β-lactam antibiotics which are derived from two amino acids. Several representatives of this group belong to the most potent and valuable agents in antibacterial chemotherapy. Penicillin/s are *N-acyl derivatives* of 6-aminopenicillanic acid (**6-APA**). The penicillin is further prepared by chemical or enzymatic cleavage of the side chain of penicillin G or V. Presently several generations have been synthesized which are in clinical use.

When the β-lactam ring is fused, it forms the base which is known as "penam". After substitution on penam, the compound which is obtained is called as "6-Aminopenicilloic acid "that on further addition of certain groups becomes the powerful antibacterial agent like penicillin. The figures are shown below.

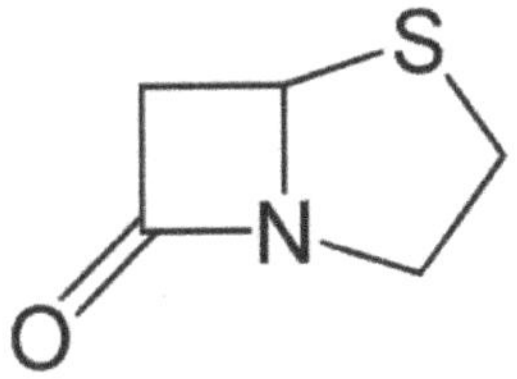

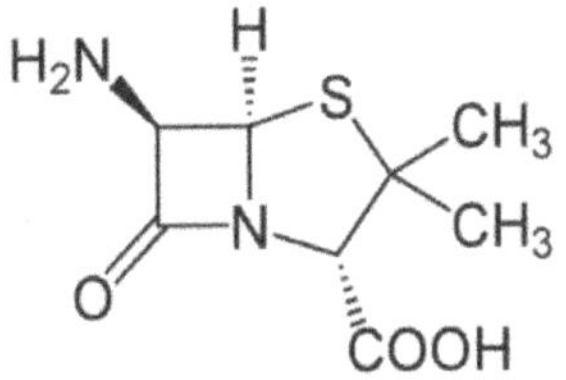

6-Aminopenicillanic acid (6-APA)

$$C_8H_{12}N_2O_3S$$

Molar mass: 216.26g/mol

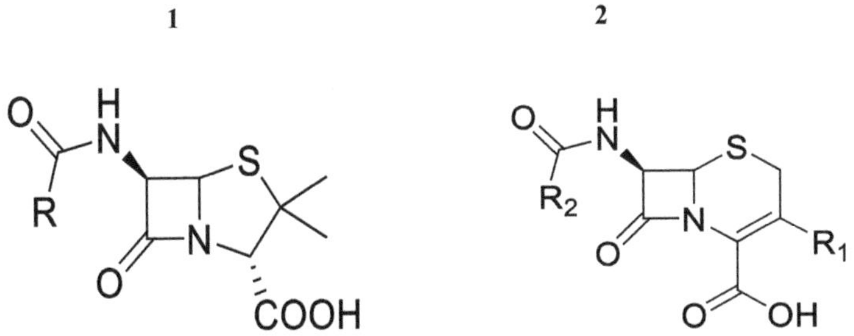

1   2

Core structure of penicillin (1) and cephalosporins (2) with β-lactam ring.

5.4.1 Cephalosporins

are formally regarded as derivatives of 7-aminocephalosporic acid (7-ACA) which is prepared by the chemical cleavage of the side chain of Cephalosporin C. This group is composed of β-lactam antibiotics which are derived from two amino acids. Presently several generations have been synthesized which are in clinical use.

7-Aminocephalosporic acid (7-ACA)
$C_{10}H_{12}N_2O_5S$
Molar mass: 272.28g/mol

5.4.2 Degradation of penicillin G and re-arrangement reactions of penicillin (in general)

5.5 Chemical synthesis of penicillin, ampicillin and amoxicillin

Synthesis of penicillin (condensed steps)

Cystein   Valine

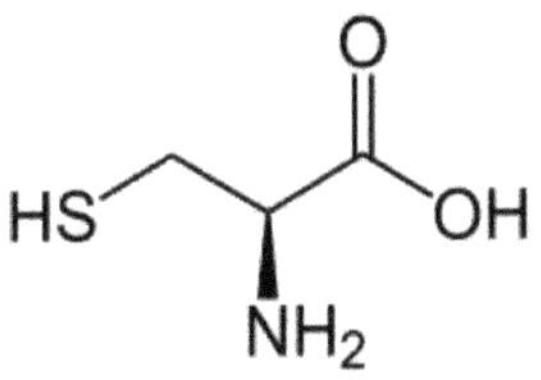

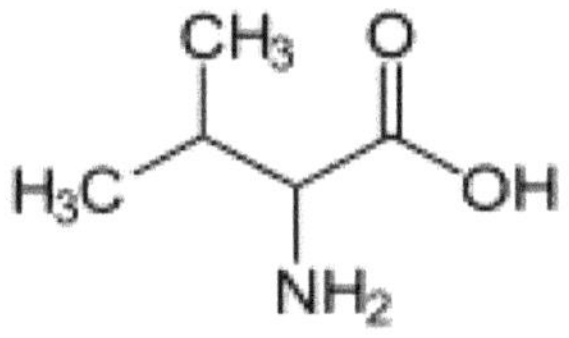

Basic structure of penicillin

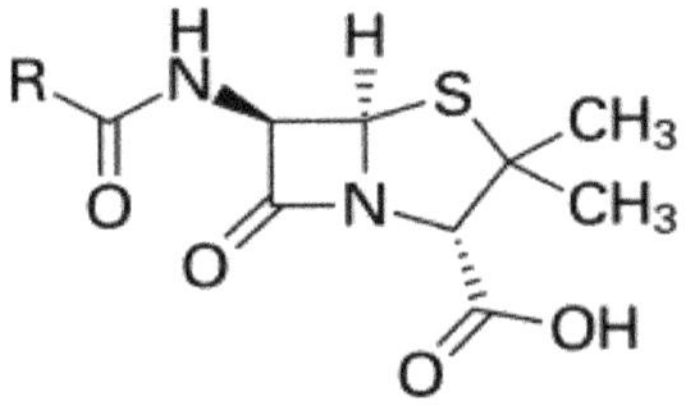

Synthesis of penicillin

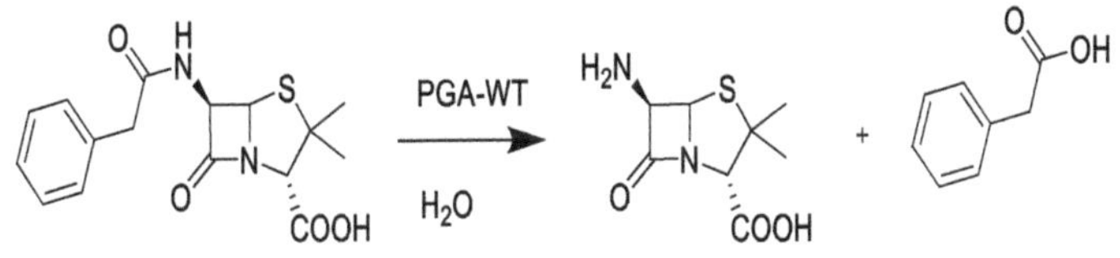

Penicillin G   6-APA   Phenylacetic acid

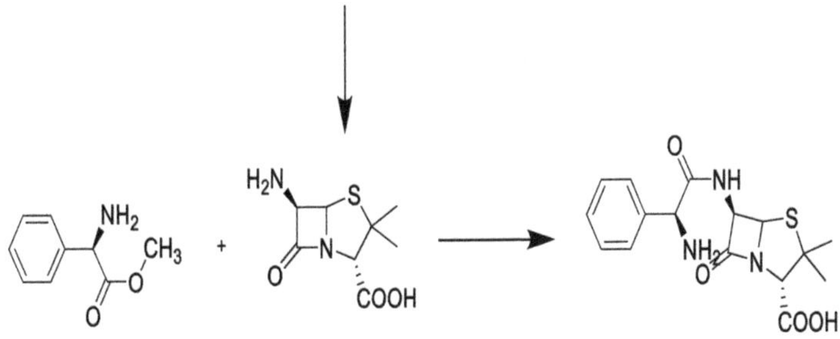

D-phenylglycine   6-APA   Ampicillin
methyl ester

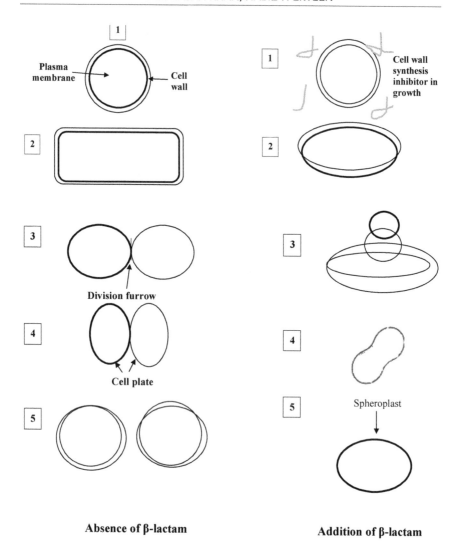

Absence of β-lactam

Addition of β-lactam

182

5.6 Broad spectrum and powerful combination

AUGMENTIN

Effective against
Gram + and gram –
bacteria

Treatment for
Skin diseases, sinusitis, urinary tract
infections, pharyngitis

Characteristics
Broad spectrum
Oral and parentral

Side effects
Rash, diarrhea, vomiting, nausea,
odema, stomatitis and fatigue

Amoxacillin + Clavulanic acid = Augmentin

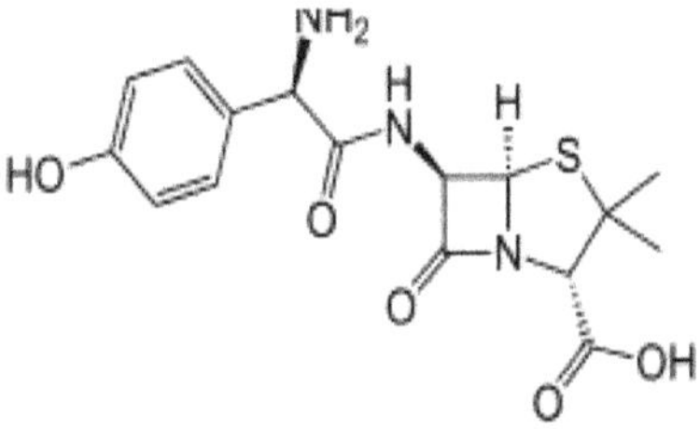

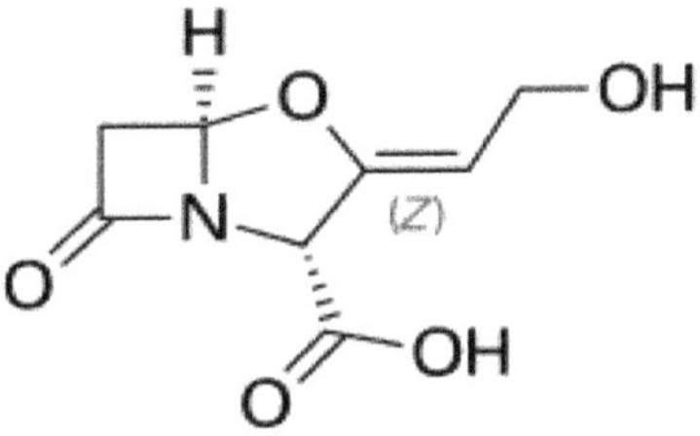

5.7 Antibiotic derived from one amino acid (individual compounds).

5.7.1 Chloramphenico

$$C_{11}H_{12}Cl_2N_2O_5$$
Molar mass
323.13g/mol

Chemistry

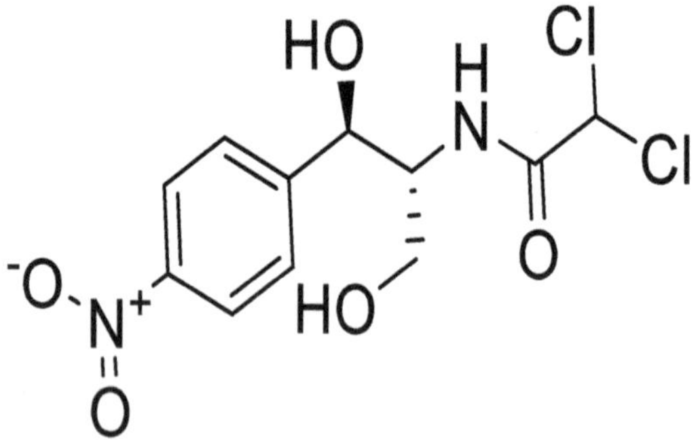

Chemical groups in Chloramphenicol molecule

This group includes the reserve broad spectrum antibiotics Chloramphenicol, thiamphenicol and azidamphenicol. This group is derived from one amino acid.

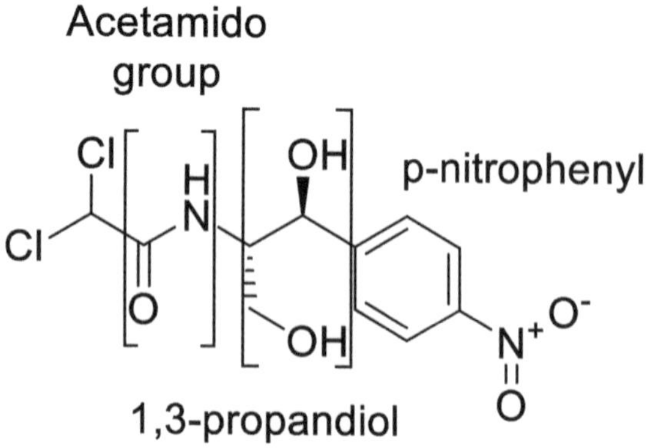

Structure activity relationship (SAR) of Chloramphenicol:

- ❏ The structure of chloramphenicol considered to be very notorious due to the presence of electro-negative NO_2 group. Whenever this group is present in any compound, the molecule becomes very toxic.
- ❏ Chloramphenicol has two asymmetric carbonatoms, therefore, it has four stereoisomers:
- ❏ *D (+) and L (-) threoisomers.*
- ❏ *D (+) and L (-) erythroiosmers.*

Bothe D and L erythroisomers are very toxic
and cannot be used in medicine.

- ❏ If the phenyl ring of chloramphenicol is replaced by heterocyclic ring, the resulting compound is less active.
- ❏ The nitro group is replaced by cyanide group (-CN), amide (-CONH), primary amine -NH_2), hydroxyl (-OH) or secondary amine (-NHR), the biological activity is reduced.
- ❏ Di-chloroacetyl group is very important for activity. Change to Bromo, the activity is reduced.
- ❏ Any change in the aliphatic chain, results deactivation.
- ❏ The hydroxic acid analogue lacks the biological activity.
- ❏ Two isomers, D-threochloramphenicol and L-threochloramphenicol are obtained, the-threo isomer is separated because L isomer is inactive therapeutically.
- ❏ The D-threo isomer (chloramphenicol) is optically and biologically active base.
- ❏ The therapeutic activity of the compound mainly lies due to the bonding of NO_2 and di-chloroacetyl groups. Any change on this group, the biological activity will be lost completely.
- ❏ The racemate is known as synthomycetin.

D-threochloramphenicol

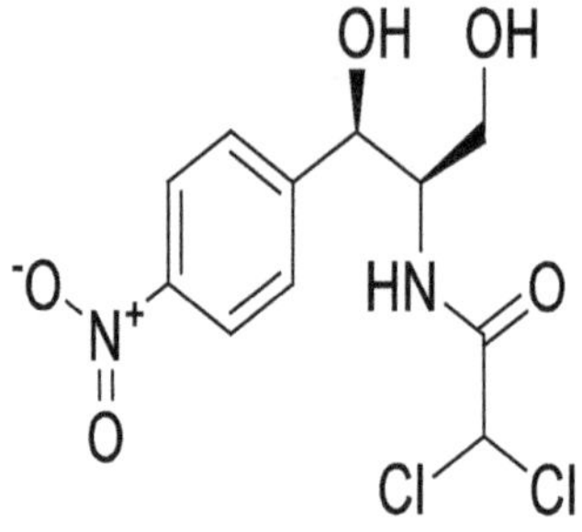

L-threochloramphenicol

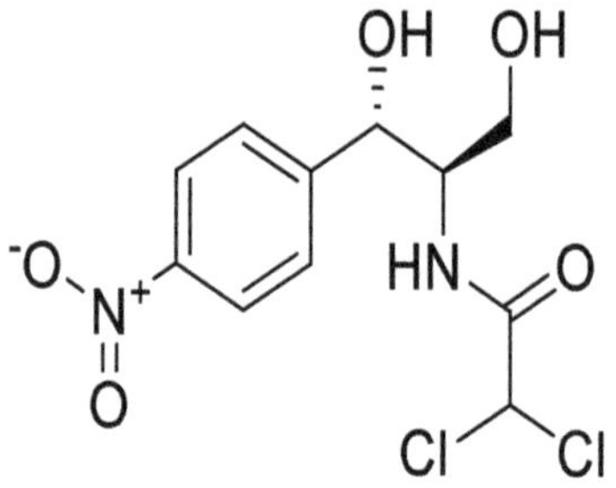

Thiamphenicol

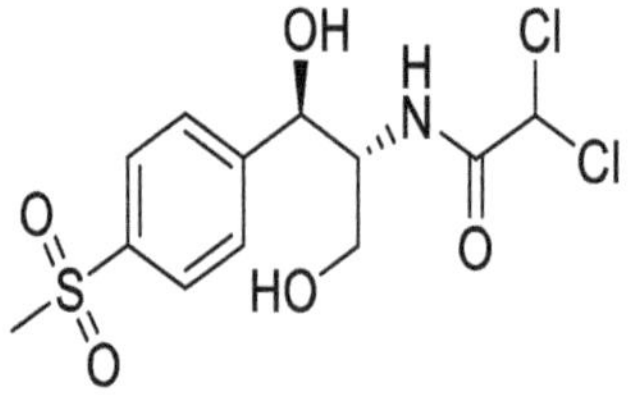

Azidamphenicol

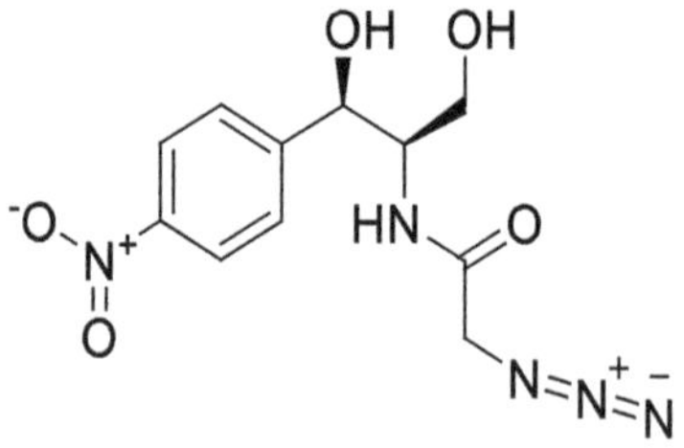

- Chloramphenicol is an antibiotic derived from one amino acid.
- The structure of chloramphenicol considered to be very notorious due to the presence of electro-negative NO2 group. Whenever this group is present in any compound, the molecule becomes very toxic.
- Chloramphenicol has two asymmetric carbon atoms therefore it has four stereoisomers:
- D (-) and L (+) threoisomers.
- D (-) and L (+) erythroiosmers.
- Both D and L erythroisomers are very toxic and cannot be used in medicine.
- Two isomers, D-threochloramphenicol and L-threochloramphenicol are obtained where the L-threo isomer is separated because L isomer is inactive therapeutically.

- The D-threo isomer (chloramphenicol) is optically and biologically active base.
- Structure 1 is suitable substitute for chloramphenicol since it does not cause irreversible haematological side effects. But is weak in asserting biological activity. Moreover, presence of N=N=N- may show enhanced toxic effects on liver.
- Structure 2 shows the absence of electro-negative nitro group, the activity is much reduced but some suitable properties like water solubility and local tolerance is better than other group of this class. It is the methyl suphonyl analogue of chloramphenicol. It is used in many countries as a veterinary antibiotic, but is available in China, Morocco and Italy for use in humans. I.M., I.V., ORAL.
- If phenyl ring is replaced by heterocyclic ring, the compound becomes less active.
- In the structure of chloramphenicol, if chlorine atoms are replaced by fluorine atoms at position 3(fluoramphenicol), (as shown in chemistry section above) the activity is reduced.
- The carbonyl group is necessary to attain the complete biological activity.
- If amino group is changed to any other group, the biological activity is reduced.
- Change in any one of the hydroxyl group, the biological activity is reduced.
- Alteration in the length of aliphatic chain, deactivation of the compound takes place.
- Oral, I.M.

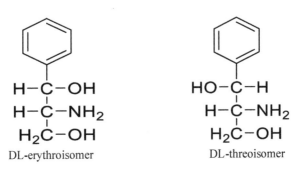

DL-erythroisomer   DL-threoisomer

- The therapeutic activity of the compound mainly lies due to the bonding of NO_2 and di-chloroacetyl groups. Any change brought the biological activity is lost completely.
- The racemate is known as synthomycetin.
- Structure 1 is considered suitable substitute for chloramphenicol since it does not cause irreversible haematological side effects. But is weak in asserting biological activity.
- Structure 2 shows the absence of electro-negative nitro group, the activity is much reduced but some suitable properties like water solubility and local tolerance is better than other group of this class. Moreover, presence of N=N=N- may show enhanced toxic effects on liver.
- If phenyl ring is replaced by heterocyclic ring, the compound becomes less active.
- In the structure of chloramphenicol, if chlorine atoms are replaced by fluorine atoms at position 3 (fluoramphenicol), the activity is reduced.
- The carbonyl group is necessary to attain the complete biological activity.
- If amino is changed to any other group, the biological activity is drastically reduced.
- Change in any one of the hydroxyl group, the biological activity is reduced.
- Alteration of the length of aliphatic chain, deactivation of the compound takes place.
- If amino is changed to any other group, the biological activity is drastically reduced.
- Change in any one of the hydroxyl group, the biological activity is reduced.
- Alteration of the length of aliphatic chain, deactivation of the compound takes place.

Metabolism

Chloramphenicol is metabolized by the liver to inactive chloramphenicol glucuronate.

Chloramphenicol Glucuronate

- Chloramphenicol is extremely lipid soluble and the absorption depends upon particle size.
- Stops the bacterial growth by stopping the production of proteins.
- Only a tiny fraction of the chloramphenicol is excreted by the kidneys unchanged.
- Examination of the structure of chloramphenicol (indicates the presence of both lipophilic (nonpolar) and hydrophilic (polar) groups and substituents.
- The presence of oxygen and nitrogen containing functional groups usually enhances water solubility.
- While lipid solubility is enhanced by non-ionizable hydrocarbon chains and ring systems.

Chloramphenicol is the example of enzymatic inactivation of antibiotic by the mechanism of acetylation by certain R- factor – carrying bacteria (resistance factor) which produces a specified "acetyltransferase" in typhoid fever.

Pharmacological uses

Chloramphenicol was the first effective broad-spectrum antibiotic by preventing peptide bond formation (interfering the synthesis of bacterial protein). Its use by mouth or by injection is only recommended when safer antibiotics cannot be used due to any reasons. It is best to treat meningitis, plague, cholera, pneumonia, typhoid fever and many other sex- linked infections, eye infections.

Adverse effects

aplastic anaemia, bone marrow depression.

Contraindications

- Chloramphenicol passes into breast milk, so should be avoided during breast feeding.
- Chloramphenicol is antagonistic with most of the cephalosporins and using both together should be avoided in the treatment of infections.
- Administration of chloramphenicol concomitantly with bone marrow depressant drugs is contraindicated, although concerns over aplastic anaemia associated with ocular chloramphenicol have largely been discounted. In young children grey baby syndrome.

Enzymatic degradation of Chloramphenicol

Synthesis of Chloramphenicol I

Synthesis of Chloramphenicol 2

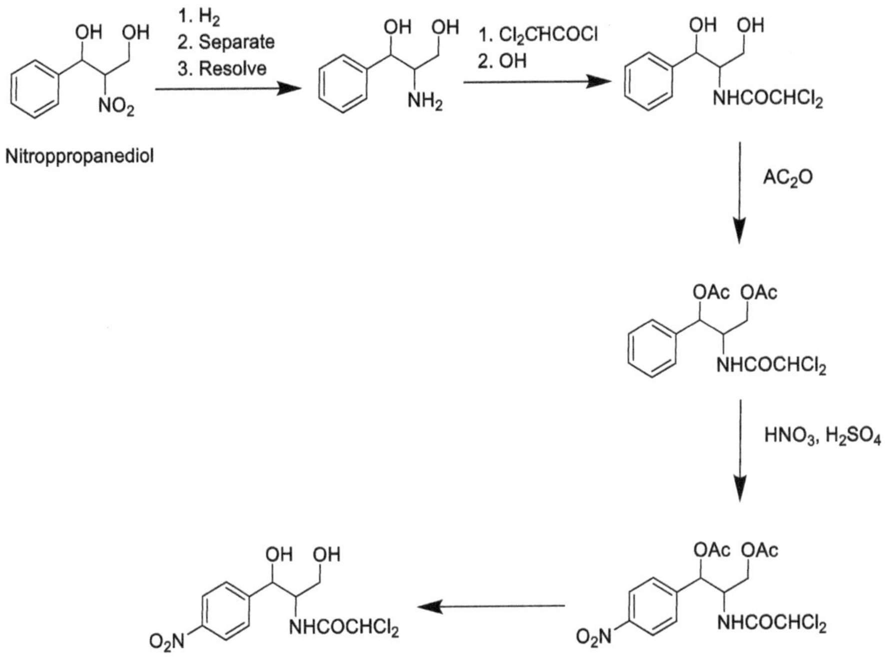

Nitroppropanediol

Reagents and conditions:
1. H$_2$
2. Separate
3. Resolve

1. Cl$_2$CHCOCl
2. OH

AC$_2$O

HNO$_3$, H$_2$SO$_4$

Synthesis of Chloramphenicol 3

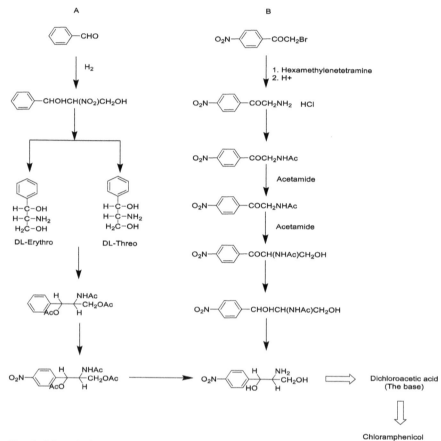

Chemical degradation

Chemical degradation

Chloramphenicol

5.8 Properties of individual important beta-lactam penicillin antibiotics

5.8.1 Chemistry of Penicillin in general

Phenoxymethylpenicillin (penicillin V) has been found to be considerably more stable than other penicillin in the presence of acid, a fact which immediately suggested its suitability for use in oral formulations. Since benzylpenicillin is rapidly destroyed by the acidic contents of the stomach, the oral use of the antibiotic is feasible only if special buffered late in the penicillin.

Some 30 different crystalline penicillin were prepared. Later, the synthesis of penicillin having various aliphatic side chains by adding the corresponding aliphatic precursors during fermentation, the basic difference among these penicillin lies in the nature of the R group. Only monosubstituted acetic formulations or insoluble salts are employed. The discovery of the superiority of penicillin V is the isolation of 6-aminopenicillanic in the penicillanic acid from penicillium chrysogenum. 6-Aminopenicillanic acid that there is no acyl side chain is present.

6-aminopenicillanic acid may represent an alternative metabolite are not precluded. 6-Aminopenicillanic acid can be acylated to obtain penicillin analogs not otherwise available or obtained under difficult conditions. Penicillin K is produced in excellent yields by penicillium chrysogenum unless phenylacetic acid is present.

Para-hydroxy-benzyl penicillin is superior to benzylpenicillin for the treatment of certain types of infections although the antibacterial spectrum of this penicillin is qualitatively similar to that of the benzyl form. Many of these have excellent antibacterial properties although, again, this activity is qualitatively similar to that of benzylpenicillin. Using precursors and the high yielding strains of Penicillia. It was possible to isolate benzylpenicillin without resorting to the cumbersome chromatographic procedures needed in making the early preparations. The acidified culture fluid is continuously introduced at the center of a rotating spiral tube while amyl or butyl acetate is fed into the periphery.

The penicillin free acids are very unstable, but organic base salts or alkali metal salts of the antibiotic are relatively stable in the dry state. Many penicillin salts can be easily crystallized. Aqueous solutions of the antibiotic are only moderately stable in the pH range 6-7 but the addition of buffer agents, especially phosphate buffer, has a preservative effect. The loss in activity of aqueous solutions is accompanied by the evolution of carbon dioxide. The chemistry of penicillin was shown to be b-dimethylcysteine. Desulfurization of the isocyanate derivative with Raney nickel gave N-phenylcarbamyl-D-valine. This reaction established the configuration of one of the three asymmetric centers of penicillin. Penicillamine is obtained from the penicillin under a variety of conditions. It may be prepared by the direct acid hydrolysis of the antibiotic with strong acid. It is degraded to penicillamine by treatment with stronger acid or by heating with mercuric chloride.

Penilloic acids are the dimer carboxylation products obtained by warming B-lactam penicilloic acids. The latter are produced by treating penicillin with alkali solution exposing the antibiotics to preparations of the enzyme penicillinase. The hydrolysis of the B-lactam group of penicillin also occurs when the antibiotic is allowed to stand in methanol solution or is treated with primary or secondary amines. The stability of the thiazolidine ring of penicillin to oxidation is attributed to the presence of the B-lactam portion, since thiazolidines known to be protected by N acylation. In case the antibiotic is degraded to penicilloic acid prior to oxidation. Ring cleavage then occurs and sulfonic acid derivative is obtained. The penilloaldehydes and intermediate penaldic acids are other key degradation products. The penilloaldehydes and penicillamine are obtained by treating penicillin with strong acid or by heating penillic acid with mercuric chloride.

(The structural representation is carried out in the latter chapters).

Many attempts have been made to cyclize penicilloic acid, but azlactone formation has invariably taken precedence over the formation of the desired B-lactam ring. The thiazolidine ring then ruptures and penicillenates obtained were isolated, only the "B"-isomer could be cyclized to the B-lactam. The natural penicillin corresponds to the a-isomer. The desired benzyl natural penicillin was obtained by cyclization of a-4-carbomethoxy-5,5-dimethyl-a-benzylsulfonamido-2-thiazolidineacetic acid hydrochloride.

(The structural synthesis of penicillin and derivativeare described in the latter chapters).

5.8.2 Degradation of penicillin in general

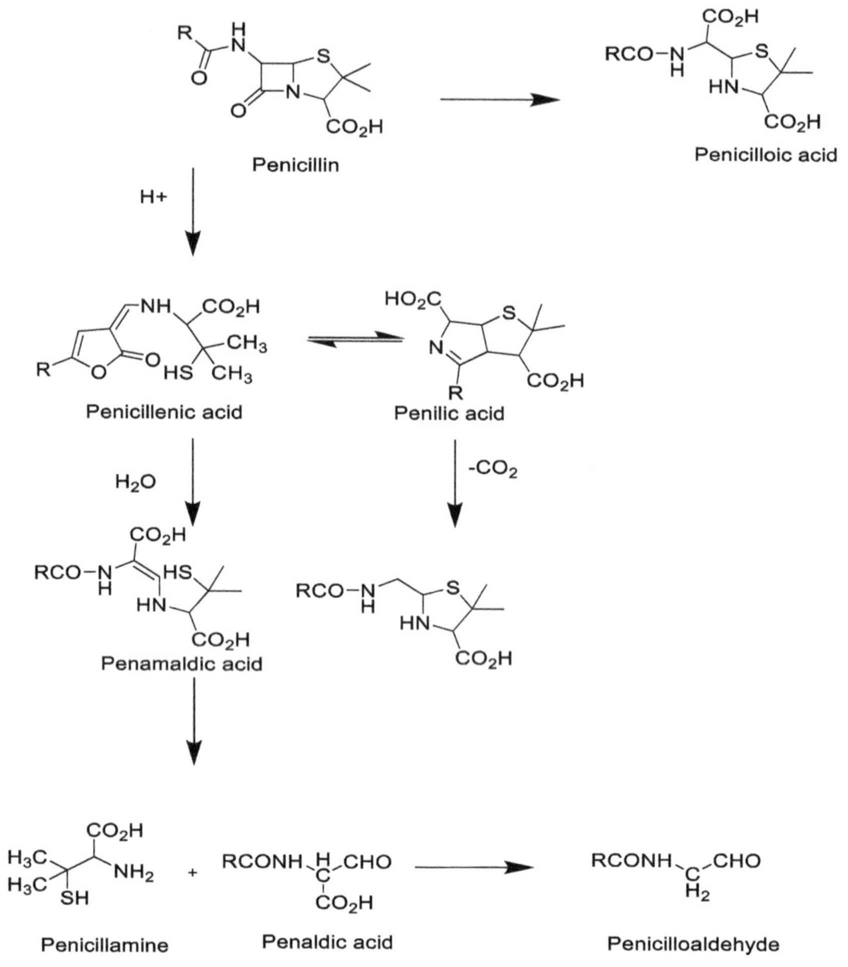
Penicillin
Penicilloic acid
H+
Penicillenic acid
Penilic acid
H2O
-CO2
Penamaldic acid
Penicillamine
Penaldic acid
Penicilloaldehyde

5.8.3 Mechanism based inhibition of β-lactamase.

5.8.4 Conversion of natural penicillin to synthetic penicillin

5.8.5 Reactions of penicillin where R= $C_6H_5CH_2$

- The chemistry of penicillin is to degrade to penicillamine which is caused by hydrogenation /acid hydrolysis of penicillin gives penicillamine and is called as β -β-dimethylcysteine.
- Desulphurization with renay nickle gives N-phenylcarbamyl-d-valine.
- Treatment with amino group, it gives amide of penicilloic acid.
- Penilloic acid after treatment with aq. mercuric chloride gives penicillamine.

Scheme for the above reactions

Penicillamine

Penicillin $\longrightarrow$

hydrogenation / acid hydrolysis of penicillin gives penicillamine which is β -β-dimethyl-cysteine

Penicllic acid

Penilloic acid

Penicilloic acid

Methyl ester

Amide / methyl penicilloic acid   =   penicillin treated with methanol to get:

Peniloaldehyde

Penaldic acid

5.8.6 Pharmacological uses and adverse reactions of penicillin in general

Systemic infections due to pneumococci, streptococci, many strains of Micrococci, clostridia, and meningococci responded dramatically to treatment with the antibiotic. Penicillin was found to be useful in the prophylactic treatment of potentially infected wounds as well as in cases where serious infections were already established. Oral formulations have been developed which include buffered tablets or tablets containing highly insoluble salts of benzylpenicillin. Penicillin V, phenoxy-methylpenicillin, which is more stable than benzylpenicillin in the acid. When a solution of penicillin is injected, 50-80% of the dose may be recovered from the urine.

When penicillin is given orally, much of the antibiotic is destroyed by the acidic environment found in the stomach. Procaine forms a highly insoluble crystalline salt with benzylpenicillin. Penicillin is outstanding among chemotherapeutic agents.

The only adverse reactions encountered in the use of penicillin are allergic in nature. Urticaria (hives) although contact dermatitis may follow topical use. Anaphylactic shock reactions occasionally accompanying the administration of the drug. Penicillin appears to be bactericidal to growing bacteria and bacteriostatic when bacteria are in the resting phase.

(Detail of adverse and toxic effects / reactions of individual compounds is discussed in latter parts

Beta-lactam   monobactam

carbacepham   oxacepham   cepham   penam   oxapenam   carbapenam

carbacephems   oxacephems X=H   cephalosporins   penicilins   clavulanic acid   carbapenems

5.9 Antibiotics derived from two amino acids (penams)

FIRST GENERATION (penicillin)
(β-lactamase sensitive)

202

(narrow spectrum)

BENZYLPENICILLIN

(Penicillin G or crystalline penicillin G)

First generation (β-lactamase sensitive)

$$C_9H_{11}N_2O_4S$$
Molar mass
334.39g/mol

Chemistry

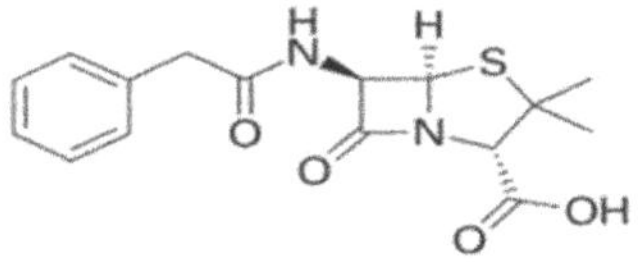

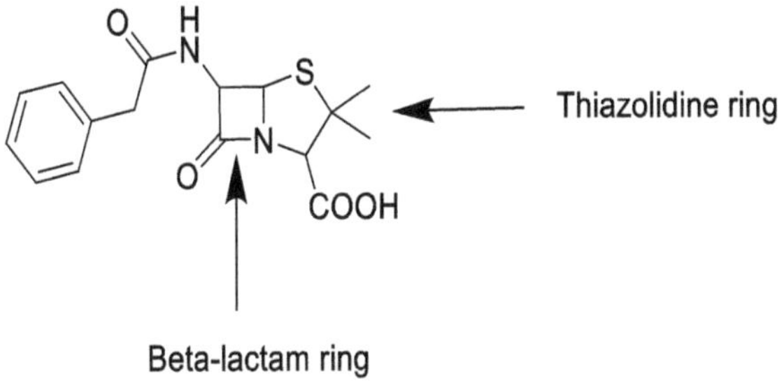

Thiazolidine ring

Beta-lactam ring

The basic structure of the penicillin consists of a 'thiazolidine ring' which is fused with β-lactam ring.

1. C 2 contains 2 methyl groups.
2. C 3 is attached with a carboxylic group.
3. In β-lactam ring, position 6 is a primary amine which has aliphatic chain consisting of a CO and CH_2 groups.

4. If CH_2 group in the aliphatic chain of Penicillin G is changed to NH_2 group, it is called as "AMPICILLIN".

5. If the terminal unsaturated 6 membered ring is attached with OH group in the point No. 7, the compound is known as "AMOXICILLIN ".

6. If the CH2 group in aliphatic chain is converted to COOH group, the compound is called as "CARBENCILLIN".

7. In case, if the CH_2 group in Penicillin G is replaced by "oxazole" group and is attached with "CHLOROBENZENE", the compound will be converted to "CLOXACILLIN".

Structure activity relationship (SAR)

❖ Beta lactam ring and R should be cyclic, aromatic or heterocyclic for minimal activity.

❖ Substitution on Alpha position of benzyl penicillin have resistance to acid hydrolysis.

❖ Increase in stability is due to electron withdrawing group on amide carbonyl group.

❖ Alpha carbon atom of an acyl group could be a part of an aromatic or heterocyclic ring.

❖ PENICILLIN G basically contains β-lactam ring fused with thiazolidine ring. These two rings contribute to the major biological activity.

❖ Position 1 is thiophene, in this ring if methyl groups are replaced, the biological activity is reduced.

❖ In thiazolidine group, if COOH group is removed or added with other inorganic or organic acid, the biological activity will be reduced drastically.

❖ CH_2 group is bonded with unsaturated 6 membered ring.

❖ If CH_2 group in the aliphatic chain of Penicillin G is changed to NH_2 group, it is called as "AMPICILLIN" (BROAD SPECTRUM ACTIVITY FOR ALL DISEASES).

❖ If the terminal unsaturated 6 membered ring is attached with OH group in the point No. 7, the compound is known as "AMOXICILLIN "which is broad spectrum but SPECIFICALLY FOR BRONCO-GENICAL SYSTEM.

❖ If the CH_2 group in aliphatic chain is converted to COOH group, the compound will be known as "CARBENCILLIN" which is broad spectrum usually used in burns).

❖ In case, if the CH_2 group in Penicillin G is replaced by "oxazole" group and further attached with "CHLOROBENZENE", the compound will be converted to

❖ "CLOXACILLIN" which is used in combination of other above drugs in septicemia.

❖ The esters of penicillin antibiotica are not bacteriostatic.

❖ The decarboxylation of the penicillin leads to the complete loss of biological activity.

❖ The addition of cyano, methoxy, nitro, fluoro and bromo groups, activity does not change but toxicity is increased.

Pharmacokinetics

Metabolism takes place in liver and excreted about 85% through kidneys. Its biological half-life is maximum about 65 hours. And can be administered by oral route, I.M., I.V.

Pharmacological uses

This has a lethal effect on bacteria. Rest as described above.

Adverse side effects

Mentioned above

Contraindications
As general described above.

Synthesis of Penicillin G (condensed)

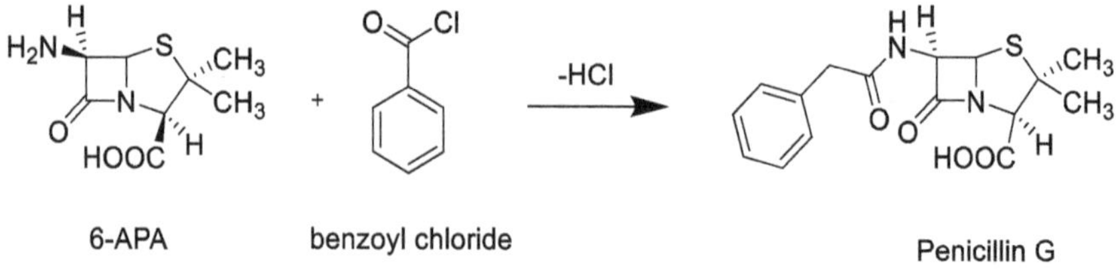

6-APA   benzoyl chloride   Penicillin G

-HCl

PENICILLIN V
(phenoxymethyl penicillin)

$$C_{16}H_{18}N_2O_5S$$
Molar mass:
350.39g/mol

Chemistry

Penicillin VK is a potassium salt of penicillin V. It is in the penicillin and beta lactam family of medications. It usually results in bactericidal.

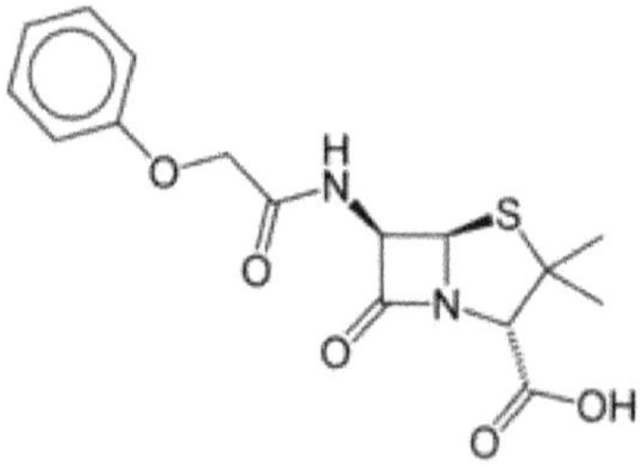

Structure activity relationship (SAR)
As mentioned above in penicillin.

Pharmacokinetics

Bioavailability is 60% (oral). It is metabolized in liver. Protein binding is about 80% and biological half- life is maximum I hour. It is excreted through kidneys and administered orally.

Pharmacological uses

It is a drug of choice against tonsillitis, pharyngitis, mild skin infections, rheumatic faver, disorders of the spleen, gingivitis.

It is not active against beta lactamase-producing bacteria but exerts bactericidal action against penicillin sensitive microorganism.

Adverse side effects

May cause transient nausea, vomiting, epigastric distress, diarrhea, constipation, acidic smell to urine.

Contraindications

Mentioned above as for penicillin.

Synthesis of Penicillin V 1

$2\lambda^3$-propan-2-yl 2-(1,3-dioxoisoindolin-2-yl)-3-oxopropanoate

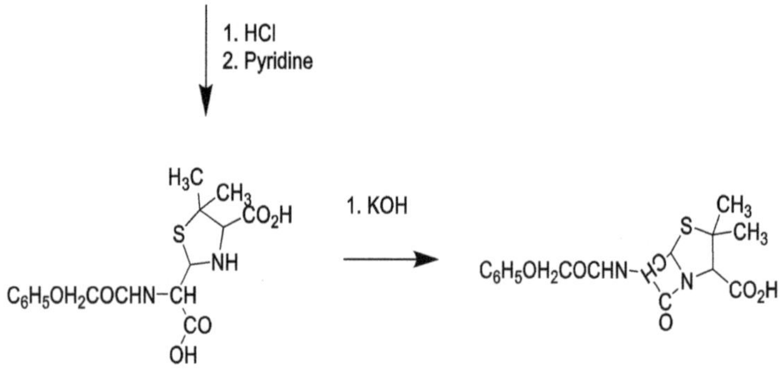

1. HCl
2. Pyridine

1. KOH

Synthesis of penicillin V 2

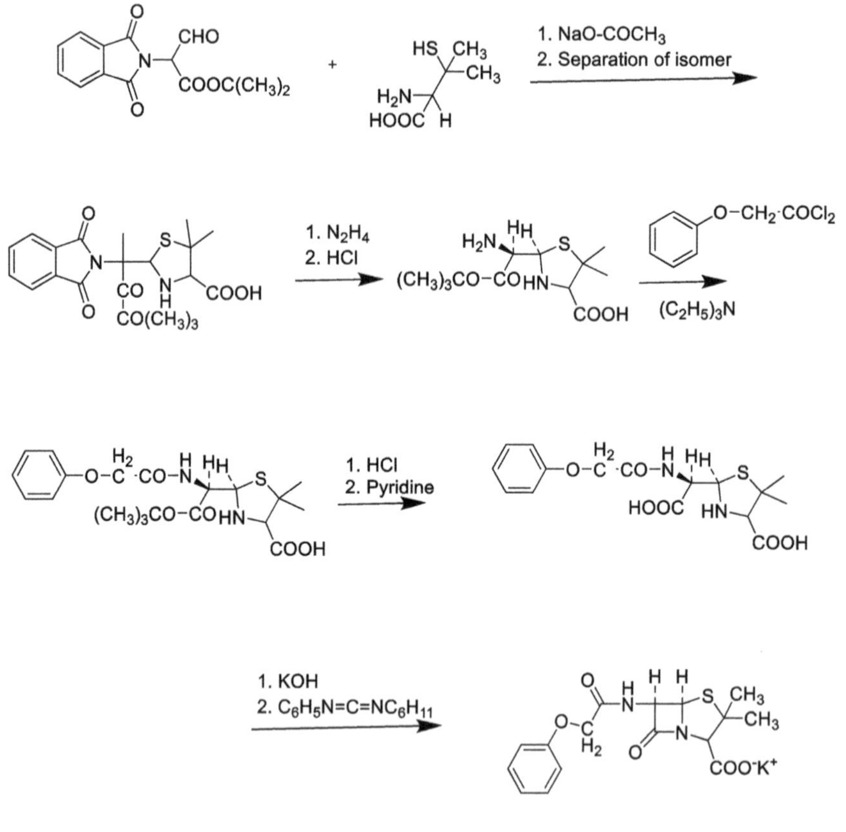

1. NaO-COCH$_3$
2. Separation of isomer

1. N$_2$H$_4$
2. HCl

1. HCl
2. Pyridine

1. KOH
2. C$_6$H$_5$N=C=NC$_6$H$_{11}$

Penicillin V

PROCAINE BENZYL PENICILLIN

(penicillin G procaine, procaine penicillin G, procaine penicillin)

Chemistry

Structure activity relationship (SAR)
Mentioned above for penicillin.

Metabolism
It is a form of penicillin which also contains benzylpenicillin and procaine.

Administered by deep i.m. injection where it hydrolyses to benzylpenicillin.

Adverse side effects
At high doses procaine penicillin can cause seizures and CNS abnormalities due to procaine present in it.

Contraindications
Mentioned above.

BENZATHINE BENZYLPENICILLIN
(benzathine penicillin G)

Chemistry

Structure activity relationship (SAR)
Mentioned above as for penicillin.

Metabolism
It is slowly absorbed into the circulation, after i.m. injection it hydrolyses to benzylpenicillin in vivo. It is the drug-of-choice when prolonged low concentrations of benzylpenicillin are required, allowing prolonged antibiotic action over 2–4 weeks after a single i.m. dose.

Pharmacological uses
Used to treat sore throat, diphtheria, syphilis and to prevent rheumatic fever. It is administered by i.m. injection.

Adverse side effects
Side effects include allergic reactions, pain. It is not recommended in those with a history of allergy from penicillin. Generally safe during pregnancy.

Contraindications
Mentioned above as for penicillin.

AZIDOCILLIN

$C_{16}H_{17}N_5O_4S$
Molar mass
375.40g/mol

Chemistry

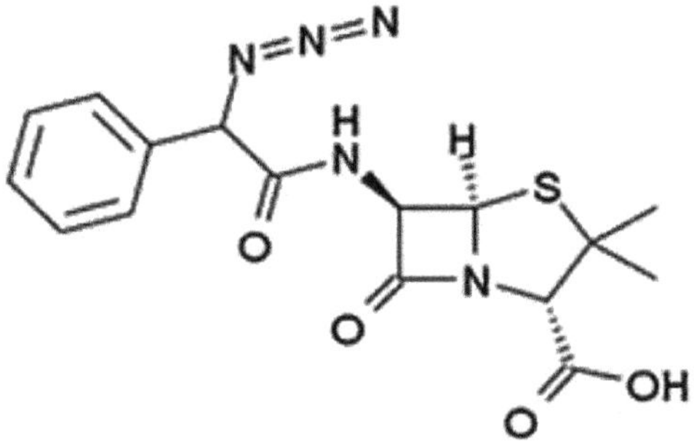

Structure activity relationship (SAR)
Mentioned above for penicillin.

Pharmacokinetics
Bioavailability: 57-64%
Metabolism: Hepatic
Biological half-life: 0.6 - 1.1 hour
Excretion:50% as active in urine
ROA: Oral, I.M., I.V.

Pharmacological uses
Mentioned above.

Adverse side effects
Mentioned above as for penicillin.

Contraindications
Mentioned above as for penicillin.

PENAMECILLIN

$C_{19}H_{22}N_2O_6S$
Molar mass
406.45 g/mol

Chemistry

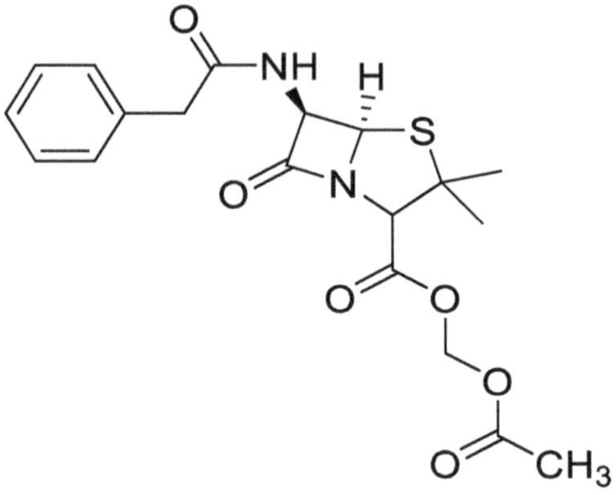

Structure activity relationship (SAR)
Mentioned above.

Metabolism
It is an acetoxymethyl ester of benzylpenicillin, is a pro-drug processed to benzylpenicillin by esterase.

Pharmacological uses
Mentioned above.

Adverse side effects
Mentioned above.

Contraindications
Mentioned above.

PROPICILLIN
$C_{18}H_{22}N_2O_5S$
Molar mass
378.45g/mol

Chemistry

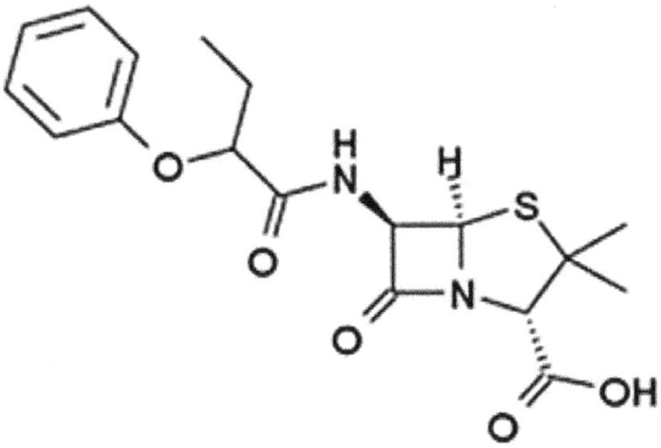

Structure activity relationship (SAR)
Mentioned above.

Metabolism
Mentioned above.

Pharmacological uses
ROA: Oral
Mentioned above.

Adverse side effects
Mentioned above.

Contraindications
Mentioned above.

PHENETICILLIN
(phenethicillin)

$C_{17}H_{20}N_2O_5S$
Molar mass
364.42 g/mol

Chemistry

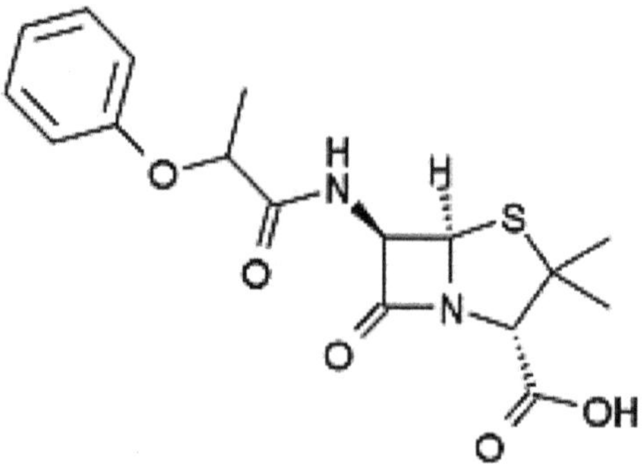

CLOMETOCILLIN
(clometacillin)

$C_{17}H_{18}C_{12}N_2O_5S$
Molar mass
433.31g/mol

Chemistry

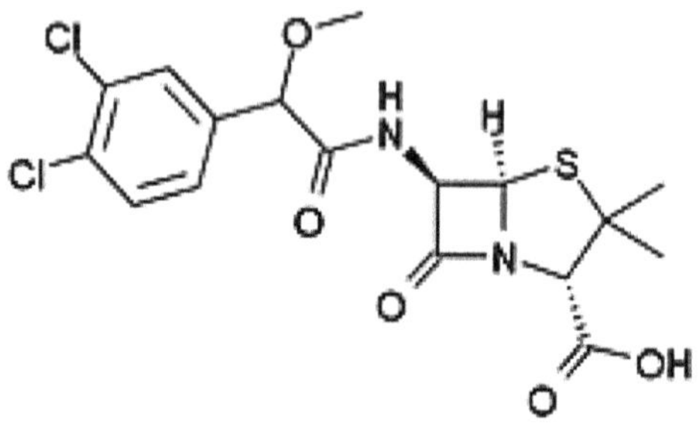

5.10 Second Generation

(β-lactamase resistant)
(narrow spectrum)

CLOXACILLIN

$C_{19}H_{18}ClN_3O_5S$
Molar mass
435.88g/mol

Chemistry

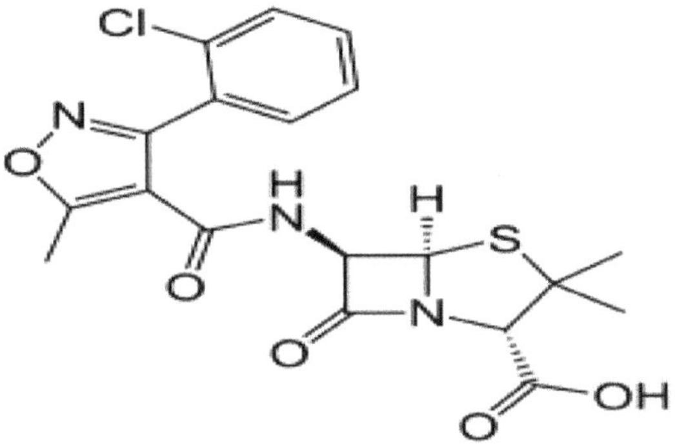

Structure activity relationship (SAR)
Mentioned above.

Pharmacokinetics
Bioavailability: 37-90%
Protein binding: 95%
Metabolism: Hepatic
Biological half- life: 30 to 60 minutes
Excretion: Renal and biliary

Pharmacological uses
ROA: Oral, I.M.

It is semisynthetic and is used against bacteria that produce β-lactamase due to its large R chain. This drug has a weaker antibacterial activity than, benzylpenicillin and is devoid of serious toxicity except for allergic reactions.

Adverse side effects

Side effects include nausea, diarrhea allergic reaction and diarrhea. It is not recommended in people who have allergy to penicillin, relatively safe in pregnancy.

Contraindications

Mentioned above.

Synthesis of Cloxacillin

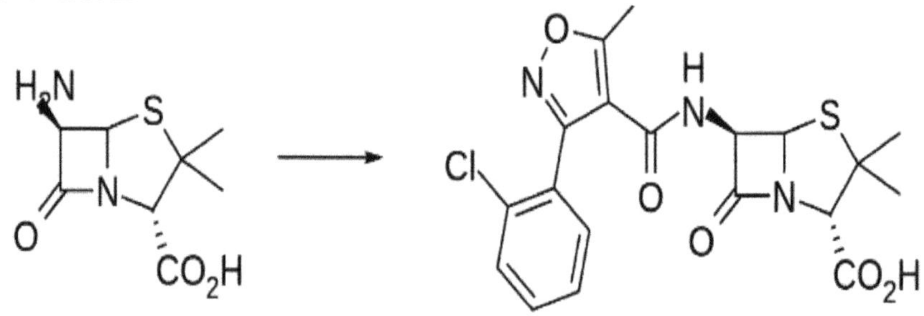

OXACILLIN

$C_{19}H_{19}N_3O_5S$
Molar mass
401.44g/mol

Chemistry

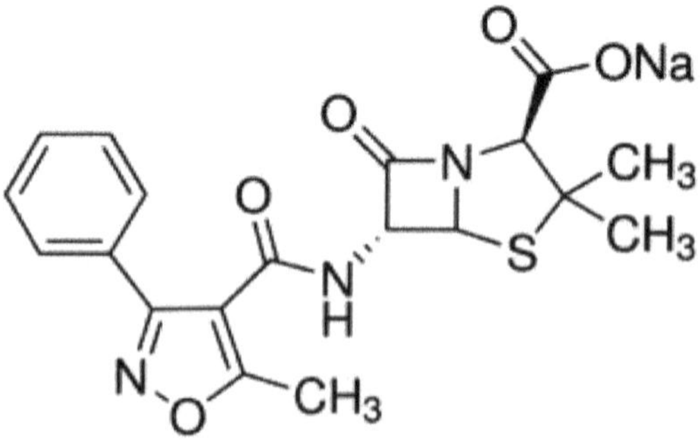

Structure activity relationship (SAR)
Mentioned above.

Metabolism
Mentioned above.

Pharmacological uses
ROA: Oral, I.M.
Mentioned above.

Adverse side effects
Mentioned above.

Contraindications
Mentioned above.

FLUCLOXACILLIN
(floxacillin)

$C_{19}H_{17}ClFN_3O5S$
Molar mass
453.88g/mol

Chemistry

Structure activity relationship (SAR)
Mentioned above.

Pharmacokinetics
Bioavailability: 50-70%
Metabolism: Hepatic
Biological half- life: 0.75- 1 hour
Excretion: Renal
ROA: Oral, I.M., I.V., intra-pleural, intra-articular.

DICLOXACILLIN

$C_{19}H_{17}Cl_2N_3O_5S$
Molar mass
470.33g/mol

Chemistry

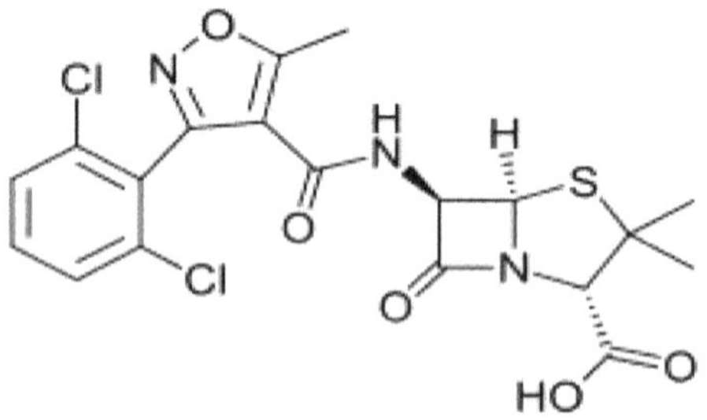

Structure activity relationship (SAR)
Mentioned above.

Metabolism
Bioavailability: 60-80% (oral)
Protein binding: 98%
Metabolism: Hepatic
Biological half- life: 0.7 hours
Excretion: Renal and biliary
ROA: Oral

Pharmacological uses
Mentioned above.

Adverse side effects

Mentioned above.

Contraindications

Mentioned above.

METHICILLIN

$C_{17}H_{20}N_2O_6S$
Molar mass
380.42g/mol

Chemistry

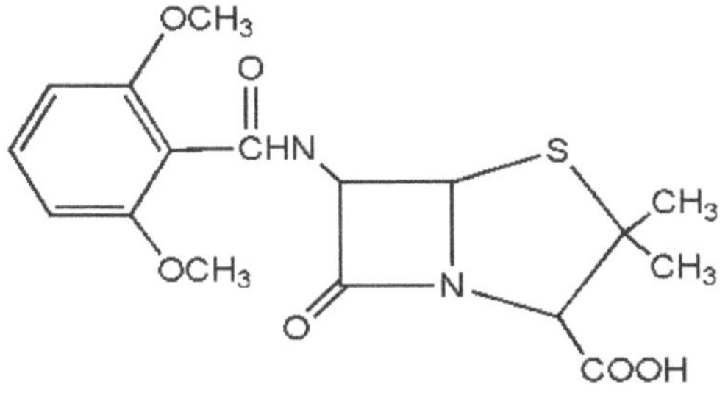

Structure activity relationship (SAR)

Mentioned above.

Pharmacokinetics

Bioavailability: Not absorbed orally

Metabolism: 20-40% hepatic

Biological half- life: 25 to 60 minutes

Excretion: Renal

ROA: i.v.

Pharmacological uses

Mentioned above.

Adverse side effects
Mentioned above.

Contraindications
Mentioned above.

NAFCILLIN

$C_{21}H_{22}N_2O_5S$
Molar mass
414.48g/mol

Chemistry

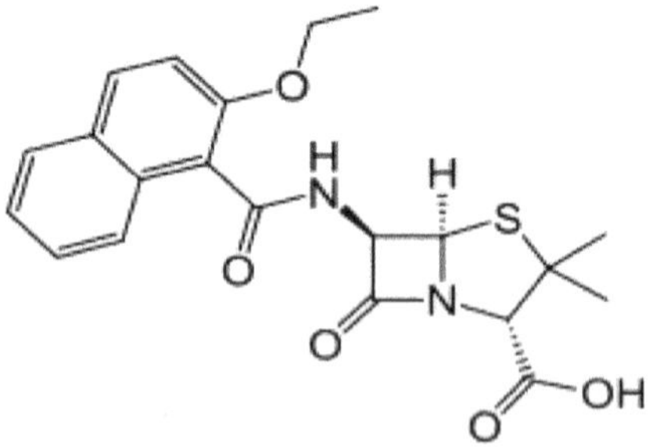

Structure activity relationship (SAR)
Mentioned above.

Pharmacokinetics
Metabolism: 30% hepatic
Protein binding: 90%
Biological half- life: 0.5 hours
Excretion: Biliary and renal
ROA: I.M., I.V.

Pharmacological uses
Mentioned above.

Adverse side effects
Mentioned above.

5.11 Third Generation (Aminopenicillin)

(extended spectrum)

AMOXICILLIN

$C_{16}H_{19}N_3O_5S$
Molar mass
365.41g/mol

Chemistry

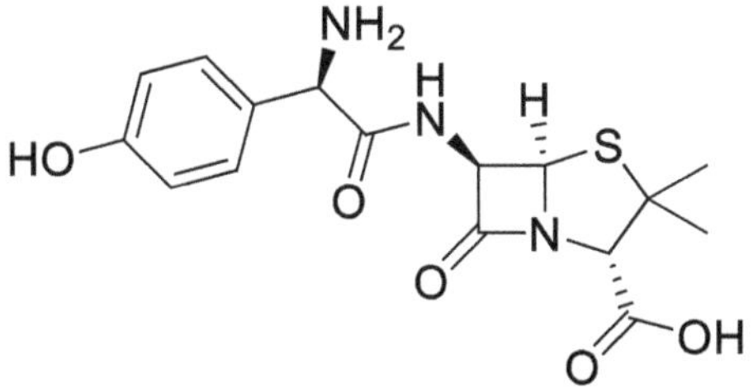

Structure activity relationship (SAR)
Mentioned above.

Pharmacokinetics
Bioavailability: 95% (oral)
Metabolism: 30% bio-transformed in liver
Biological half- life: 61.3 minutes
Excretion: Renal
ROA: Oral, i.v.

Pharmacological uses

- Amoxicillin is used in the treatment of the number of infections, including otitis. Pneumonia, skin infections, urinary tract infections, respiratory infections, H. pylori.

221

- Amoxicillin (α-amino-p-hydroxybenzyl penicillin) is a semisynthetic derivative of penicillin with a structure similar to ampicillin but with better absorption when taken by mouth, thus yielding higher concentrations in blood and in urine. Amoxicillin diffuses easily into tissues and body fluids.
- Penetration into the central nervous system increases in meningitis. It will cross the placenta and is excreted into breastmilk in small quantities.
- It is excreted into the urine and metabolized by the liver. It has an onset of 30 minutes and a half-life of 3.7 hours in newborns and 1.4 hours in adults.
- Amoxicillin attaches to the cell wall of susceptible bacteria and results in their death. It also is a bactericidal compound. It is effective against streptococci, pneumococci, enterococci, Hemophilus influenzae, Escherichia coli, Proteus mirabilis, Neisseria meningitidis, Neisseria, Shigella, Borrelia burgdorferi, and Helicobacter pylori.

Adverse side effects

- Include nausea and rash and diarrhea
- Its use in pregnancy and breastfeeding is safe.
- Rarer adverse effects include mental changes, lightheadedness, insomnia, confusion, anxiety, sensitivity to lights and sounds, and unclear thinking. Immediate medical care is required upon the first signs of these adverse effects.
- Any other symptoms that seem even remotely suspicious must be taken very seriously. However, more mild allergy symptoms, such as a rash, can occur at any time during treatment, even up to a week after treatment has ceased.

Interactions

Amoxicillin may interact with these drugs:

Warfarin, methotrexate, typhoid vaccine, oral contraceptives, allopurinol and probenecid.

Enzymatic synthesis of Amoxicillin

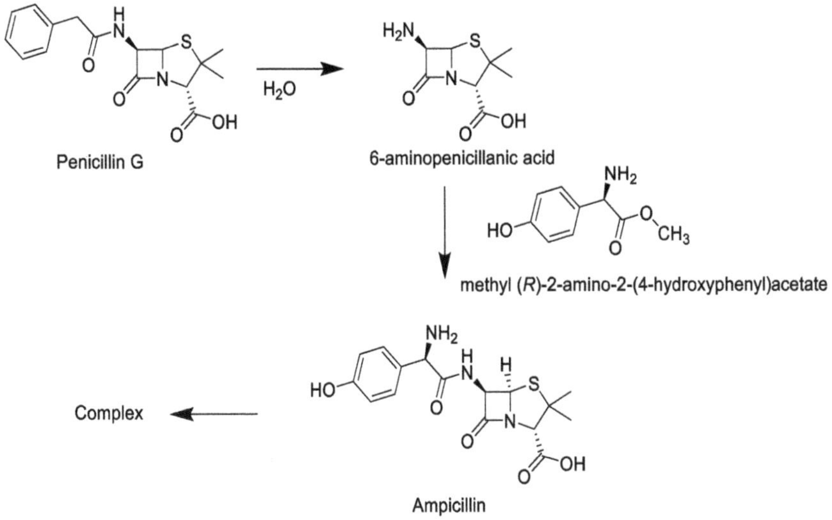
Penicillin G
H_2O
6-aminopenicillanic acid
methyl (R)-2-amino-2-(4-hydroxyphenyl)acetate
Complex
Ampicillin

Synthesis of Amoxicillin 1

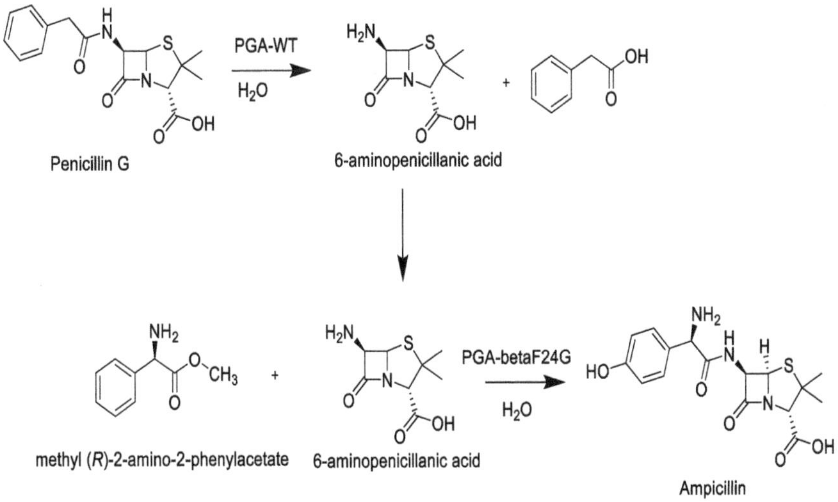
PGA-WT
H_2O
Penicillin G
6-aminopenicillanic acid
PGA-betaF24G
H_2O
methyl (R)-2-amino-2-phenylacetate
6-aminopenicillanic acid
Ampicillin

AMPICILLIN

$$C_{16}H_{19}N_3O_4S$$
Molar mass
349.41g/mol

Chemistry

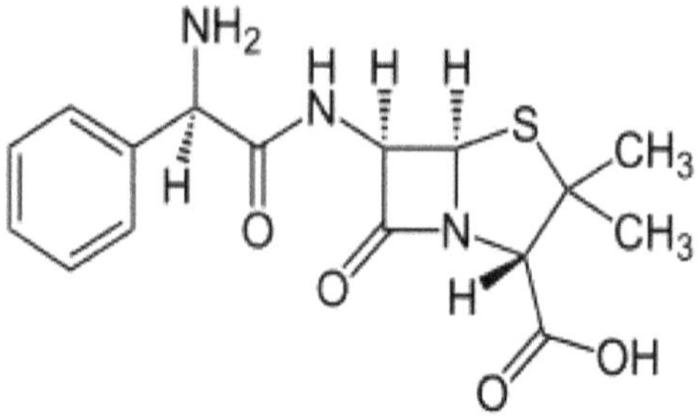

Structure activity relationship (SAR)
As mentioned above

Pharmacokinetics
Bioavailability: 40% (oral)
Metabolism: 12-50%
Protein binding: 15-25%
Biological half- life: 1 hour
Excretion: 70-85% (renal)
ROA: Oral, I.V.

Pharmacological uses
Mentioned above.

Adverse side effects
Mentioned above.

Contraindications
Mentioned above

224

Synthesis of Ampicillin 1

Ampicillin

Synthesis of Ampicillin 2

Penicillin G → 6-aminopenicillanic acid

methyl (R)-2-amino-2-phenylacetate + 6-aminopenicillanic acid → Ampicillin

PIVAMPICILLIN
(ampicillin pivaloyloxymethyl ester)

$$C_{22}H_{29}N_3O_6S$$
Molar mass
463.55g/mol

Chemistry

Structure activity relationship (SAR)
As mentioned above

Pharmacokinetics
Excretion:76% renal

226

ROA: Oral

Pharmacological uses
As above.

Adverse side effects
As above.

Contraindications
As above

HETACILLIN

$C_{19}H_{23}N_3O_4S$
Molar mass
389.47g/mol

Chemistry

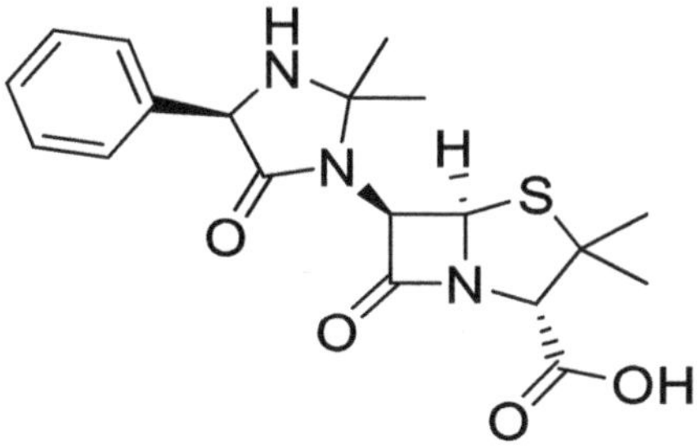

Structure activity relationship (SAR)
As above.

Metabolism
As above.

Pharmacological uses
It is meant for veterinary use. ROA: I.M.
As above

Adverse side effects
As above.

Contraindications
As above.

BACAMPICILLIN
$C_{21}H_{27}N_3O_7S$
Molar mass
465.52 g/mol

Chemistry

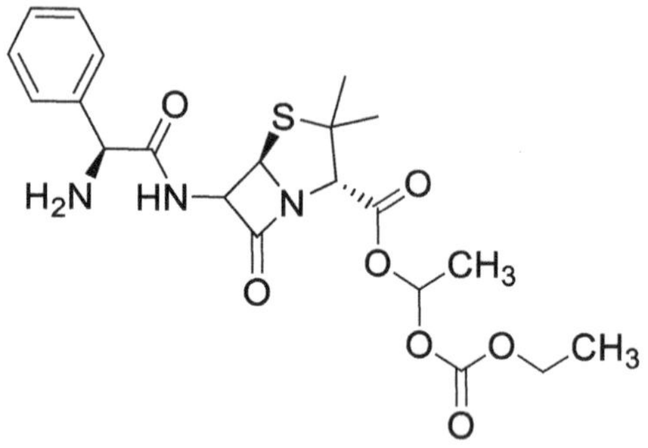

Structure activity relationship (SAR)
- It is a pro-drug of ampicillin with improved oral bioavailability.
- Semi-synthetic antibiotic related to penicillin.

Metabolism
As above

Pharmacological uses
ROA: Oral
As above

Adverse side effects
As above

Contraindications

As above

METAMPICILLIN

$C_{17}H_{19}N_3O_4S$
Molar mass
361.42 g/mol

Chemistry

It is prepared by the reaction of ampicillin with formaldehyde and is hydrolyzed in aqueous solution with the formation of ampicillin.

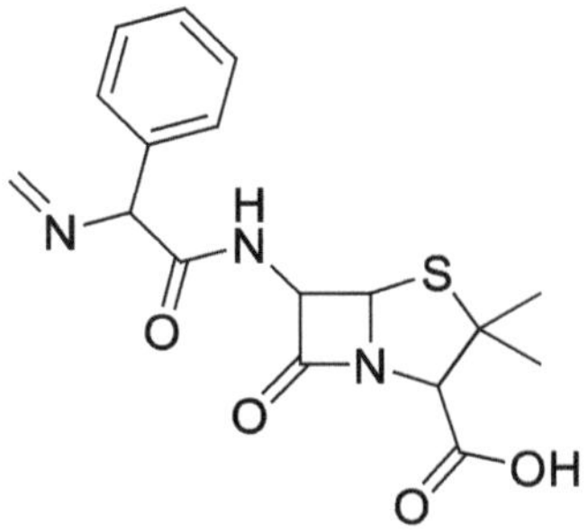

Structure activity relationship (SAR)
As above

Metabolism
Hydrolysis is rapid under acid conditions, e.g., in the stomach, less rapid in neutral media, and incomplete is solutions such as human serum.

Pharmacological uses
As above

Adverse side effects
As above

TALAMPICILLIN

$$C_{24}H_{23}N_3O_6S$$
Molar mass
481.52 g/mol

Chemistry

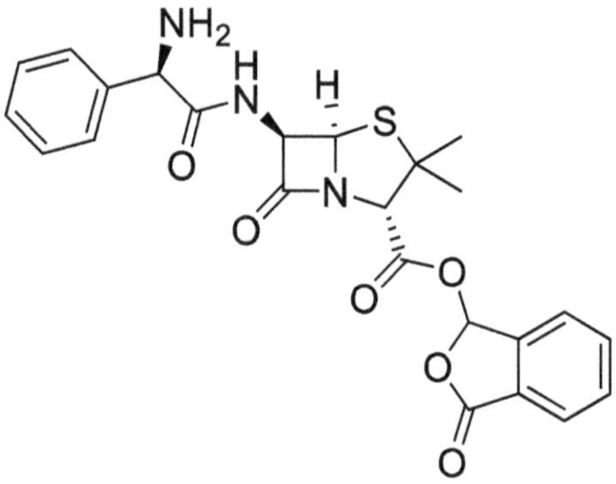

Metabolism

It is an acid stable pro-drug that was administered orally.

EPICILLIN

$$C_{16}H_{21}N_3O_4S$$
Molar mass
351.420 g/mol

Chemistry

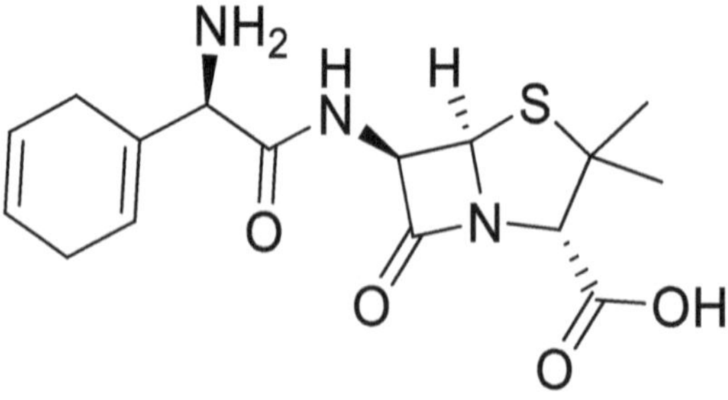

230

5.12 Fourth Generation

(Carboxypenicillins)
(extended spectrum)

TICARCILLIN

$C_{15}H_{16}N_2O_6S_2$
Molar mass
384.43g/mol

Chemistry

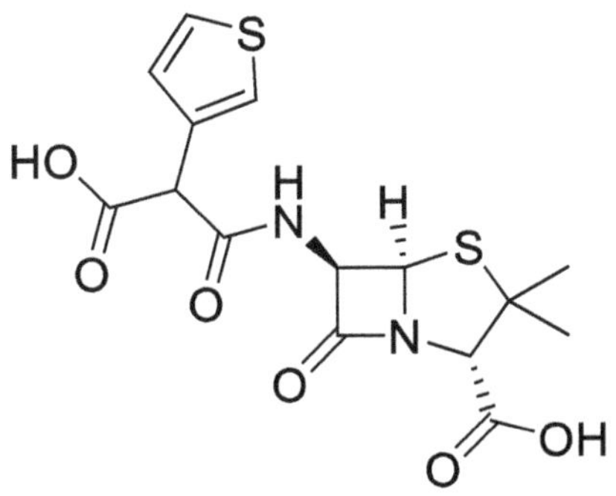

Structure activity relationship (SAR)
As above

Pharmacokinetics
Protein binding: 45%
Biological half- life: 1.1 hours
Excretion: Renal
ROA: i.v.

Pharmacological uses
As above

Adverse side effects
As above

Contraindications

As above

CARBENCILLIN

$C_{17}H_{18}N_2O_6S$
Molar mass
378.40g/mol

Chemistry

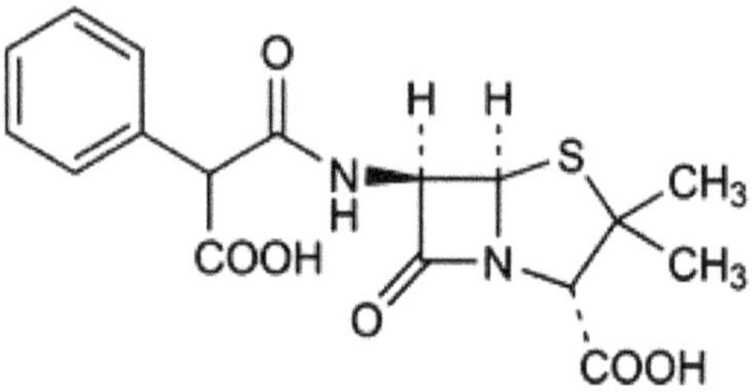

Pharmacokinetics

Bioavailability: 30-40%

Protein binding: 30-60%

Metabolism: Minimal

Biological half- life: 60 minutes

Excretion: Renal 30-40%

ROA: Oral, parenteral

CARINDACILLIN

$C_{26}H_{26}N_2O_6S$
Molar mass
494.55 g/mol

Chemistry

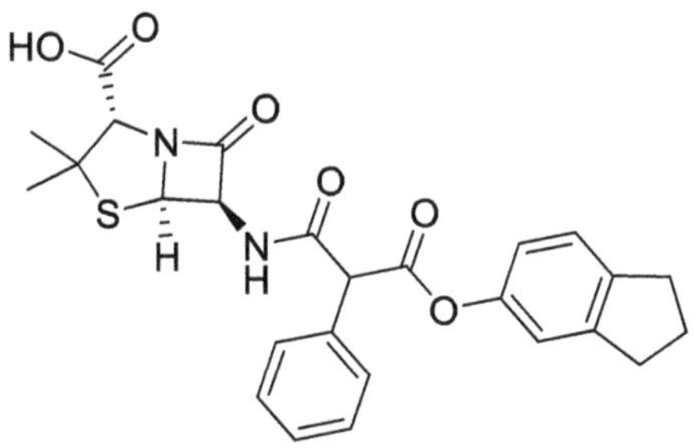

Structure activity relationship (SAR)
As above

Metabolism
As above

Pharmacological uses
Pro-drug of carbenicillin and administered orally as the sodium salt.

Adverse side effects
As above

Contraindications
As above

TEMOCILLIN

$C_{16}H_{18}N2O_7S_2$
Molar mass
414.45 g/mol

Chemistry

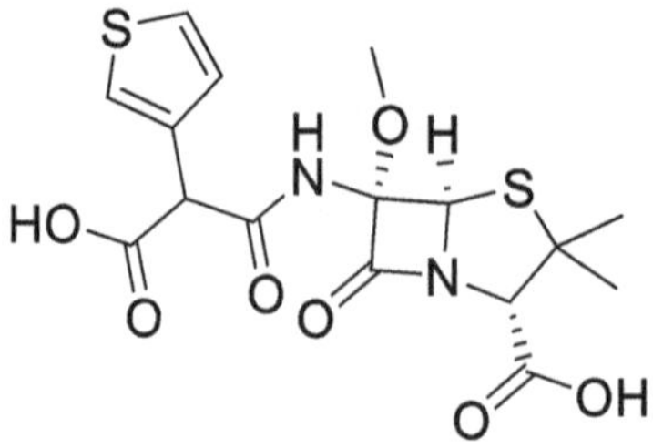

Metabolism

Temocillin is β-lactamase-resistant penicillin.

Pharmacological uses

It is used primarily for the treatment of multiple drug-resistant bacteria.

It is not active against gram-ive bacteria.

5.13 Fourth Generation

(Ureidopenicillins)
(extended spectrum)

MEZLOCILLIN

$C_{21}H_{25}N_5O_8S_2$
Molar mass
539.58g/mol

Chemistry

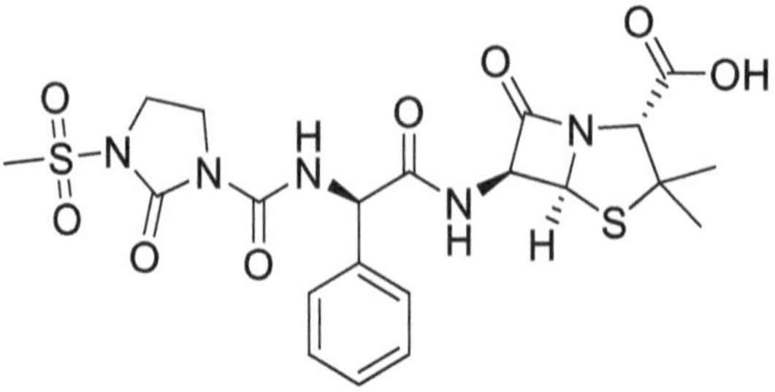

Structure activity relationship (SAR)
As above

Pharmacokinetics
Protein binding: 16-59%
Metabolism: Hepatic 20-30%
Biological half- life: 1.3-4.4 hours
Excretion: Renal 50% and biliary
ROA: i.m, i.v.

PIPERACILLIN

$C_{23}H_{27}N_5O_7S$
Molar mass
517.55g/mol

Chemistry

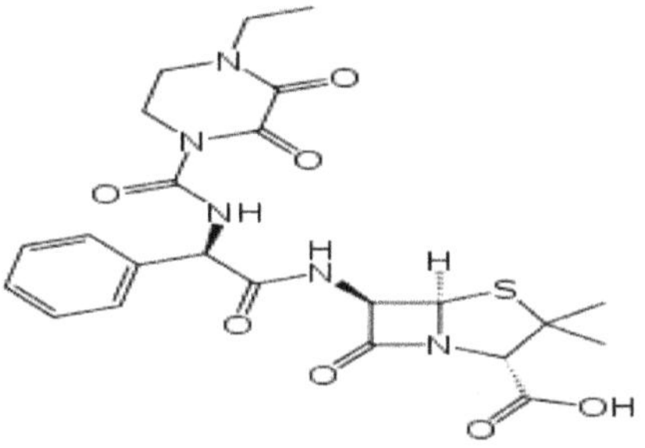

AZLOCILLIN
(acylampicillin)

$C_{20}H_{23}N_5O_6S$
Molar mass
461.49g/mol

Chemistry

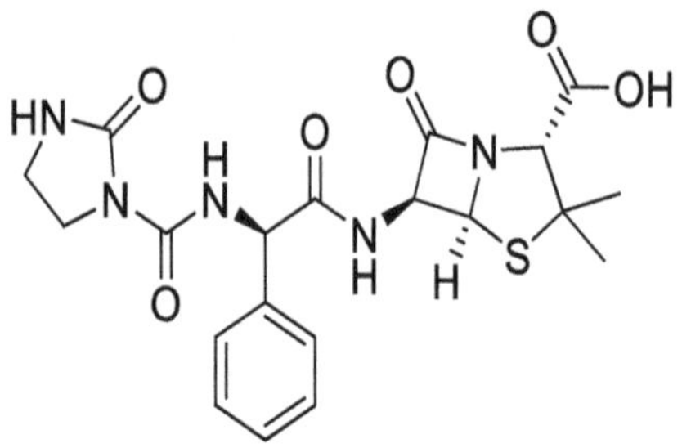

5.14 Fourth Generation

(Miscellaneous)
(extended spectrum)

SULBENICILLIN
(sulphocillin)

$C_{16}H_{18}N_2O_7S_2$
Molar mass
414.45g/mol

Chemistry

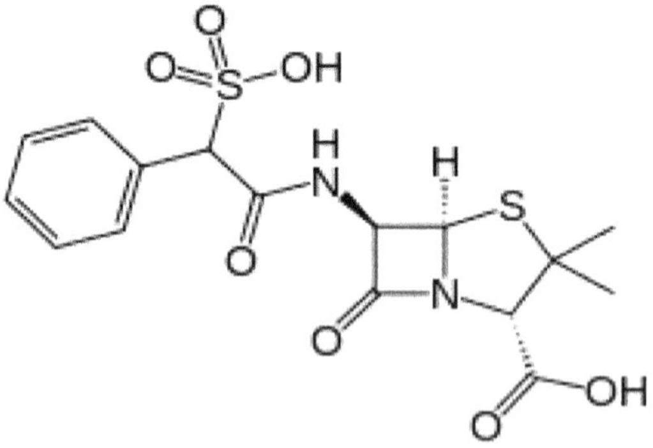

MECILLINAM
(amdinocillin)

$C_{15}H_{23}N_3O_3S$
Molar mass
325.43 g/mol

Chemistry

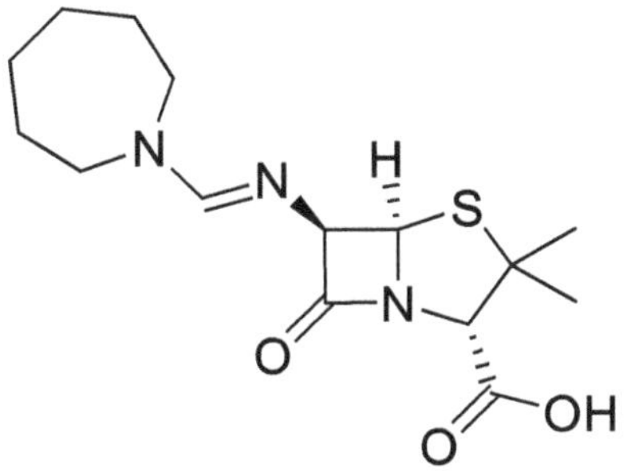

Structure activity relationship (SAR)

As above

Metabolism

Mecillinam has very low oral bioavailability.

Pharmacological uses

It is used primarily in the treatment of urinary tract infections. Also
been used to treat typhoid fever. ROA: I.M., I.V. Mecillinam is used in
the treatment of infections due to susceptible gram-negative bacteria.

Contraindications

As above

PIVMECILLINAM
(pivaloyloxymethyl ester of mecillinam)

$C_{21}H_{33}N_3O_5S$
Molar mass
439.57 g/mol

Chemistry

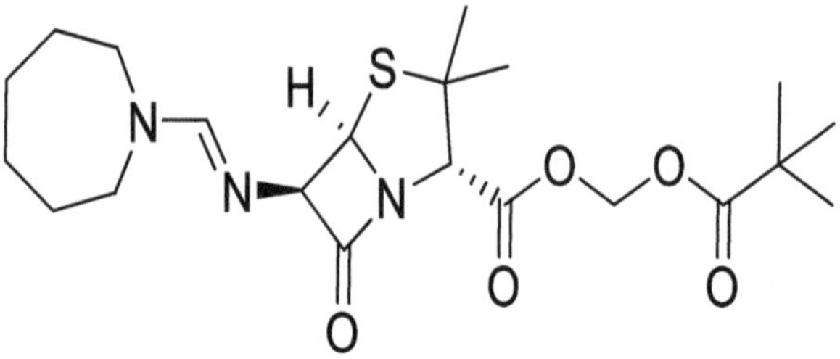

Structure activity relationship (SAR)
It is an orally active pro-drug of mecillinam.

Pharmacikinetics
Bioavailability: Low
Protein binding: 5 to 10% (as mecillinam)
Metabolism: is hydrolyzed to mecillinam
Half-life: 1 to 3 hours
Biliary, mostly as mecillinam

Pharmacological uses
Pivmecillinam is only considered to be active against Gram +ive and is used primarily in the treatment of lower urinary tract infections.

5.15 Penems

FIRST GENERATION (penicillin)

(narrow spectrum)

FAROPENEM

$C_{12}H_{15}NO_5S$
Molar mass
285.32 g/mol

Chemistry

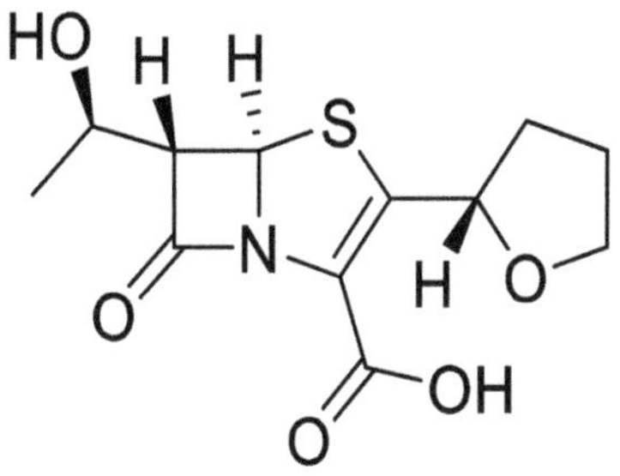

Pharmacological uses

Acute bacterial sinusitis, pneumonia, chronic bronchitis, urinary tract infections, ROA: Oral, acute bacterial sinusitis, uncomplicated skin and skin structure infections.

RITIPENEM

$C_{10}H_{12}N_2O_6S$
Molar mass
288.3 g/mol

Chemistry

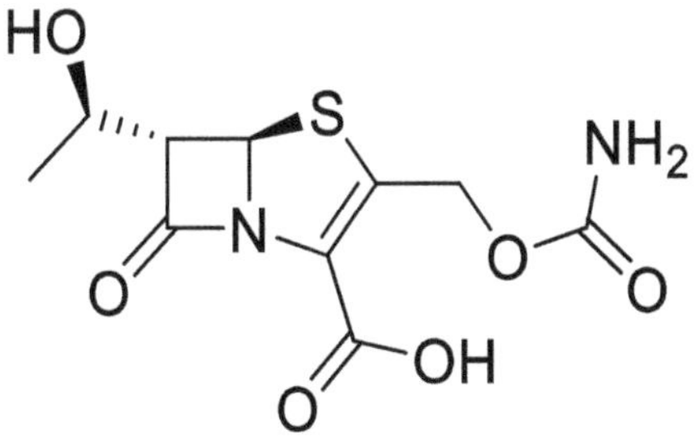

CARBAPENEMS

PENICILLINS

Synthesis of carbapenem in general

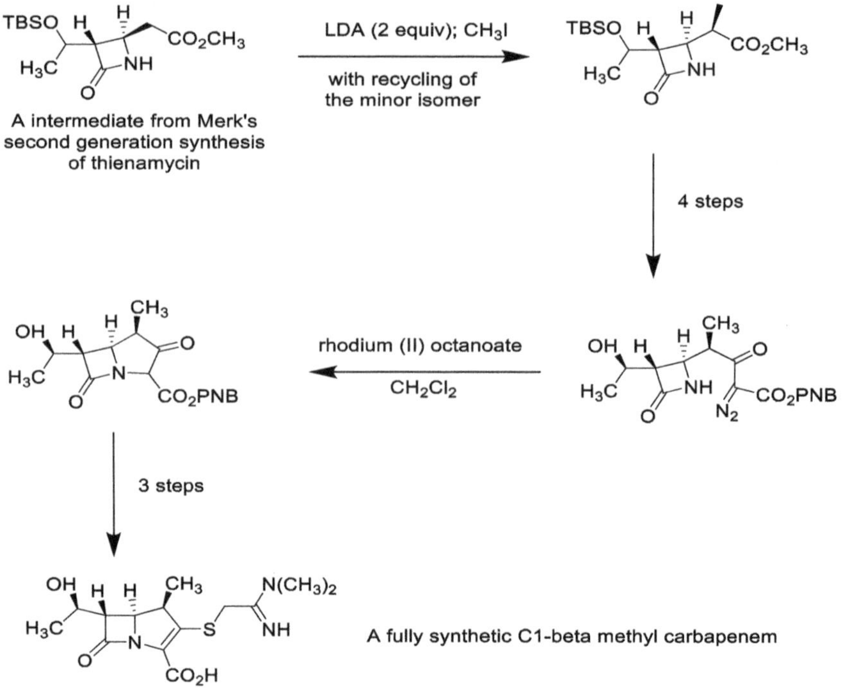

A intermediate from Merk's second generation synthesis of thienamycin

LDA (2 equiv); CH$_3$I

with recycling of the minor isomer

4 steps

rhodium (II) octanoate

CH$_2$Cl$_2$

3 steps

A fully synthetic C1-beta methyl carbapenem

ERTAPENEM

C$_{22}$H$_{25}$N$_3$O$_7$S
Molar mass
475.52g/mol

Chemistry

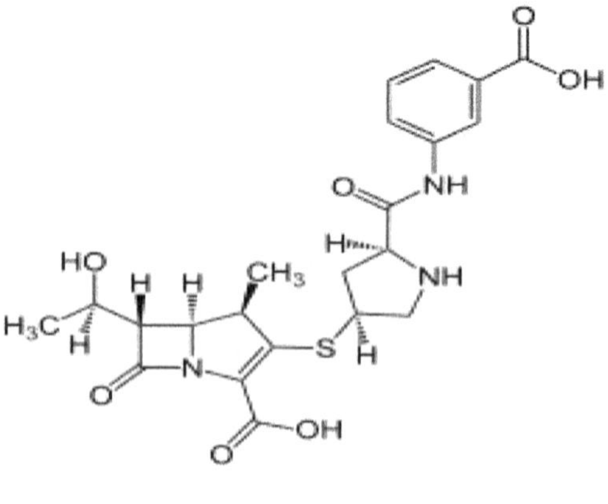

Pharmacological uses:
It has been designed to be effective against Gram-positive, anaerobic and Gram-ive bacteria.
ROA: I.M., I.V.

DORIPENEM

$$C_{15}H_{24}N_4O_6S_2$$
Molar mass
420.51 g/mol

Chemistry

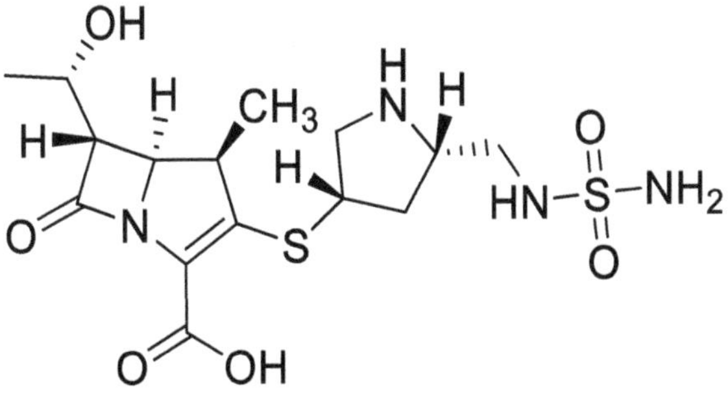

Pharmacokinetics
Doripenem is metabolized by the enzyme de-hydropeptidase-I into an inactive ring-opened metabolite.
Excretion: Renal
Ultra-broad-spectrum injectable.
ROA: I.M., I.V.

IMIPENEM
(primaxin)

$$C_{12}H_{17}N_3O_4S$$
Molar mass
299.35g/mol

Chemistry

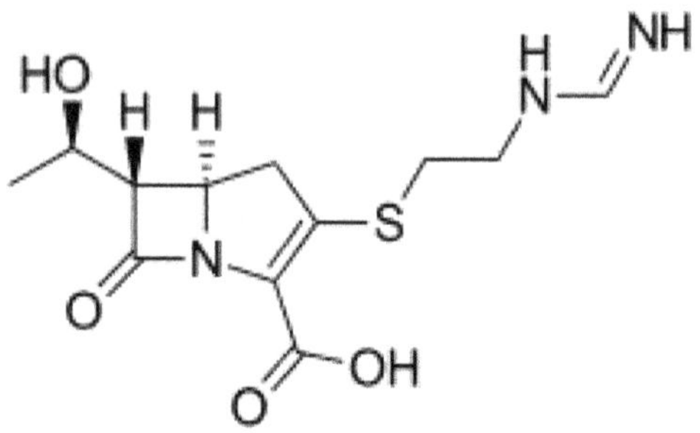

Pharmacokinetics
Protein binding: 20%
Metabolism: Renal
Biological half- life: 38-68 minutes
Excretion: Urine 70%
ROA: I.V.

MEROPENEM

$C_{17}H_{25}N_3O_5S$
Molar mass
383.46g/mol

Chemistry

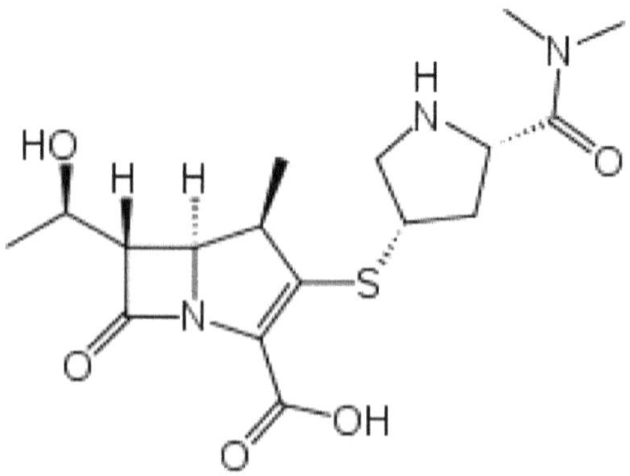

Structure activity relationship (SAR)
As above

Pharmacokinetics
Bioavailabilty: 100%
Protein binding: 2%
Metabolism: Renal
Biological half- life: 60 minutes
Excretion: Renal
ROA: I.V.

Pharmacological uses
It is effective against Gram-positive, anaerobic and Gram-ive
bacteria, used to treat meningitis, pneumonia, sepsis and anthrax. is
highly resistant to degradation by β-lactamases or cephalosporinases.

BIAPENEM

$C_{15}H_{18}N_4O_4S$
Molar mass
350.40g/mol

Chemistry

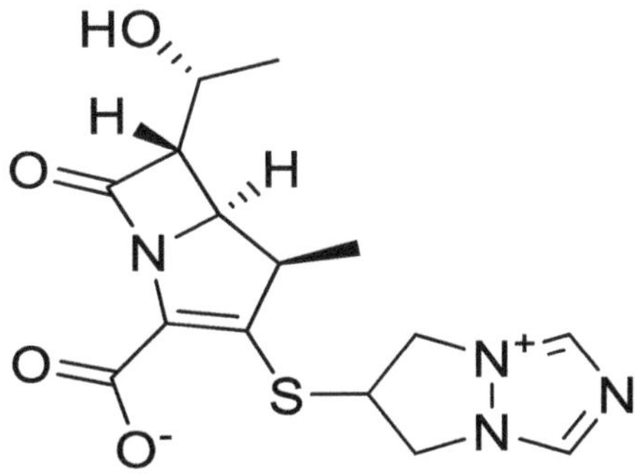

Pharmacological uses
It has in vitro activity against anaerobes.

ROA: I.V.

THIENAMYCIN
(thienpenem)

$C_{11}H_{16}N_2O_4S$
Molar mass
272.32 g/mol

Chemistry
zwitterion at pH 7.

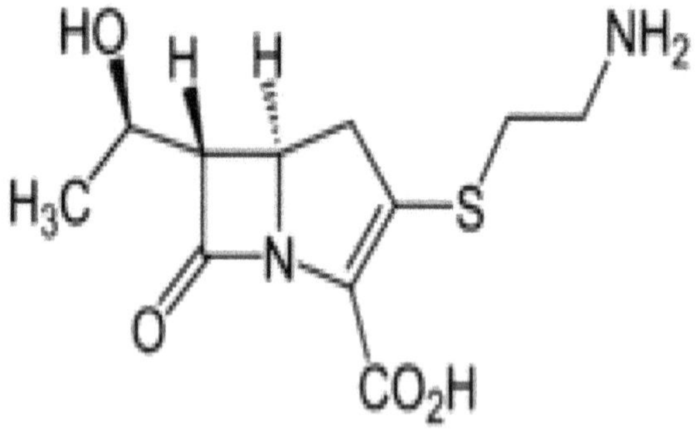

Metabolism
Extremely unstable and decomposes in aqueous. solution.

De-hydropeptidase is an enzyme found in the kidneys and is responsible for degrading.

Pharmacological uses
has excellent activity against both Gram-positive and Gram-negative bacteria and is resistant to bacterial β-lactamases or cephalosporinases.

PANIPENEM
(betamipron)
(Carbenin)

Chemistry

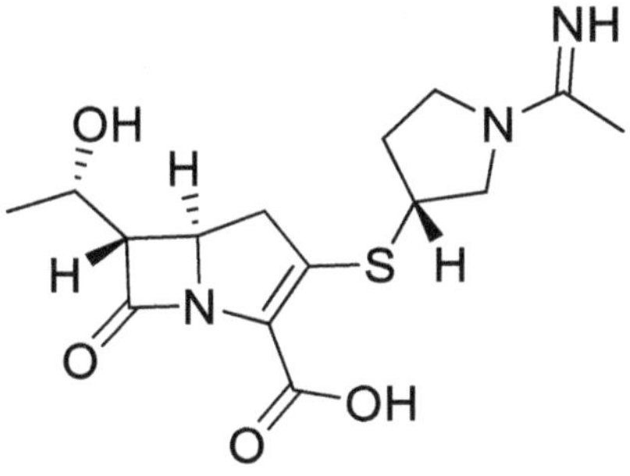

Pharmacological uses

It is the renal inhibitor. Panipenem uptake into the renal tubule and prevent nephrotoxicity.

5.16 β-Lactamase Inhibitor

CLAVULANIC ACID

$C_8H_9NO_5$
Molar mass
199.162 g·mol^{-1}

Chemistry

β-lactamases or cephalosporinases.

Clavulanic acid is biosynthesized from the amino acid and the sugar and looks structurally similar to penicillin, but the biosynthesis of this molecule involves a different pathway and set of enzymes.

Pharmacokinetics
β-lactamases or cephalosporinases based.
Bioavailabilty: 100% well absorbed.
Metabolism: Hepatic extensive
Biological half- life: 60 minutes
Excretion: Renal 30-40%
ROA: Oral, I.V.

Pharmacological uses
Potassium clavulanate" is combined with amoxicillin (described above), trade names Augmentin, Pyelonephritis during pregnancy, amoxicillin or amoxicillin-clavulanate potassium is preferred, is a suicide inhibitor. Used in veterinary as well.

Adverse side effects
The use of clavulanic acid with penicillin has been associated with an increased incidence of jaundice.

Contraindications
As above

Synthesis of Clavulanic acid

Biosynthesis of Clavulanic acid

5.17 General list of compounds from Cephalosporin group of antibiotics

Historical background

The cephalosporins are B-lactam antibiotics isolated from Cephalosporium species or prepared semi-synthetically. Cephalosporin C turned out to be a close congener of penicillin N, containing a dihydrothiazine ring instead of the thiazolidine ring of the penicillin. However, the discovery that the a-aminoaadipoyl side chain could be removed to efficiently produce 7-aminocephalosporanic acid (7-ACA)" prompted investigations that led to semisynthetic cephalosporins of medicinal value. The relationship of 7-ACA and its acyl derivatives to 6-APA and the semisynthetic penicillin is obvious.

Nomenclature

The chemical nomenclature of the cephalosporins is more complex than even that of the penicillins use of the fused ring system which is designated by Chemical Abstract. The trivialized forms of nomenclature of the type that have been applied to the penic are not consistently applicable to cephalosporins, although some derivatives of cephalosporanic acids, because of variation in the substituent at the 3-position cephalosporins have been aimed as acids. 7-ACA nucleus have resulted from acylation of the different acids or nucleophilic substitution.

However, the presence of an allylic acetoxyl function in the 3-position provides a reactive site at which various 7-acylaminocephalosporanic acid structures can easily be varied by nucleophilic displacement reactions. In the preparation of semisynthetic cephalosporins, the following improvements are sought:

- ❖ increased acid stability:
- ❖ improved pharmacokinetic properties, particularly better oral absorption:
- ❖ broadened antimicrobial spectrum:
- ❖ increased activity against resistant microorganisms (as a result of resistance to enzymatic destruction, improved penetration, increased receptor affinity:
- ❖ decreased allergenicity:
- ❖ increased tolerance after parenteral administration.

5.18 First Generation

Biological description

Gram-positive: Activity against penicillinase-producing, methicillin susceptible (though they are not the drugs of choice for such infections). No activity against methicillin-resistant staphylococci or Gram-negative: have no activity against indole-positive Proteus, or Serratia.

Cephacetrile, (Cefadroxyl), (Cephalexin; Keflex), (Cephaloglycin), (Cephalonium), (Cephaloradine), (Cephalothin; Keflin), (Cefadryl), Cefatrizine, (Cephazolin: Kefzol) (Cephradine; Velosef) AND MANY OTHERS

5.19 Second Generation

Biological description

Gram-positive: Less than first-generation. Gram-negative: Greater than first-generation.

(Ceclor, Distaclor, Keflor, (Raniclor), (Monocid), (Cefproxil; Cefzil), (Altacef, Zefu, Zinnat, Zinacef, Ceftin, Biofuroksym, Xorimax) AND MANY OTHERS

The following cephems are also sometimes grouped with second-generation cephalosporins:

(Lorabid), (Zefazone), (Cefotan), (Mefoxin), (Pansporin) AND MANY OTHERS

5.20 Third Generation

Biological description

Gram-positive: Some members of this group (in particular, those available in an oral formulation and those with anti-pseudomonal activity) have decreased activity against gram-positive organisms. Activity against staphylococci and streptococci less active with the third-generation compounds than with the first-and second-generation compounds. Gram-negative:

Third generation cephalosporins have a broad spectrum of activity and further increased activity against gram-negative organisms. They are also able to penetrate in the CNS and useful against meningitis caused by pneumococci, meningococci, H. influenzae, and penicillin-resistant N. gonorrhoeae. Since August 2012, the third-generation cephalosporin, ceftriaxone, is the only recommended treatment for gonorrhea in addition to azithromycin or doxycycline for concurrent Chlamydia treatment). Cefixime is no more recommended as a first-line treatment due to evidence of decreasing susceptibility.

**(Sefdin, Omnicef), (Zifi, Suprax), (Claforan),
(Convenia), (Vantin), (Cedax), (Naxcel, Excenel),
(Cefizox), (Rocephin), Antipseudomonal
activity: (Cefobid, Meezat, Fortum),**

**This following cephem is also sometimes grouped
with the third generation cephalosporins:
(moxalactam)**

5.21 Fourth Generation

Biological description

Gram-positive: They are extended-spectrum agents with similar activity against Gram-positive organisms as first-generation cephalosporins. Gram-negative: Fourth generation cephalosporins are zwitterions. They also have a greater resistance to β-lactamases than the third generation cephalosporins. Many can cross the blood brain barrier. Cefiderocol has been called a fourth-generation cephalosporin.

(Maxipime), (Fetroja), (Cefrom)

This following cephem is also sometimes grouped with fourth generation cephalosporins:

Oxacephems, Flomoxef
AND MANY OTHERS

5.22 Fifth Generation

Biological description

Ceftobiprole has been described as "fifth-generation" cephalosporin, though acceptance for this terminology is not universal. Ceftobiprole has anti-pseudomonal activity and appears to be less susceptible to development of resistance. Vancomycin-resistant enterococci that ceftobiprole has. Ceftaroline has activity against the treatment of complicated intra-abdominal infections and complicated urinary tract infections.

Ceftobiprole, Ceftaroline, Ceftolozane
AND SOME OTHERS

5.23 Miscellaneous Others

Biological description

Nitrocefin is a chromogenic cephalosporin substrate
which is used for detection of β-lactamases.

**These cephems have progressed far enough to be named,
but have not been assigned to a particular generation:**

**Cefalorm, Cefaparole, Cefcanel, Cefedrolor,
Cefempidone, Ceftrizole, Cefivitril
AND MANY OTHERS**

5.24 Antibiotics derived from two amino acids.

CEPHALOSPORIN

FIRST GENERATION

(Moderate spectrum)

Chemistry in general
The cephalosporins are a class originally derived from which was
previously known as "Cephalosporium".

Pharmacological uses
Cephalosporins are indicated for the treatment of infections caused
by bacteria. Cephalosporins are active predominantly against Gram
+ive bacteria. The antibiotic may be used for patients who are allergic
to penicillin. The drug is excreted in the urine.

Side effects
Common adverse reactions are diarrhea, nausea, rash, electrolyte
disturbances, and pain and inflammation at injection site. Overall, the

research shows that all beta lactams have the intrinsic hazard of very serious hazardous reactions in susceptible patients. Consumption of alcohol after taking cephalosporin orally or intravenously is contraindicated, and in severe cases can lead to death.

Resistance

Resistance to cephalosporin antibiotics can involve either reduced affinity of existing PBP components or the acquisition of a supplementary β-lactam-insensitive PBP.

Degradation of Cephalosporins in general

Fragmentation and fragment products

Classification

The classification of cephalosporins into "generations" is commonly practied, although the exact categorization is often imprecise. For example, the fourth generation of cephalosporins is not recognized as such in Japan. In Japan, cefaclor is classed as a first-generation cephalosporin, though in the United States it is a second-generation one; and cefbuperazone, cefminox, and cefotetan are classed as second-generation cephalosporins. Cefmetazole and cefoxitin are classed as third generation cephems. Flomoxef and latamoxef are in a new class called oxacephems.

Most first-generation cephalosporins were originally spelled "ceph-" in English-speaking countries. Fourth generation of cephalosporins were considered to be "a class of highly potent antibiotics that are among medicine's last defenses against several serious human infections".

Fifth generation cephalosporins, however, are effective against MRSA.

CEPHALORIDINE
(cefaloridine)

$$C_{19}H_{17}N_3O_4S_2$$
Molar mass
415.49g/mol

Chemistry and SAR in general

☐ Cephaloridine is a cephalosporin compound with pyridinium-1-ylmethyl and 2-thienylacetamido side groups. Cephaloridine (or cefaloridine) is a first-generation semisynthetic derivative of antibiotic cephalosporin C.

☐ Cephaloridine was briefly popular because it is tolerated intramuscularly and attained higher and more sustained levels in blood than cephalothin. However, it binds to proteins to a much lesser extent.

- Cephalosporin structure basically contains thiopyran ring fused with β-lactam ring.
- Position 3 is occupied by a terminal acetyl group.
- Position 4 is a carboxylic acid.
- At C 7, usual NH_2 group is present which is linked with an aliphatic chain.
- Aliphatic chain contains three molecules of CH_2 groups.
- At the terminal, primary amine and a carboxylic group is attached.
- In Cephalosporin C, replacement of entire (CH_2) 3 group with a complete ring and change of acetyl group at C 3 with methyl group, the compound is changed to "CEPHALEXIN".
- Changing acetyl group at C 3 to pyridine and terminal aliphatic chain is replaced by a carbonyl and thiophene, the compound becomes "CEPHALORIDINE".
- In the structure of cephalosporin C, the terminal chain at C 7, is replaced by a thiophene but position C 3 remains unchanged (acetylated), the compound is called to be "CEPHALOTHIN".

Cephalexin   Cephalosporin

Cephaloridine   Cephalothin

Metabolism
Excretion: Renal

Cephaloridine is easy absorbed after intramuscular injection and poorly absorbed from the gastrointestinal tract.

Cephaloridine is excreted in the urine without undergoing metabolism. It inhibits organic ion transport in the kidney. This process is preceded by the lipid peroxidation. When side-group leaves, the β-lactam ring is destabilized by intramolecular electron shifts. Thus, the leaving group creates a reactive product.

Pharmacological uses
Cephaloridine was used to treat patients with urinary tract infections and in the treatment of various lower respiratory tract infections. Cephaloridine was very effective to cure pneumococcal pneumonia.

Adverse side effects
Cephaloridine can cause kidney damage in humans since it is actively taken up from the blood by the proximal tubular cells via an organic anion transporter (OAT) in the basolateral membrane. The cationic group (pyridinium ring) of the compound probably inhibits the efflux through the membrane.

Contraindications
Complications caused by the use of cephaloridine include seizures, coma, chronic kidney failure, acute kidney failure and death. Vitamin D supplements and sodium bicarbonate (to correct the acid-base disturbance).

257

Synthesis of cephaloridine

Cephaloridine can be synthesized from Cephalothin and pyridine by deacetylation. This can be done by heating an aqueous mixture of cephalothin, thiocyanate, pyridine and phosphoric acid for several hours. After cooling, diluting with water, and adjusting the pH with mineral acid, cephaloridine thiocyanate salt precipitates. This can be purified and converted to cephaloridine by pH adjustment or by interaction with ion-exchange resin.

CEPHALOSPORIN C

$C_{16}H_{21}N_3O_8S$
Molar mass
415.42g/mol

Chemistry

Structure activity relationship (SAR)

Cephalosporin C is the product of the biosynthesis pathway of third generation cephalosporins. This is done by exchanging the acetyl CoA into DAC. To achieve cephalosporin C as the end product, there are 6 genes reported to be in control of the pathway.

Mechanism

Cephalosporin C acts by inhibiting penicillin binding proteins.

Pharmacological uses

Cephalosporins are used to treat bacterial infections such as respiratory tract infections, skin infections and urinary tract infections.

Adverse side effects

Itching, swelling, dizziness, trouble breathing, severe stomach cramps, fever, fast heartbeat.

Inhibition of β-lactamase by Cephalosporins

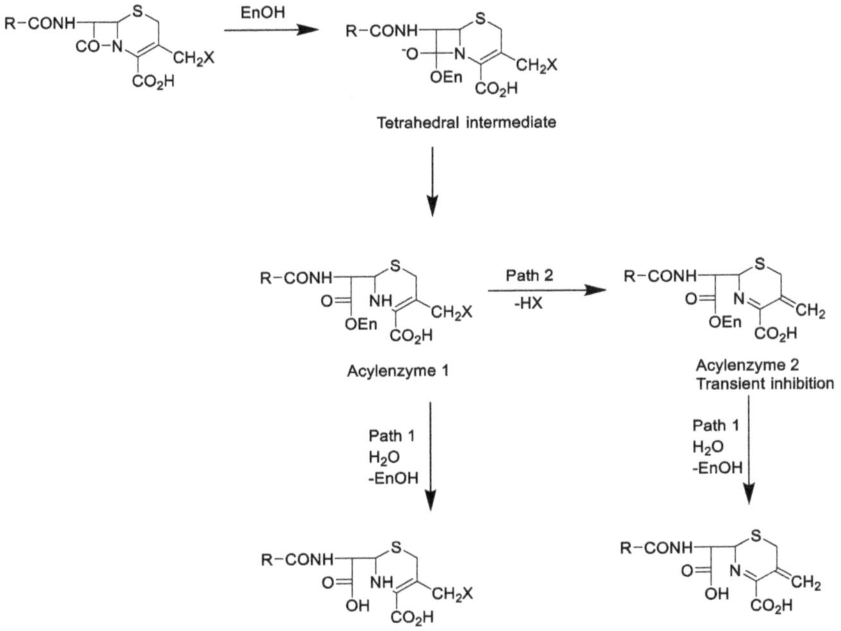

Tetrahedral intermediate

Acylenzyme 1

Acylenzyme 2
Transient inhibition

Path 2
-HX

Path 1
H_2O
-EnOH

Path 1
H_2O
-EnOH

CEPHALOTHIN

$C_{16}H_{16}N_2O_6S_2$
Molar mass
396.44g/mol

Chemistry

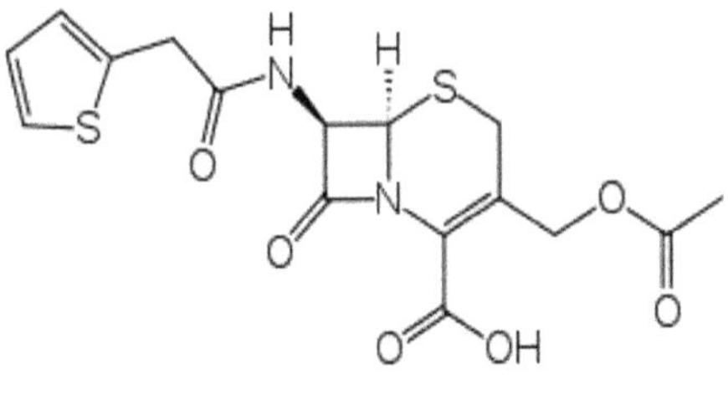

Pharmacokinetics
Protein binding: 65-80%
Metabolism: Hepatic
Biological half- life: 30-60 minutes
Excretion: Hepatic
ROA: I.V.

Pharmacological uses
As mentioned above.

Adverse side effects
As above

Synthesis of cephalothin

Cephalothin

CEPHALEXIN

$C_{16}H_{17}N_3O_4S$
Molar mass
347.39g/mol

Chemistry

Structure activity relationship (SAR)
As above

Pharmacokinetics
Bioavailability: absorbed
Protein binding: 15%

Metabolism
80% excreted unchanged in urine within 6 hours of administration.
Biological half- life: 0.6-1.2 hours
Excretion: Renal
ROA: Oral

Pharmacological uses
Cefalexin can treat certain bacterial infections, including those of the middle ear, bones, skin, joints and urinary tract infections and in pneumonia. It is a useful alternative to penicillin in patients with penicillin intolerance. Cefalexin is a beta-lactam antibiotic of the cephalosporin family. It is bactericidal and acts by inhibiting synthesis of the peptidoglycan layer of the bacterial cell wall.

Common side effects
Include cause of diarrhea, is not harmful in pregnancy or breast feeding. It can be used in children and those over 65 years of age. The most common adverse effects of cefalexin, are gastrointestinal (stomach area) disturbances and hypersensitivity reactions reactions

include rash, itching, swelling, trouble breathing, or red, blistered, swollen, or peeling skin.

Synthesis of Cephalexin 1

| Cephalexin | Maleic anhydride | Cephalexin ProD 1 |

| Cephalexin | Succinic anhydride | Cephalexin ProD 1 |

Synthesis of Cephalexin 2

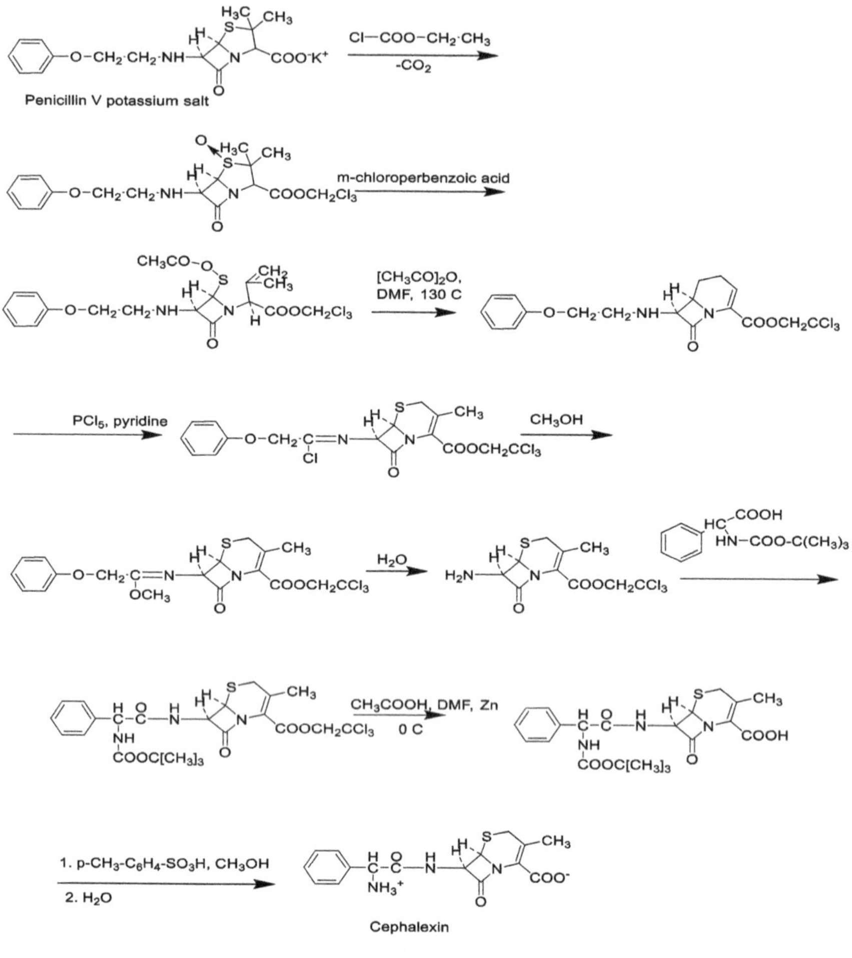

Penicillin V potassium salt

$$Cl-COO-CH_2\cdot CH_3 \xrightarrow{-CO_2}$$

m-chloroperbenzoic acid

$[CH_3CO]_2O$, DMF, 130 C

PCl$_5$, pyridine

CH$_3$OH

$$\begin{array}{c} HC-COOH \\ HN-COO-C(CH_3)_3 \end{array}$$

H$_2$O

CH$_3$COOH, DMF, Zn   0 C

1. p-CH$_3$-C$_6$H$_4$-SO$_3$H, CH$_3$OH

2. H$_2$O

Cephalexin

CEPHALOGLYCIN

$C_{18}H_{19}N_3O_6S$
Molar mass
405.43g/mol

Chemistry

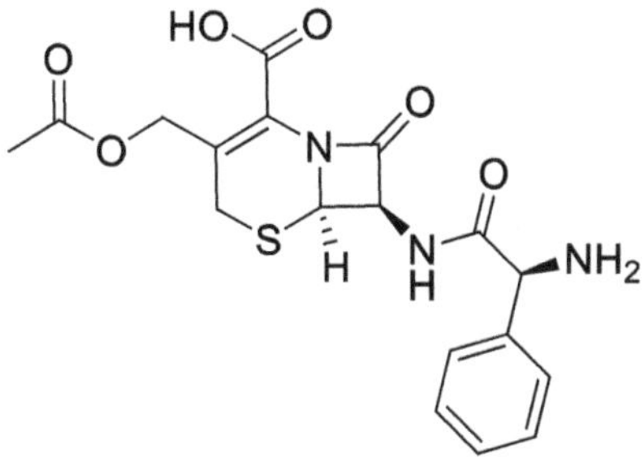

Structure activity relationship (SAR)

As above

Metabolism

As above

Pharmacological uses

As above

Adverse side effects

As above

Contraindications

As above

CEFAZOLIN
(cefazoline)
(cephazolin)

$C_{14}H_{14}N_8O_4S_3$
Molar mass
454.51 g/mol

Chemistry

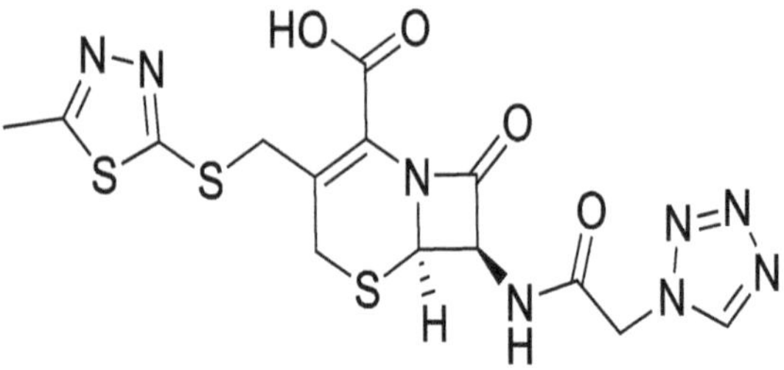

Structure activity relationship (SAR)
As above

Pharmacokinetics
Biological half- life: 1.8 hours by I.V. and 2.0 hours by I.M.
Excretion: Renal unchanged
ROA: I.M., I.V.

Pharmacological uses
> Indicating general safety for use in pregnancy, Skin infections, biliary tract infections, bone and joint infections, genital infections and blood infections.
> Cefazolin inhibits cell wall biosynthesis.

Adverse side effects
As above.

5.25 Second Generation

(moderate spectrum)
CEFACLOR

$C_{15}H_{14}ClN_3O_4S$
Molar mass
367.81g/mol

Chemistry

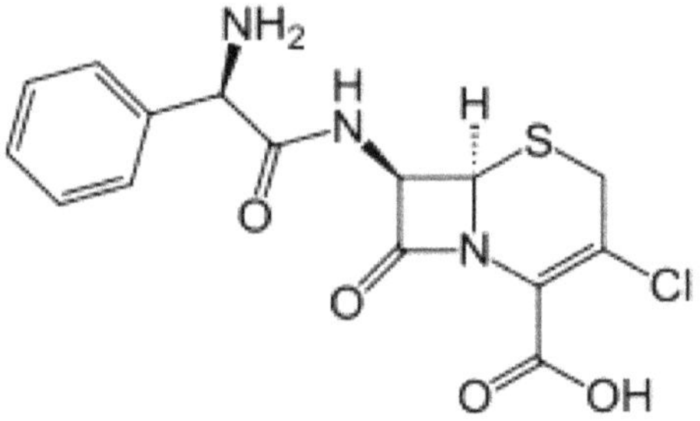

Structure activity relationship (SAR)

As above

Pharmacokinetics

Bioavailability: absorbed
Protein binding:15-40%
Biological half-life:0.6-0.9 hours
Excretion: Renal
ROA: Oral, I.M., I.V.

Pharmacological uses

Used for the treatment of biliary tract infections, peritonitis and urinary tract infections. Excretion being principally renal. Cefaclor is active against gram + ive and gram -ive bacteria.

Spectrum of activity

Cefaclor is frequently used against bacteria responsible for causing skin infections, otitis media, urinary tract infections, and others.

Adverse side effects

- Hypersensitivity. Penicillin-sensitive patients will also be allergic to the cephalosporins, often overestimated. Allergic reactions may present as, for example, rashes, itching, fever.
- Other side effects include gastrointestinal disturbances (e.g. diarrhea, nausea and vomiting, abdominal discomfort,

267

disturbances in liver enzymes, transient hepatitis and cholestatic jaundice and Stevens-Johnson syndrome.

Contraindications

- Cefaclor is passed into the breast milk in small quantities but is generally accepted to be safe.
- Cefaclor is not known to be harmful in pregnancy.
- Cautions include known sensitivity to beta-lactam antibacterial, such as penicillin (Cefaclor should be avoided if there is a history of immediate reaction); renal impairment (no dose adjustment required, although manufacturer advises caution):

CEFAMANDOLE
(cephamandole)

$$C_{18}H_{18}N_6O_5S_2$$
Molar mass
462.51g/mol

Chemistry

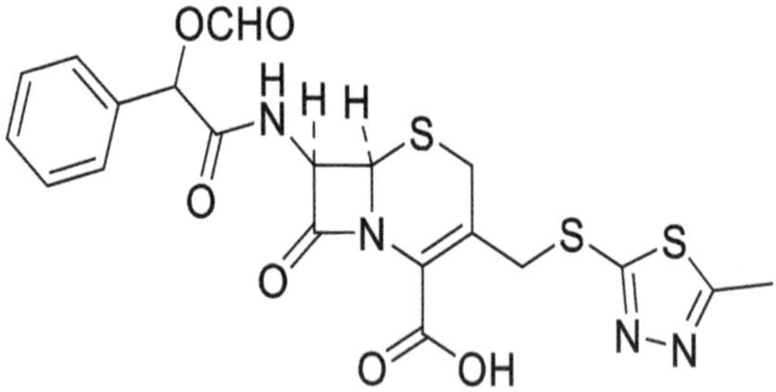

Pharmacokinetics
Protein binding: 75%
Biological half-life: 48 minutes
Excretion: Renal (unchanged)
ROA: I.M., I.V.

Pharmacological uses

Is a prodrug.

Synthesis of Cefamandole nafate

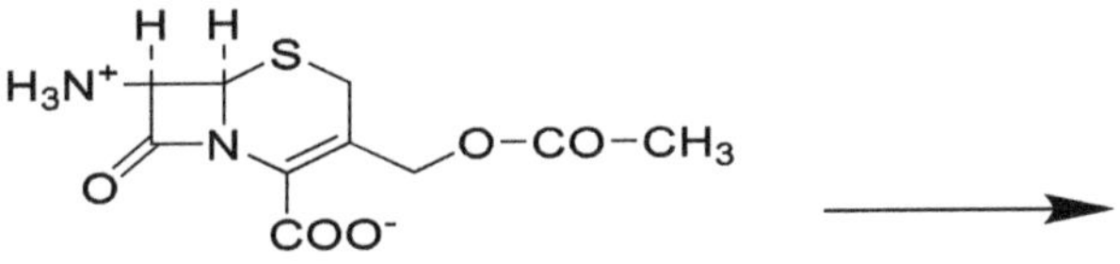

(6R,7R)-3-(acetoxymethyl)-7-
ammonio-8-oxo-5-thia-1-
azabicyclo[4.2.0]oct-2-ene-2-
carboxylate

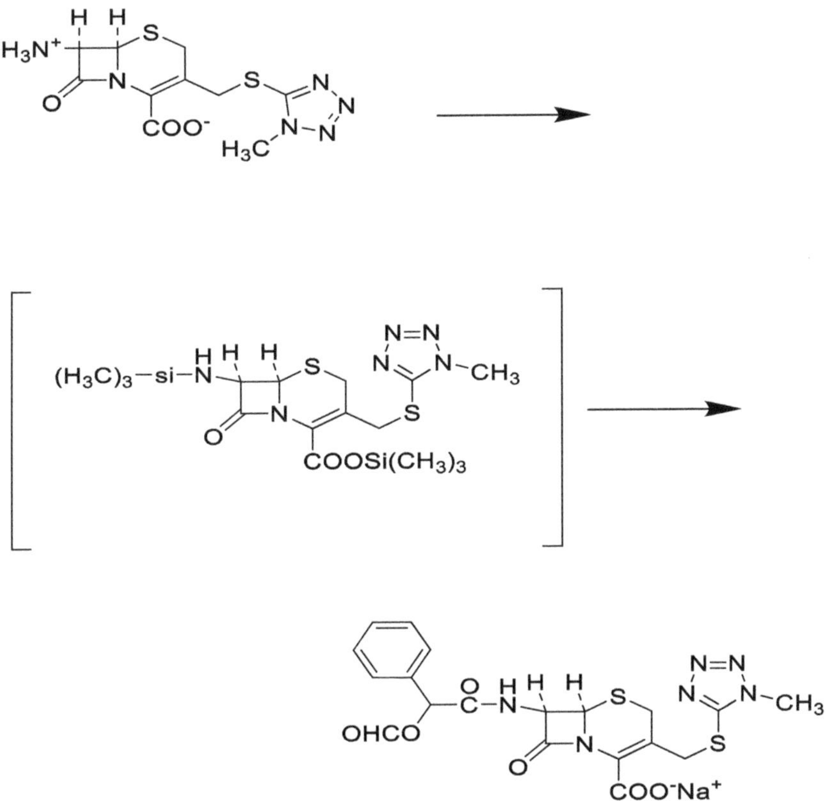

CEPHUROXIME

$C_{16}H_{16}N_4O_8S$
Molar mass
424.39g/mol

Chemistry

Structure activity relationship (SAR)
As above

Pharmacokinetics
Bioavailability: 37% on an empty stomach, up to 52% if taken after food
Biological half- life: 80 minutes
Excretion: 66-100% by urine unchanged
ROA: Oral, I.M., I.V.

Pharmacological uses
A systematic review found high quality evidence that injecting the eye with cefuroxime after cataract surgery will lower the chance of developing endophthalmitis after surgery.

Adverse side effects
Common side effects include nausea, diarrhea, allergic reactions, and pain at the site of injection.

Contraindications

As above.

Synthesis of Cephuroxime

Cefuroxime, a second-generation cephalosporin antibiotic, was synthesized from 7-amino cephalosporinic acid (7-ACA) and (Z)-2-methoxyimino-2-(furyl-2-yl) acetic acid ammonium salt (SMIA) as starting materials. The total yield of cefuroxime synthesized via the 4-step scheme was 42%. The novel feature of this study was the use of oxalyl chloride activating reagent which replaced phosphoryl chloride in the activation of SMIA. The result showed that the yield was 90% in the reaction time of 1.5 hours. Especially, this synthesis can be considered as a green process because the water only contained NH4Cl, CO and CO2 non-toxic compounds.

CEPHONICID
(cephalosporin)

$$C_{18}H_{18}N_6O_8S_3$$
Molar mass
542.57g/mol

Chemistry

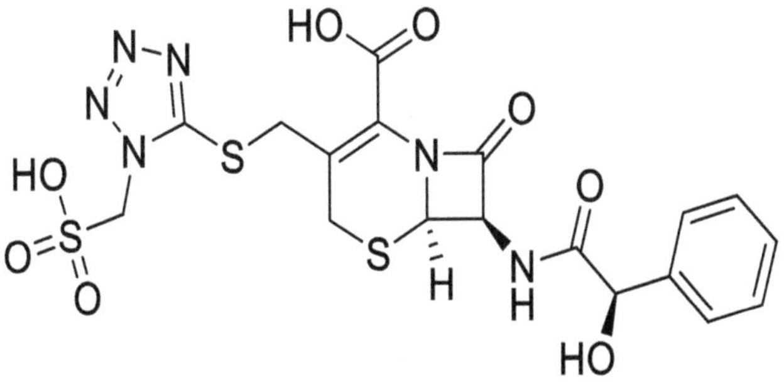

Pharmacokinetics

Semisynthetic I.M.

CEFOTETAN

$C_{17}H_{17}N_7O_8S_4$
Molar mass
575.62/mol

Chemistry

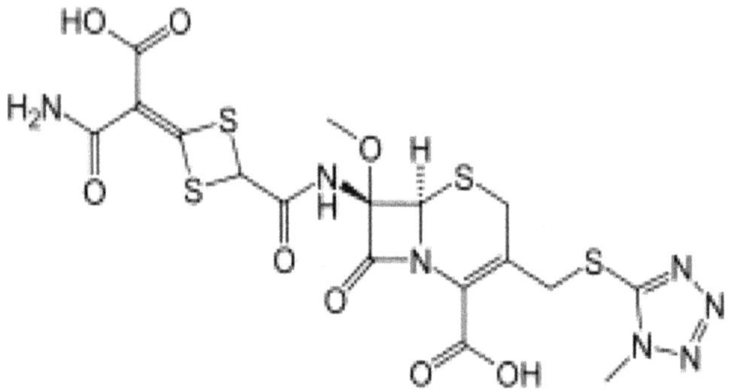

CEFOXITIN

$C_{16}H_{17}N_3O_7S_2$
Molar mass
427.45/mol

Chemistry

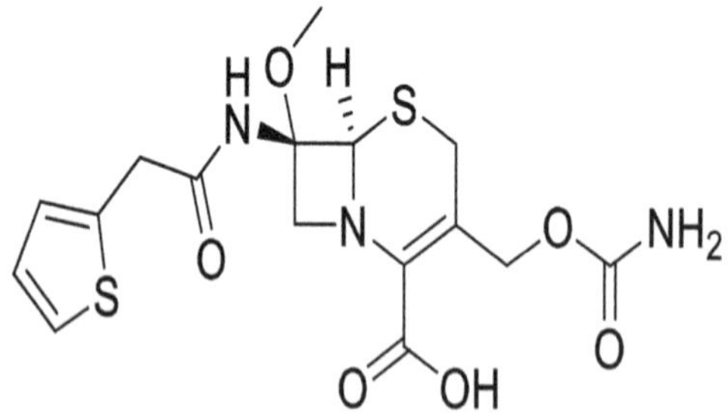

Structure activity relationship (SAR)
As above

272

Pharmacokinetics

Biological half-life: 41-59 minutes
Excretion: Urine 85%
ROA: I.V.

Pharmacological uses

- Escherichia coli: 0.2 μg/ml – 64 μg/ml
- Haemophilus influenzae: 0.5 μg/ml – 12.5 μg/ml
- Streptococcus pneumoniae: 0.2 μg/ml – 1 μg/m
- Skin infections, primarily due to Staphylococcus, Urinary tract infections, Bronchitis, Tonsillitis, Gonorrhea.

Adverse side effects

- local tenderness or pain at the site of injection, skin color change, mild diarrhea, mild nausea, vaginal discharge and itching and swelling of feet or legs.

Contraindications

Patients with colitis, kidney disease, or liver disease are also advised not to take cefoxitin.

5.26 Third Generation

(broad spectrum)

CEPHTIZOXIME

$C_{13}H_{13}N_5O_5S_2$
Molar mass
383.41g/mol

Chemistry

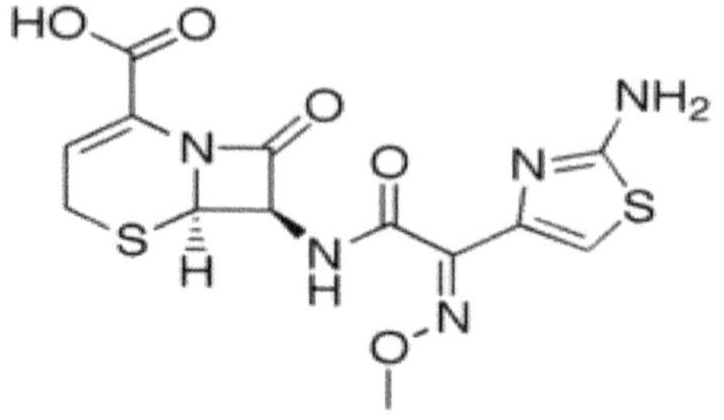

Synthesis of Cephtizoxime

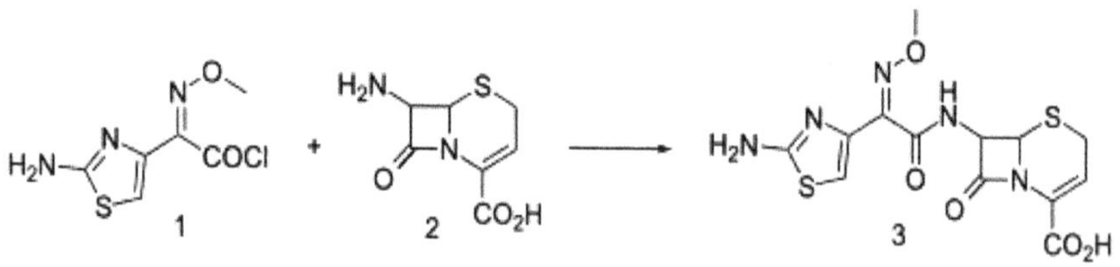

CEPHTRIAXONE

$$C_{18}H_{18}N_8O_7S_3$$
Molar mass
554.58g/mol

Chemistry

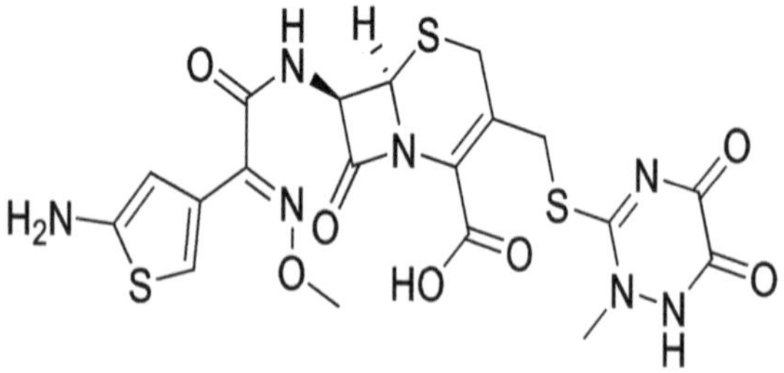

Structure activity relationship (SAR)

The stability of this configuration results in increased activity of ceftriaxone against otherwise resistant Gram-negative bacteria.

274

Pharmacokinetics

Biological half- life: 5.7-8.7 hours

Excretion: 33–67% kidney, 35–45% biliary

ROA: I.M., I.V.

Pharmacological uses

acute bacterial skin and skin structure infections, intra-abdominal infections, surgical prophylaxis.

Adverse side effects

There is tentative evidence that ceftriaxone is relatively safe during pregnancy and breastfeeding.

Contraindications

As above

CEPHIXIME

$C_{16}H_{15}N_5O_7S_2$
Molar mass
453.45g/mol

Chemistry

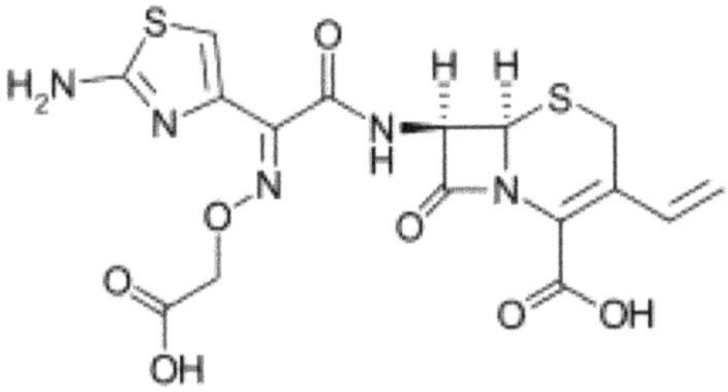

Structure activity relationship (SAR)

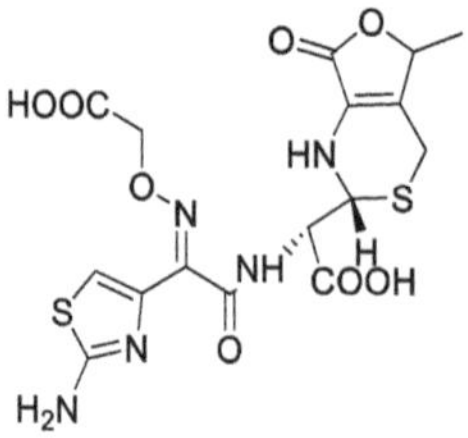

A Impurity

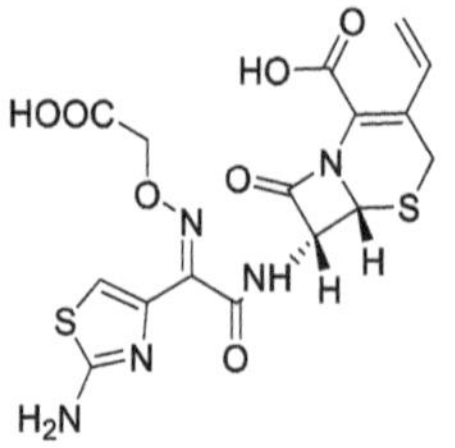

Cefixime

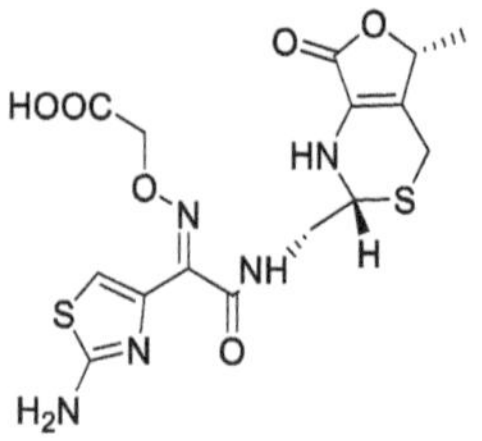

B Impurity

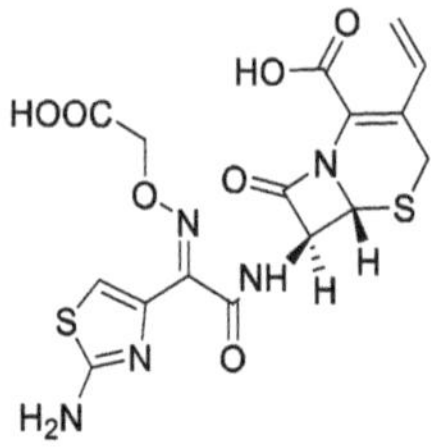

C Impurity

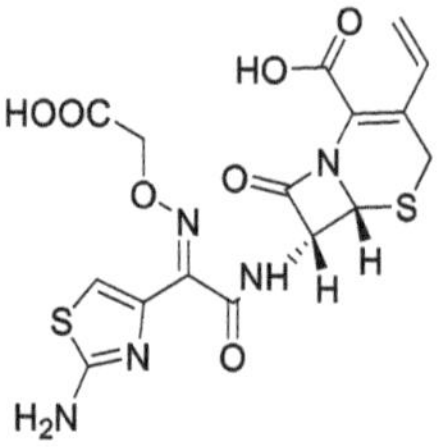

D Impurity

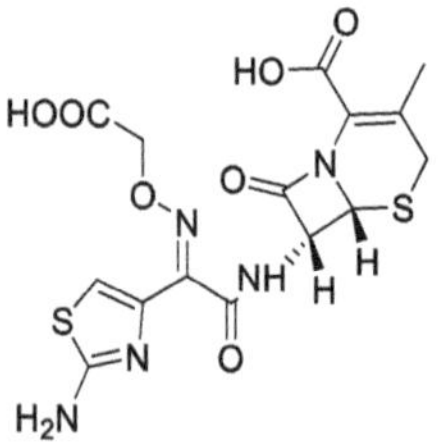

E Impurity

Pharmacokinetics

Bioavailability: 40-50%, Protein binding:60%, Biological half- life: 3-4 hours

Excretion: Kidney and biliary, ROA: Oral

Pharmacological uses

As above

Adverse side effects

As above

MOXALACTAM
(latamoxef)

$C_{20}H_{20}N_6O_9S$
Molar mass
520.47g/mol

Chemistry

Pharmacokinetics

Protein binding: 35-50%

Biological half- life: 2 hours

Excretion: Mostly renal unchanged and biliary

ROA: I.M, I.V.

Synthesis of Moxalactam

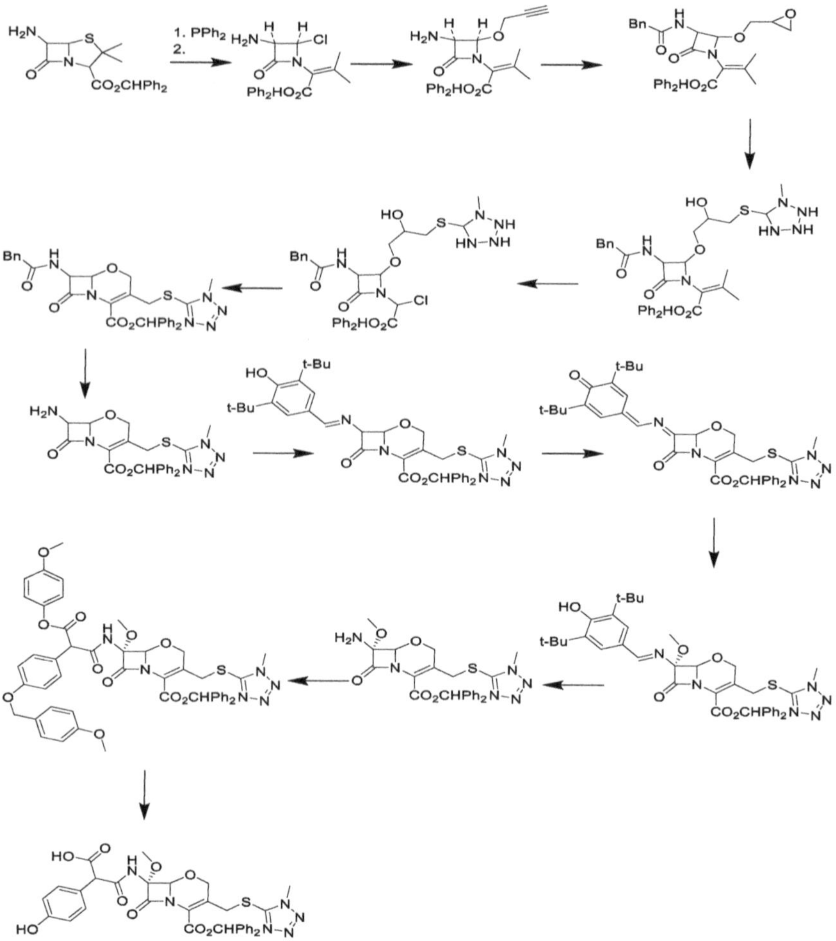

CEFOTAXIME

$C_{16}H_{17}N_5O_7S_2$
Molar mass
455.47 g/mol

Chemistry

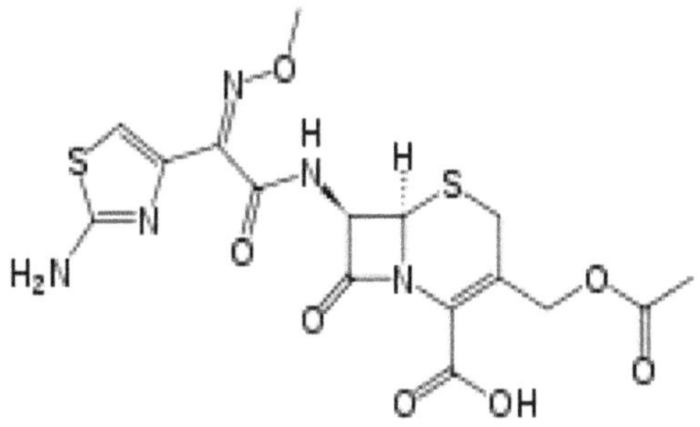

Metabolism

Metabolism: Liver
Protein binding: 21-29%
Biological half- life: 0.8-1.4 hours
Excretion: Kidney (50-59-8%)
ROA: Oral, I.M., I.V.

Pharmacological uses

☐ It is widely used to treat plant tissue infections with Gram-
negative bacteria, in humans against numerous gram +ive
and gram -ive bacteria, pneumonia, Genitourinary system
infections and Gynecologic infections, endometritis, and pelvic
cellulitis and CNS infections like meningitis, pneumoniae.

Synthesis of Cefotaxime 1

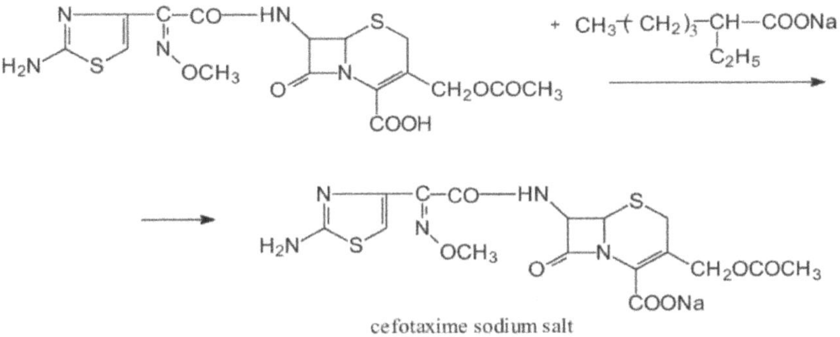

cefotaxime sodium salt

279

Synthesis of Cefotaxime 2

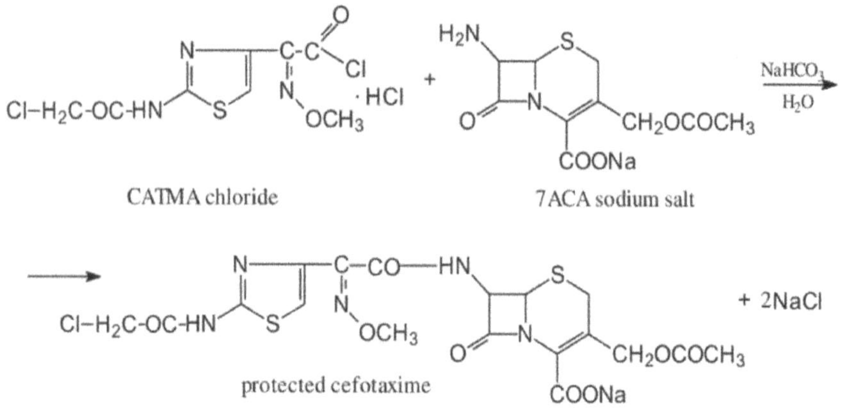

CATMA chloride   7ACA sodium salt

protected cefotaxime

+ 2NaCl

CEFPODOXIME

$C_{15}H_{17}N_5O_6S_2$
Molar mass
427.46g/mol

Chemistry

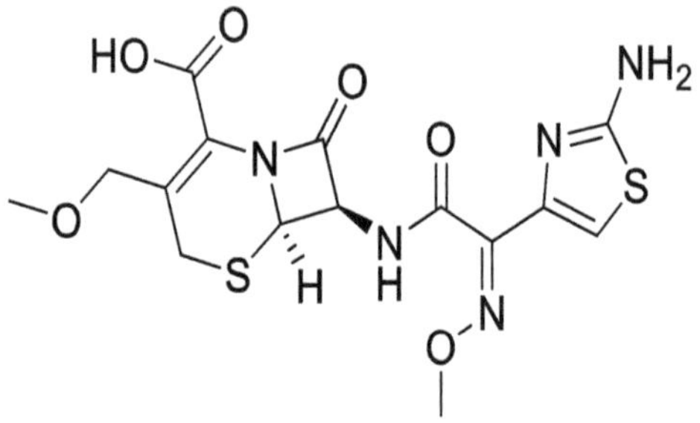

Metabolism
Bioavailability: 50%
Protein binding: 21-29%
Biological half- life: 2 hours
Excretion: Renal (unchanged)
ROA: Oral

Pharmacological uses

ORAL veterinary use as well. It is indicated in community acquired pneumonia, uncomplicated skin and skin structure infections, and uncomplicated urinary tract infections.

CEFTAZIDIME

$$C_{22}H_{22}N_6O_7S_2$$
Molar mass
446.58g/mol

Chemistry

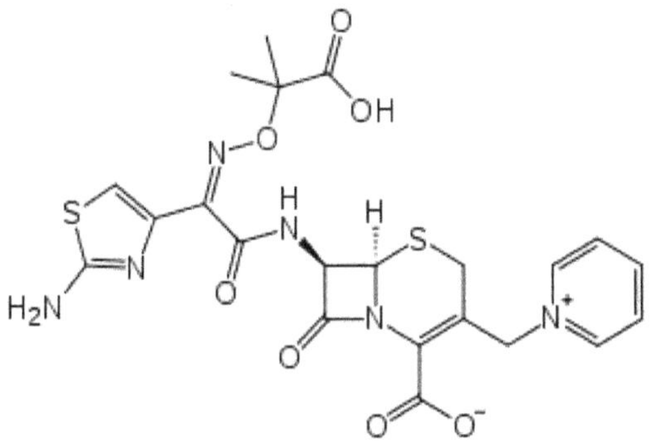

Structure activity relationship (SAR):

As above

Metabolism

Bioavailability: 91% I.M.
Protein binding: 60%
Biological half- life: 1.6-2 hours
Excretion: Kidney (90-96%)
ROA: Ora

Pharmacological uses

Gastrointestinal symptoms, including diarrhea, nausea, vomiting, and abdominal pain, were reported in fewer than 2% of patients.

Side effects
As above

CEFTRIAXONE

$$C_{18}H_{18}N_8O_7S_3$$
Molar mass
554.58g/mol

Chemistry

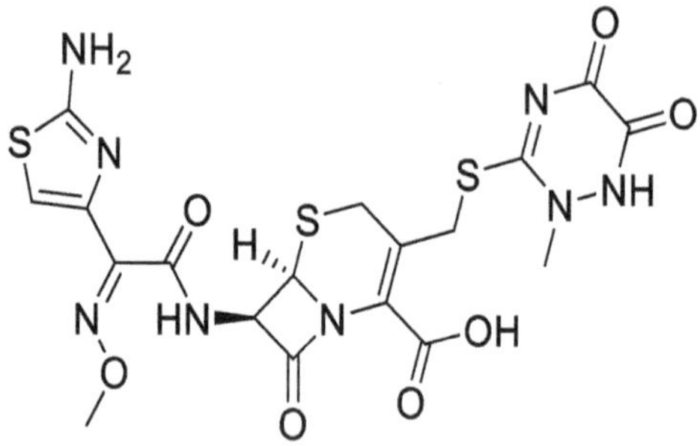

Metabolism
Protein binding: 60%
Biological half- life:5.8-8.7 hours
Excretion: Kidney (33-67%) and biliary (35-45%)
ROA: Oral, I.V., I.M.

Pharmacological uses
Skin and skin structure infections, urinary tract infections gonorrhea
and Breastfeeding

Adverse side effects
Diarrhea (2.7%), Local reactions—pain, tenderness, irritation (1%).
Rash (1.7%). Some less frequently reported adverse events itchiness,
fever, chills, nausea, vomiting, headache and dizziness.

Synthesis of Ceftriaxone

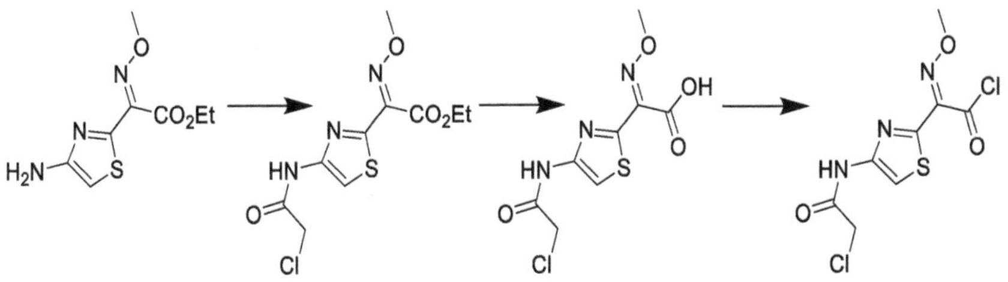

5.27 Fourth Generation

(broad spectrum)

CEFIPIME

$C_{16}H_{15}N_5O_7S_2$
Molar mass
453.45g/mol

Chemistry

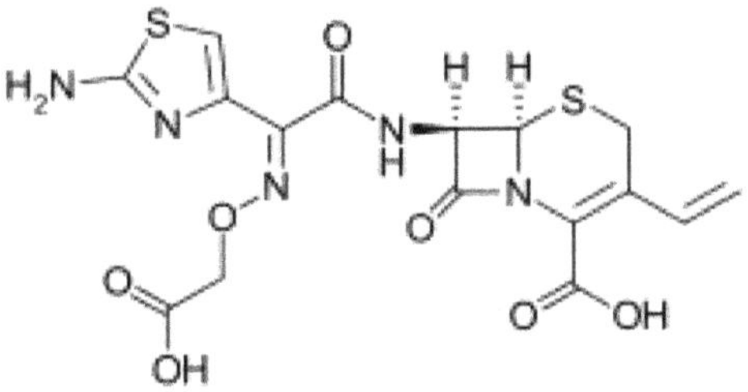

Metabolism
Bioavailability: 40-50%
Protein binding: 60%
Biological half-life: 3-4 hours
Excretion: Kidney and biliary
ROA: Oral

CEFPIROME

$$C_{22}H2_2N_6O_5S_2$$
Molar mass
514.58g/mol

Chemistry

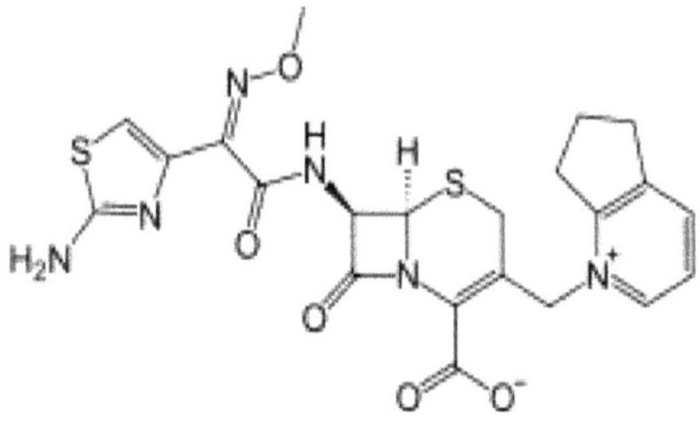

5.28 Fifth Generation

(broad spectrum)

CEFTAROLINE FOSAMIL

$$C_{24}H_{25}N_8O_{10}PS_4$$
Molar mass
744.74g/mol

Chemistry

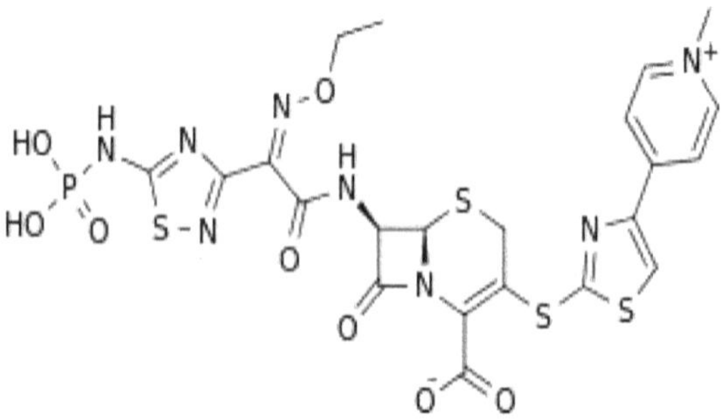

284

Metabolism

Protein binding: 20%

Biological half- life: 2-5 hours

Excretion: Urine 88% and faces 6%

ROA: I.V.

CEFOZOPRAN

$C_{19}H_{17}N_9O_5S_2$
Molar mass
515.52g/mol

Chemistry

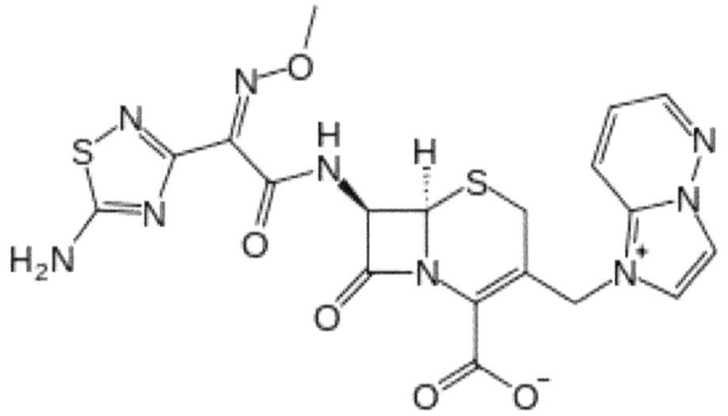

CEFTOBIPROLE

$C_{20}H_{22}N_8O_6S_2$
Molar mass
534.57g/mol

Chemistry

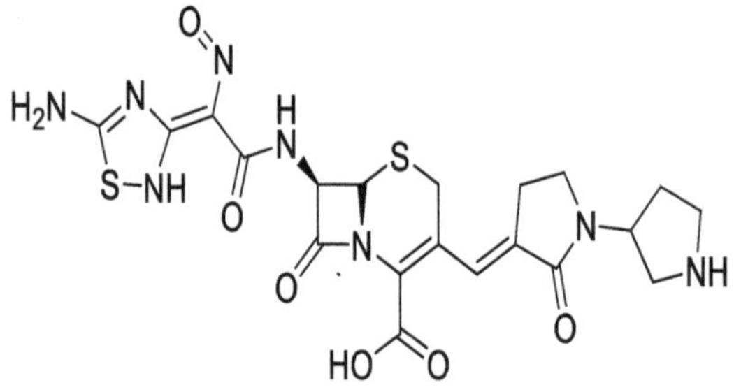

Metabolism

Ceftobiprole has been approved for the treatment of adult patients with hospital acquired pneumonia.

CEFTOLOZANE
(combined with Tazobactam)
(Tazobactam (penicillinate sulfone β-lactamase inhibitor)

$$C_{23}H_{30}N_{12}O_8S_2$$
Molar mass:
666.689 g/mol g·mol−1

Chemistry

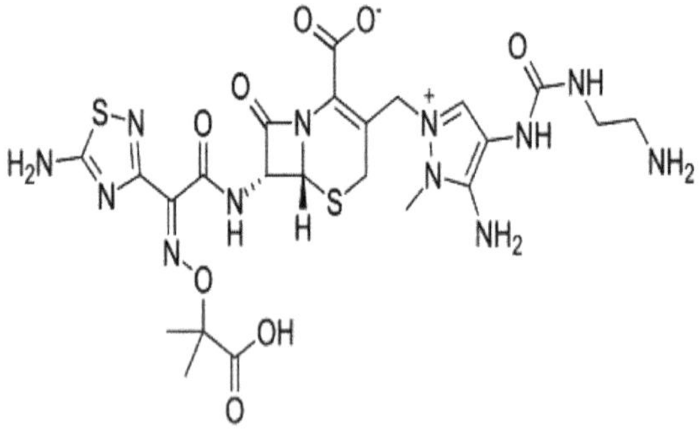

Structure activity relationship (SAR)

  i. Affording increased activity against gram-negative organisms
  ii. Dimethylacetic acid moiety that contributes to enhanced activity against *Pseudomonas aeruginosa*.

iii. The addition of a bulky side chain (a pyrazole ring) at the 3-position prevents hydrolysis of the β-lactam ring via steric hindrance.

Metabolism

The metabolism and excretion of ceftolozane is similar to those of most β-lactam antimicrobial agents.

Pharmacological uses

It is indicated for the treatment of complicated intra-abdominal infections in adults.

Adverse side effects

The most common AEs reported with ceftolozane/tazobactam were headache (5.8%), constipation (3.9%), hypertension (3%), nausea (2.8%), and diarrhea (1.9%).

CHAPTER 6

TETRACYCLINES

6.1 General characters of Tetracyclines

Among most important broad-spectrum antibiotics are members of the tetracycline family such as tetracycline, demeclocycline, meclocycline, methacyclin, rolitetracycline, oxytetracycline, doxycycline, and minocycline have been introduced possessing antibiotic activity. Several Tetracyclines are obtained by fermentation procedures from Streptomyces species or by chemical transformations of the natural products. Their chemical identities have been established by degradation studies and confirmed by the synthesis of three members or the group. The important members of the group are derivatives of an octahydro-naphthacene, a hydrocarbon system that comprises four six-membered rings. It is from this tetracyclic system that the group name is derived. The semi-synthetic modifications of certain substituents on the tetracycline skeletol has led to the derivatives which possess improved chemotherapeutic properties.

Antibiotics of the tetracycline group are active against gram-positive and gram-negative bacteria. Chlortetracycline was first isolated from Streptomyces aureofaciens. Tetracycline was prepared in 1953 by catalytic reduction of chlortetracycline. Later studies have led to the preparation of various tetracycline derivatives by fermentation or hemi-synthesis. Their Structures are shown in the following figures.

Three biochemically distinct mechanisms of resistance to tetracyclines have been described.

6.1.1   Permissable substitution of tetracyclines

The molecule of tetracycline retains its antimicrobial activity when Substitution is made at positions 5 to 9. See figure 1.2. Replacing the carbox-amido at position 2 by acetyl, the activity is decreased. Even by replacing one of the hydrogens of carbox-amido by another group, the activity is reduced. When any replacement is made at other positions, the activity is lost.

6.1.2   Ionization of tetracyclines

The tetracyclines in neutral or slightly acidic conditions (pH 3 to 7) are zwitterions. The tetracyclines are amphoteric and have two acid and one basic functional group. The basicity of tetracycline is due to the presence of the dimethylamino group at C4. The groups responsible for the acidity of tetracycline hydrochloride is shown in figures below. The pka values of tetracyclines were determined by Stephens et al. and Benet et al.

6.1.3   Transformation of tetracyclines

In certain conditions the tetracyclines undergo transformation. Not all the tetracyclines undergo all the transformations. Tetracyclines in solution at pH 2 to 6 epimerises at C-4 resulting in 4-epitetracyclines, reduces the epimerisation process strongly Antibiotic activity of Tetracyclines down to 2 to 5%. This epimerisation is an equilibrium. Oxytetracycline and doxycycline are relatively stable towards C-4 epimerisation probably due to the hydrogen bonding of the hydroxyl group at C-5 with the C-4 dimethylamino group.

The mechanism of epimerisation is represented in figures below. Due to the presence of a tertiary hydroxyl group at C-6 in Tetracycline, Chlortetracycline and Oxytetracycline, acid degradation takes place resulting in the formation of anhydroderivatives. Overaged tetracycline preparations degrading to 4-epianhydrotetracycline show a definite toxicity to renal tubular function (Fanconi syndrome). The absence of hydroxyl at C-6 in Doxycycline and Metacycline excludes the possibility of acid degradation. The anhydro-derivative of oxytetracycline rearranges in acidic hydroxylic media to two isomers, α-apooxytetracycline and β-apooxytetracycline. Chlortetracycline in aqueous basic medium leads to the formation of isochlor-tetracycline which epimerises to 4-epiisochlortetracycline.

Glycylcyclines and Fluorocyclines are new classes of antibiotics derived from tetracycline. These tetracycline analogues are specifically designed to overcome two common mechanisms of tetracycline resistance, namely resistance mediated by acquired efflux pumps and /or ribosomal protection. Tetracyclines are among the cheapest classes of antibiotics available and have been used extensively in prophylaxis and in treatment of human and animal infections, as well as at subtherapeutic levels in animal feed as growth promoters.

6.1.4   Different compounds of Tetracycline group of antibiotics with their origin and half-life

No.	Name of compound	Origin	Half-life
1.	Tetracycline	Natural	6-8 hours (short acting)
2.	Chlotetracycline	Natural	6-8 hours (short acting)
3.	Oxytetracycline	Natural	6-8 hours (short acting)
4.	Demeclocycline (declomycin)	Natural	12 hours (intermediate acting)
5.	Lymecycline	Semi-synthetic	6-8 hours (short acting)
6.	Meclocycline	Semi-synthetic	6-8 hours (short acting)
7	Methacycline (metacycline)	Semi-synthetic	12 hours (intermediate acting)
8.	Minocycline	Semi-synthetic	+16 hours (long acting)
9.	Rolitetracycline	Semi-synthetic	6-8 hours (short acting)
10.	Doxycycline	Semi-synthetic	+16 hours (long acting)
11.	Tigecycline (Glycecyclines)	Synthetic	+16 hours (long acting)
12.	Eravacycline	Newer	+16 hours (long acting)
13.	Sarecycline	newer	+16 hours (long acting)
14.	Omadacycline	newer	+16 hours (long acting)

6.2 Acid–base equilibria for tetracycline

The balance of lipophilicity to hydrophilicity in tetracyclines is affected by pH, such a property is usually a clue that there are functional groups in the molecule under investigation which are ionizable at physiological pH values. Each tetracycline has at least one readily ionizable amine group (at C4) and two enol groups (at C3 and C12) that are also relatively easily ionized. First- and second-generation tetracyclines have three pKa values in the physiological pH range (generally around 3.2, 7.6, and 9.6) – the two enol groups, at C3 and C12, are the most acidic (and so have the lower pKa values). The pKa of the phenol group at C10 (~12) means that it is not ionized at physiological pH values. The acid–base equilibria for tetracycline, which are typical of the tetracycline antibiotics, are demonstrated below.

pH <2.5: Fully protonated form predominates
Overall charge: +1

pH 4.0–7.0: Zwitterionic, neutral, form predominates
Overall charge: 0

pH>8.0: Second enol group deprotonates
Overall charge: –1

pH >12.5: Fully deprotonated form predominates
Overall charge: –3

pH 10.0–11.5: Tertiary amine deprotonates
Overall charge: –2

Half-life of some therapeutically important tetracyclines

Short acting half-life 6-8 hours	Intermediate acting half-life 12 hours	Long acting half life 16-18 hours
Tetracycline	Demeclocycline	Doxycycline
Oxytetracycline	Methacycline	Minocycline
Chlortetracycline		

pka values of clinically important Tetracycline hydrochloride units and three acidity constants in aqueous solution at 25 C°

Type	pka_1	pka_2	Pka_3
Tetracycline	3.3	7.7	9.5
Chlortetracycline	3.3	7.4	9.3
Demeclocycline	3.3	7.2	9.3
Oxytetracycline	3.3	7.3	9.1
Doxycycline	3.4	7.7	9.7
Minocycline	2.8	7.8	9.3

Naturally occuring	Semisynthetic	Pro-drugs
Tetracycline	Doxycycline	Rolitetracycline
Chlortetracycline	Lymecycline	Lymelicycline
Demeclocycline	Meclocycline	Pipacycline
		Guamecycline

First generation	Second generation	Third generation	New third generation

6.3 Biosynthesis of Tetracyclines

The biosynthesis of tetracycline antibiotics is related to the bacterial synthesis of fatty acids through the bacterial type II polyketide synthase pathway, consisting of a well-studied set of enzymes, although the synthesis of tetracyclines is unique to certain bacteria. The biosynthetic pathways to tetracycline and oxytetracycline are the most studied.

Enzymes involved in Tetracycline biosynthesis.

Enzyme	Function
OxyA	Ketosynthase
OxyB	Chain length factor
OxyC	Acyl carrier protein
OxyJ	Ketoreductase
OxyK	Aromatase
OxyN	Cyclase
OxyF	C-methyltransferase
OxyE	Flavin-dependent monooxygenase
OxyL	NADPH-dependent dioxygenase
OxyQ	Aminotransferase
OxyT	N, N-dimethyltransferase
OxyS	Monooxygenase hydroxylates stereospecifically at C6
Cts4	Halogenase

6.4 Chemical synthesis of Tetracyclines in general

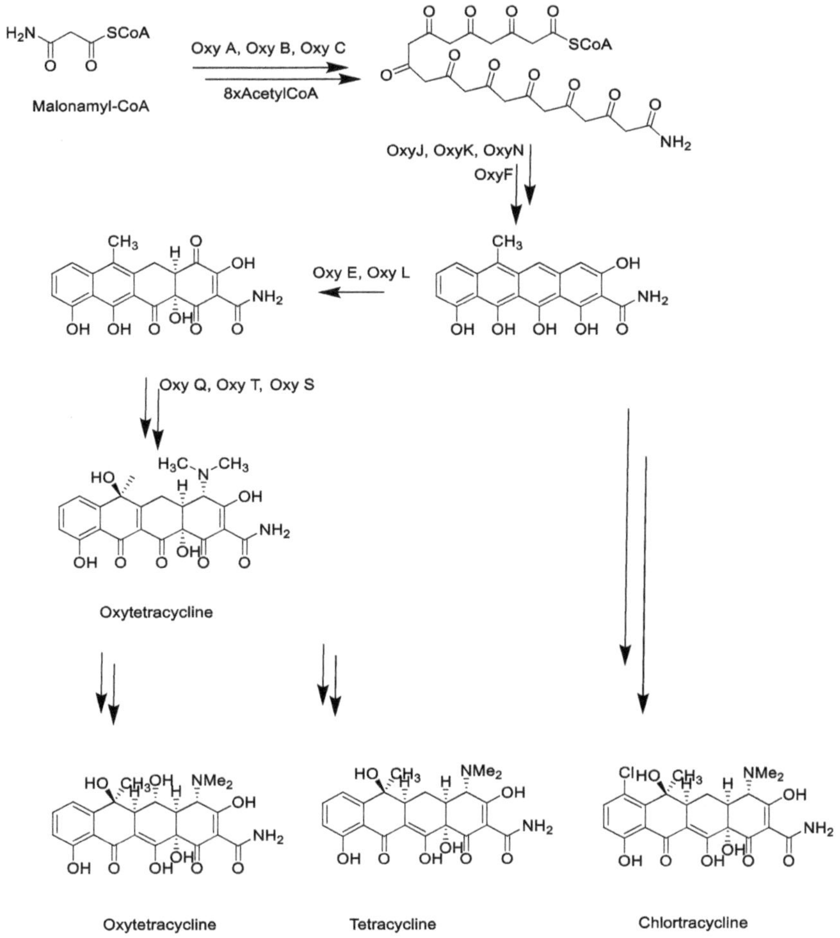

Malonamyl-CoA

Oxy A, Oxy B, Oxy C

8xAcetylCoA

OxyJ, OxyK, OxyN
OxyF

Oxy E, Oxy L

Oxy Q, Oxy T, Oxy S

Oxytetracycline

Oxytetracycline

Tetracycline

Chlortracycline

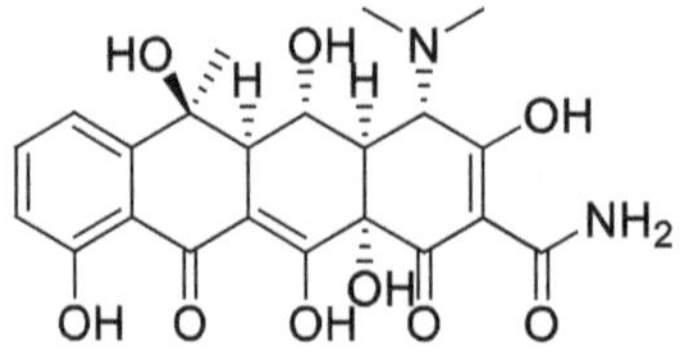

Oxytetracycline

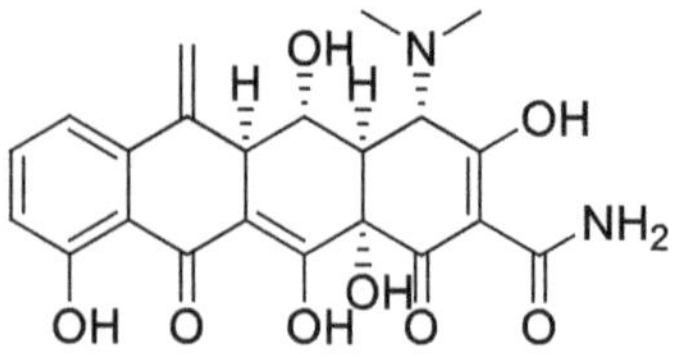

Metacycline

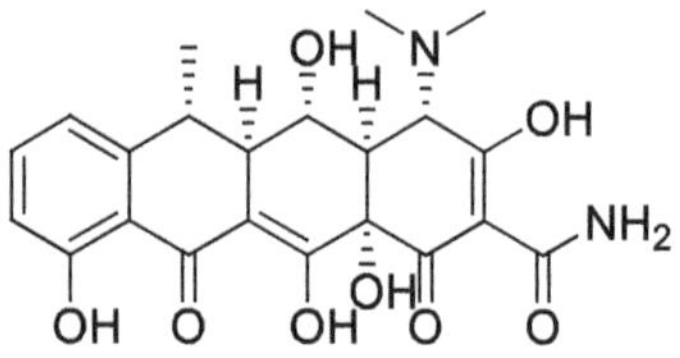

Doxycycline

6.5 Bioavailability of Tetracyclines in general

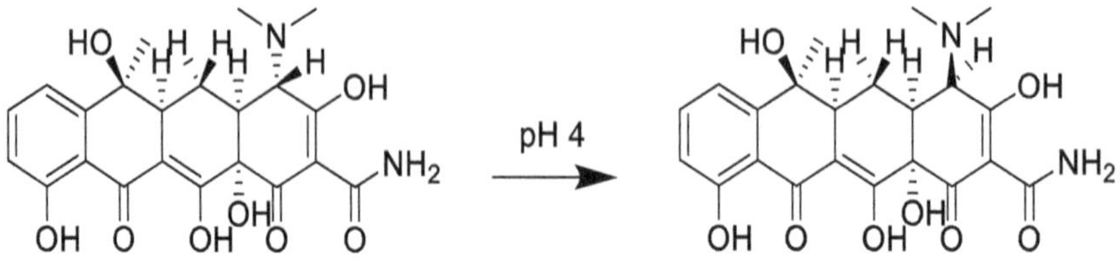

Tetracycline

Epitetracycline

Acid-catalysed dehydration of chlortetracycline and improved stability of demethylchlortetracycline (demeclocycline) is shown below.

Lymecycline is a prodrug form of tetracycline that is hydrolyzed at acidic and neutral pH *in vivo* to tetracycline, formaldehyde (methanal), and the amino acid lysine after oral and parenteral administration (*In vivo* hydrolysis of lymecycline to form tetracycline (as shown below). Interestingly, it has lower oral bioavailability than the parent compound, tetracycline.

Lymecycline → in vitro hydrolysis → Tetracycline

6.6   Formation of metal chelates

✓ Stable chelate complexes are formed by the tetracyclines with many metals as calcium, magnesium and iron.
✓ These chelates are usually insoluble in water.
✓ The tetracyclines are distributed into the milk of lactating mothers and will cross the placental barrier inti fetus.

Metal

metal binding site

Zwitterionic tetracycline predominates
at physiological pH

Chelation of divalent metal ions via
C11 and C12 oxygen atoms
Overall [Tet-Mg]$^+$ predominates

6.7 Permissible changes in the structure

6.8 Structure activity relationship

☐ Tetracyclines are composed of a rigid skeleton of 4 fused rings. The rings structure of tetracyclines is divided into an upper modifiable region and a lower non modifiable region.

☐ An active tetracycline requires a C10 phenol as well as a C11-C12 keto-enol substructure in conjugation with a 12a-OH group and a C1-C3 diketo sub-structure.

☐ Removal of the dimethylamine group at C4 reduces antibacterial activity. Replacement of the carboxyl-amine group at C2 results in reduced antibacterial activity but it is possible to add substituents to the amide nitrogen to get more soluble analogs like the prodrug, Lymecycline.

☐ The simplest tetracycline with measurable antibacterial activity is 6-deoxy-6-demethyltetracycline and its structure is often considered to be the minimum pharmacophore for the tetracycline class of antibiotics. C5-C9 can be modified to make derivatives with varying antibacterial activity.

☐ The presence of 2-amino and 4-dimethylaminos are essential for its physiological activity.

☐ Demthyl tetracyclines are more stable to acids and alkalies.

☐ The 4-epi, 5-epi derivatives of tetracyclines are inactive biologically.

☐ Introduction of bromine at 7 position, makes the compounds six times more active biologically but more toxic as well.

☐ Methacycline is obtained from oxytetrcycline and is more active physiologically than parent compound.

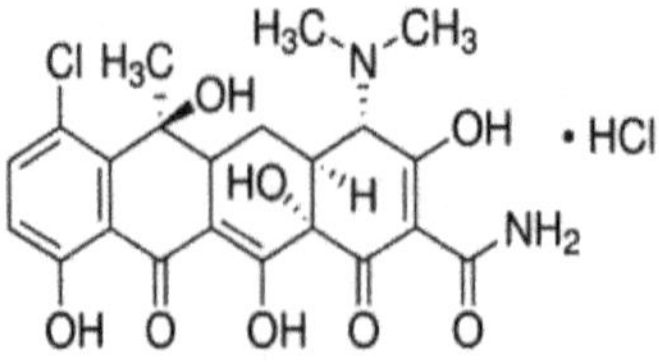

Chlortetracycline

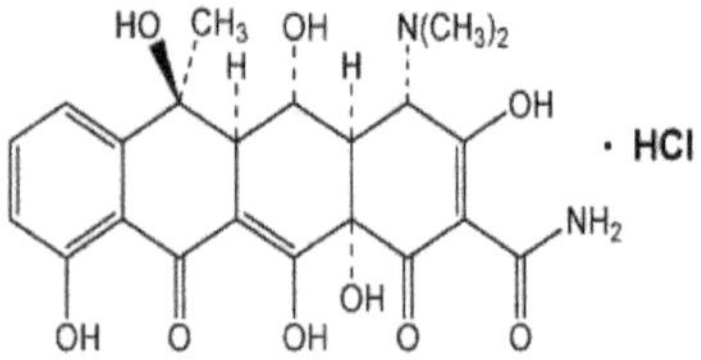

Oxytetracycline

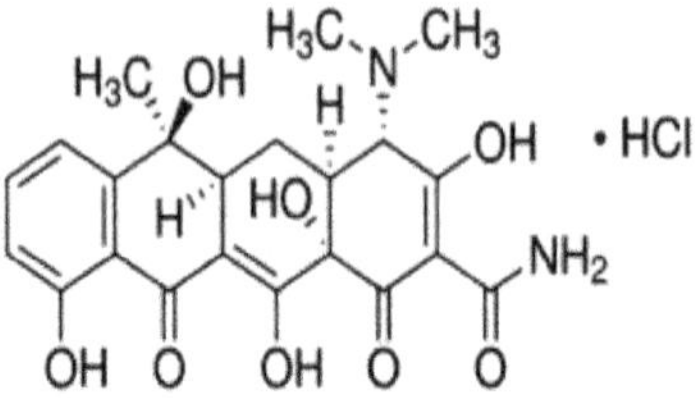

Tetracycline

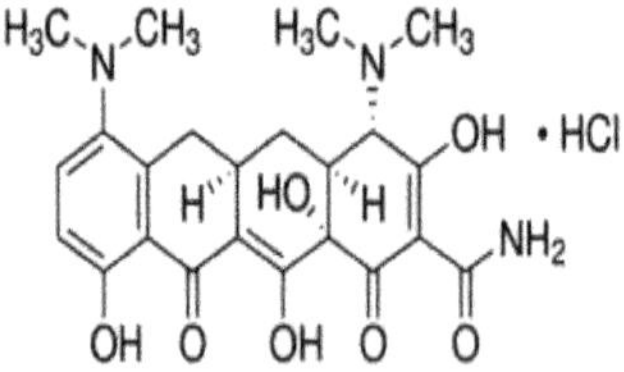

Minocycline

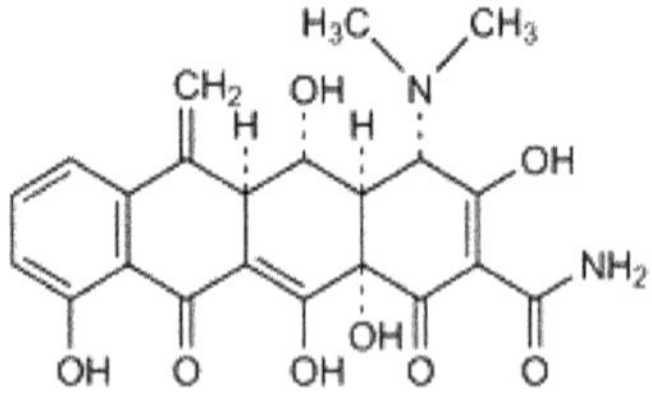

Metacycline
(methacycline)

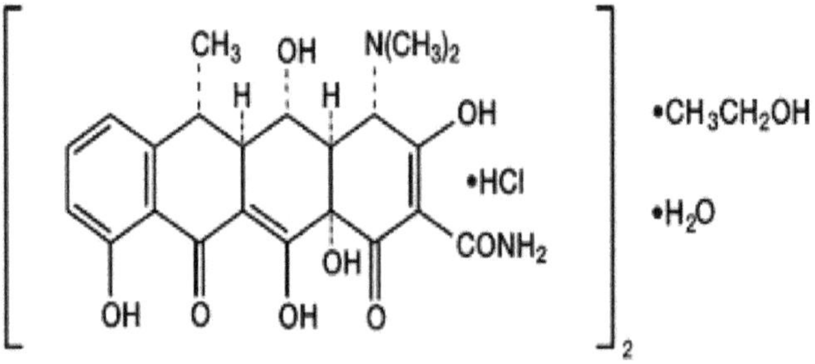

Doxycycline hyclate

Demeclocycline
(declomycin)

Eravacycline

6.9 Pharmacological uses

Tetracyclines are generally used in the treatment of infections of the urinary tract, respiratory tract, and the intestines. Doxycycline is also used as a for malaria treatment and prophylaxis, as well as treating elephantitis. Very rarely, severe headache and vision problems may be signs. Likelihood of causing teeth discoloration in the fetus as they develop in infancy. For this same reason, tetracyclines are contraindicated for use under 8 years of age. All the clinically used medicinal compounds belonging to the tetracycline family acts as bacteriostatic.

Contraindications

Tetracycline use should be avoided in pregnant or lactating women, and in children with developing teeth because they may result in permanent staining (dark yellow-gray teeth with a darker horizontal band that goes across the top and bottom rows of teeth), and possibly affect the growth of teeth and bones. In tetracycline preparation, stability must be considered in order to avoid formation of toxic epi-anhydrotetracyclines.

General information about the use of the tetracycline antibiotics group is problematic:

Discolor permanent teeth (yellow-gray-brown), from prenatal period through childhood and adulthood.

Be inactivated by Ca2+ so are not to be taken with milk, curd and other dairy products.

Absorption of tetracyclines has been reported to be impaired by milk products, aluminum hydroxide gels, sodium bicarbonate, calcium and magnesium salts, laxatives containing magnesium and iron preparations.

Interfere with methotrexate (antineoplastic drug) by displacing it from the various protein-binding sites. Caution should be exercised in long-term use when breastfeeding.

Adverse reactions of Tetracycline in general

- Kidney toxicity
  renal tubular acidosis (Fanchoni syndrome)
- Local tissue toxicity
  (venous thrombosis)
- Photosensitization
  (to sunlight or ultra- violet light)

- Vestibular reactions
(dizziness, vertigo, nausea and vomiting)

6.10 Mechanism of action of Tetracyclines in general

Tetracycline antibiotics inhibit the initiation of translation in variety of ways by binding which is made up of 16S rRNA and 21 proteins.

Pharmacokinetics of Tetracyclines in general

Usually administered orally. Absorption adequate but incomplete (except Doxycycline, Minocycline which is 90-100%). Absorbed in upper small intestine and best in absence of food.

Food, di / trivalent cations (Ca, Mg, Fe, Al) impair absorption. Protein binding is 40-80%. Distributed well (except cerebrospinal fluid. Cross placenta and excreted in milk.

Excretion= bile 10-40% (enterohepatic) and kidneys 10-50%. (exception of Doxycycline which is largely metabolized in the liver.

6.11 Properties of individual important compounds of tetracycline group of antibiotics

CHLORTETRACYCLINE

$$C_{22}H_{23}ClN_2O_8$$
Molar mass
478.88g/mol

Chemistry

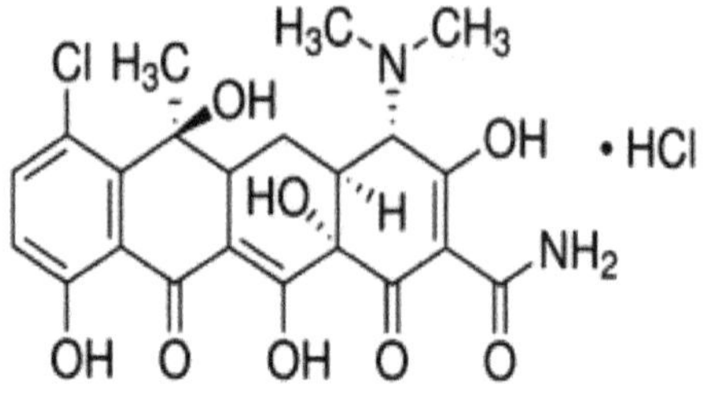

Chemistry of Chlortetracycline (scheme 1)

Chlortetracycline (CTC) is the oldest antibiotic of the tetracycline Group. It was First isolated from Streptomyces aureofaciens by Duggar in 1948. CTC like other tetraclines, undergoes epimerization at position C-4 forming 4-epichlortetracycline (ECTC). Due to the hydroxyl group at C-6, CTC is liable to acid degradation forming anhydro-chlortetracycline (ACTC). ACTC further epimerizes at position C-4 resulting in the formation of 4-epianhydrochlortetracycline (EACTC). CTC is not stable in alkaline medium. This results in the formation of isochlor-tetracycline (ISOCTC) which further epimerizes to 4-epiisochlortetracycline (BISOCTC) as shown in figure below. Tetracycline (TC) and 6-demethylchlortetracycline (DMCTC) may also be present as impurities in CTC samples. Therefore, a good method for the purity control purpose is supposed to separate TC, DMCTC, ISOCTC, EACTC, ACTC, ECTC and CTC. The separation of the 4-epimers ETC, EISOCTC, EDMCTC and of 6-demethyltetraxycline (DMTC) is of minor importance since they can be considered as impurities of impurities.

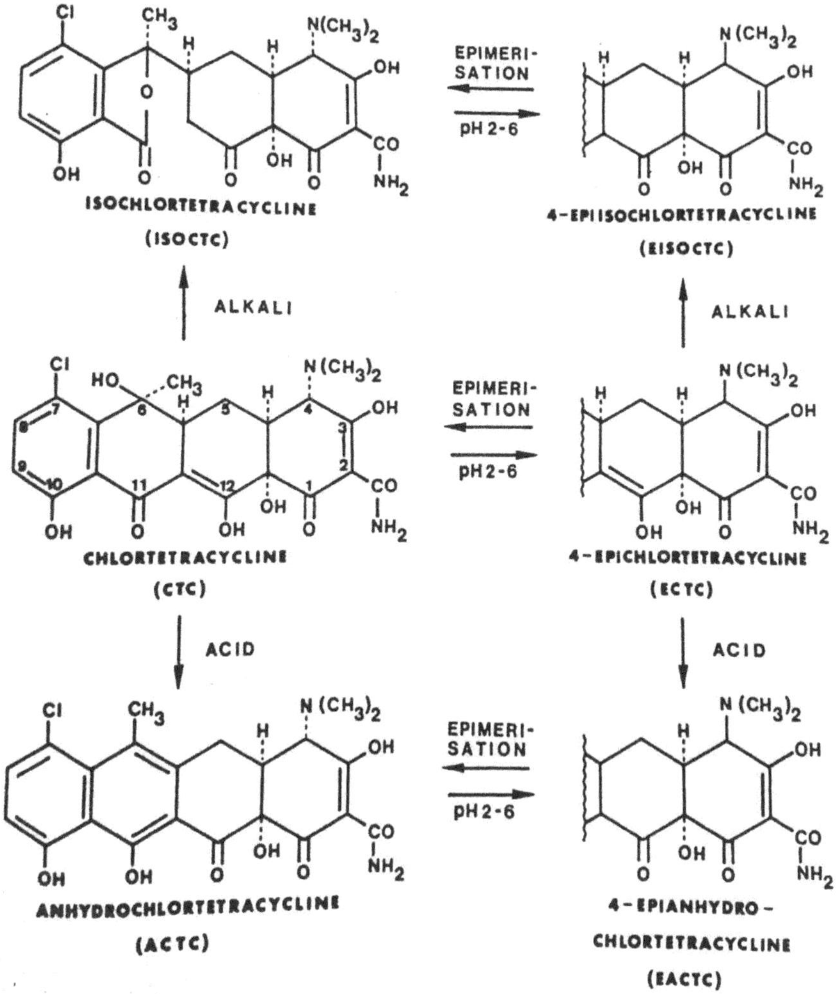

The above structures have been copied from the Ph. D.
thesis of the main author, drawn by stencils in 1988)

Chemistry of Chlortetracycline (scheme 2)

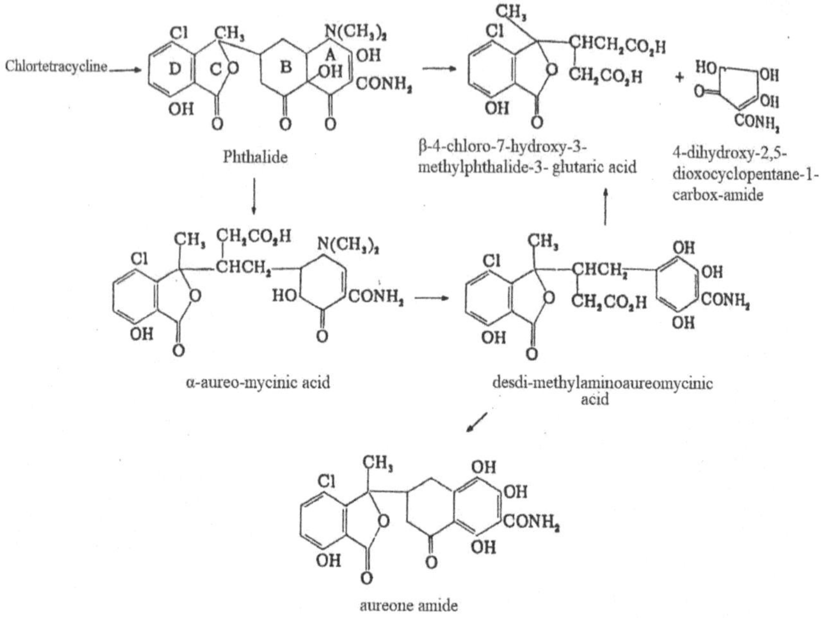

Phthalide

β-4-chloro-7-hydroxy-3-methylphthalide-3- glutaric acid

4-dihydroxy-2,5-dioxocyclopentane-1-carbox-amide

α-aureo-mycinic acid

desdi-methylaminoaureomycinic acid

aureone amide

(The above structures have been copied from the Ph. D. thesis of the main author, drawn by stencils in 1988)

Structure activity relationship (SAR) of CTC

- Chlortetracycline is the first tetracycline to be identified having four rings with broad spectrum biological activity.
- The molecule is 'amphoteric' (having acidic and basic functions at one time).
- The molecule is not stable in basic medium.
- Position 4 is occupied by dimethyl amino group and is basic in character.
- Biological activity is mainly due to position 4.
- Position 2 is the carbox-amido group.
- Change of cabox-amido group at position 2, may reduce the activity and increase the toxicity.

306

- Position 6 is occupied by hydroxyl group in the back of the ring and methyl group in front of the ring.
- Position 7 is a halogen 'Cl'. If this Cl is replaced by any other halogen, biological activity is reduced.
- Adding some other methyl group/s at position 7 increases bacterial spectrum with prolonged activity.
- Positions 1-3 and 10-12 are acidic in character.
- Degradation of the molecule (about 50% degradation of the molecule) takes place due to the presence of hydroxyl groups at position 6.
- Position 4 is responsible for epimerization.
- Replacing one or both the methyl groups at position 4, biological activity is lost completely.
- Change at position 7, the biological activity does not change but changes the spectrum of activity.

Metabolism

Bioavailability: 30% (oral). Metabolism: 75% in liver. Protein binding: 50-55%. Biological half- life: 5.6 -9 hours. Excretion: Renal and biliary. ROA: Oral, I.V., topical

Pharmacological uses

Chlortetracycline may increase the neuromuscular blocking activities of atracurium besilate.

Chlortetracycline becomes dangerous past its expiration date.

OXYTETRACYCLINE

$$C_{22}H_{24}N_2O_9$$
Molar mass
460.43g/mol

Chemistry

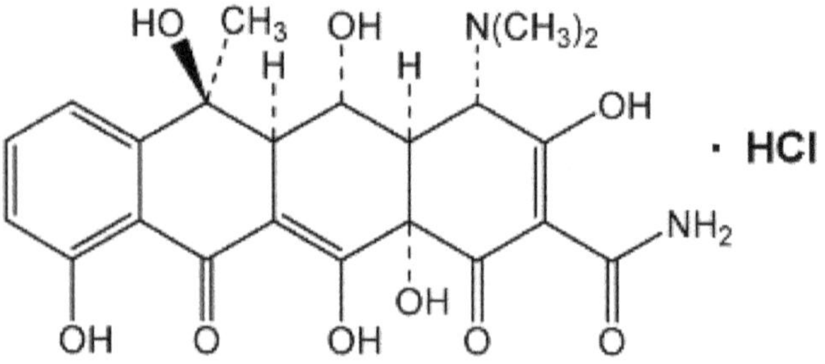

(The above structure has been copied from the Ph. D. thesis of the main author, drawn by stencils in 1988)

Chemistry of Oxytetracycline

Oxytetracycline (OTC) was first isolated from Streptomyces rimosus. Later on, many other microorganisms were found to produce OTC Streptomyces alboflavus, Streptomyces aureofacien, Streptomyces armillatus. OTC is extensively used in therapy as well as in agriculture. OTC as other tetracyclines undergoes epimerization at position C-4 resulting in the formation of 4-epioxytetracycline (EOTC). This epimerization is in equilibrium but due to the presence of hydroxyl group at position C-5, the epimerization rate is low as in the case of doxycycline (DOX). The presence of a hydroxyl group at C-6 enables acid degradation, resulting in the formation of anhydro-oxytetracycline (AOTC). This anhydro-derivative rearranges in acid hydroxylic media to two following isomers:

- α-apooxytetracycline (α-APOTC)
- β-apooxytetracycline (β-APOTC).

The alkaline treatment of AOTC also leads to the formation of α -APOTC and β-APOTC. In 1960, Hochstein et al described another related compound, 2-acetyl-2-decarboxamidooxytetracycline ADOTC. It is a fermentation impurity which is practically inactive therapeutically. Tetracycline (TC) is also described as a fermentation impurity of OTC. Therefore, a good analytical method for the purity control is supposed to separate EOTC, OTC, ADOTC, TC, AOTC, α and β-APOTC as described in the Figure below:

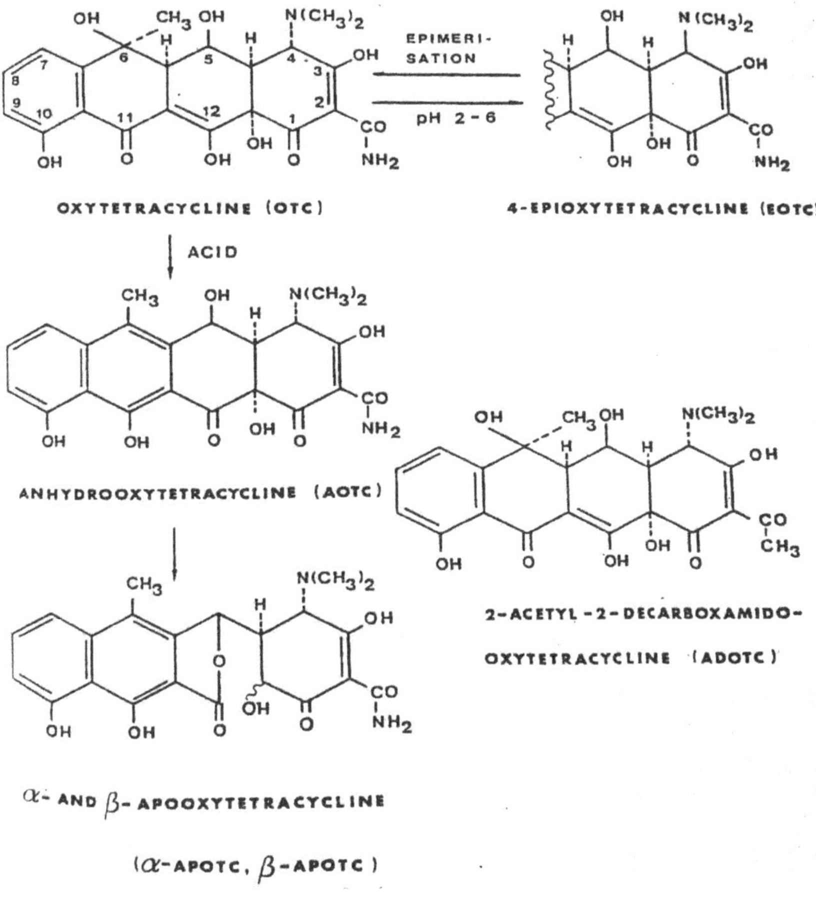
EPIMERI-
SATION
pH 2-6
OXYTETRACYCLINE (OTC)
4-EPIOXYTETRACYCLINE (EOTC)
ACID
ANHYDROOXYTETRACYCLINE (AOTC)
2-ACETYL-2-DECARBOXAMIDO-
OXYTETRACYCLINE (ADOTC)
α- AND β- APOOXYTETRACYCLINE
(α-APOTC, β-APOTC)

(The above structures have been copied from the Ph. D. thesis of the main author, drawn by stencils in 1988)

Structure activity relationship (SAR) of OTC

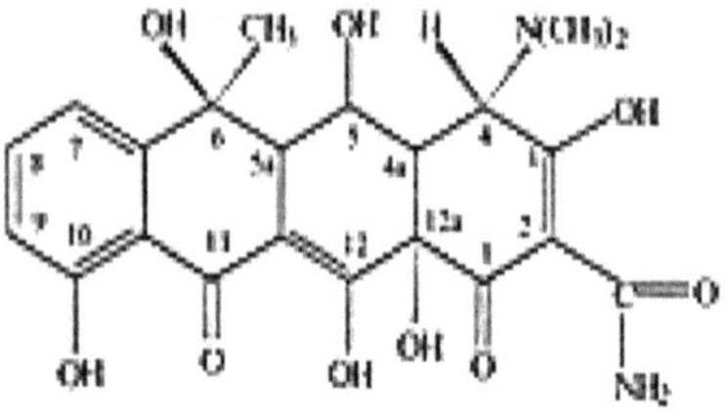

OTC

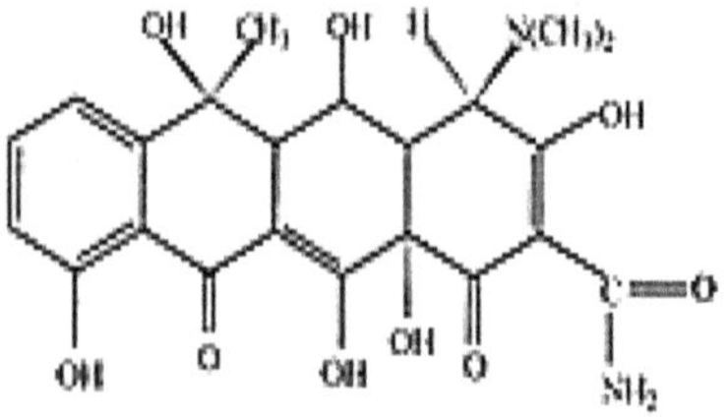

EOTC

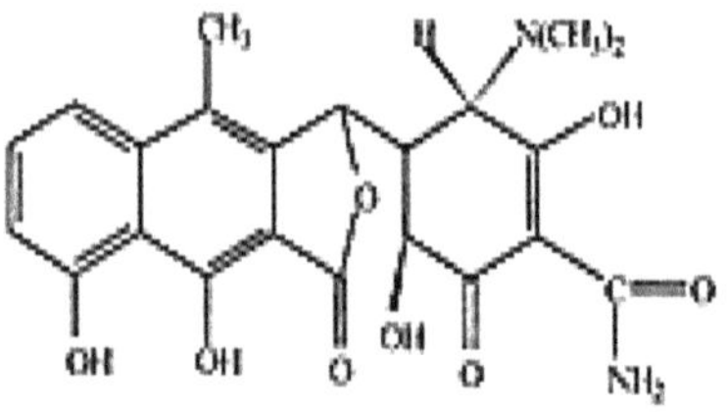

α-Apo-OTC

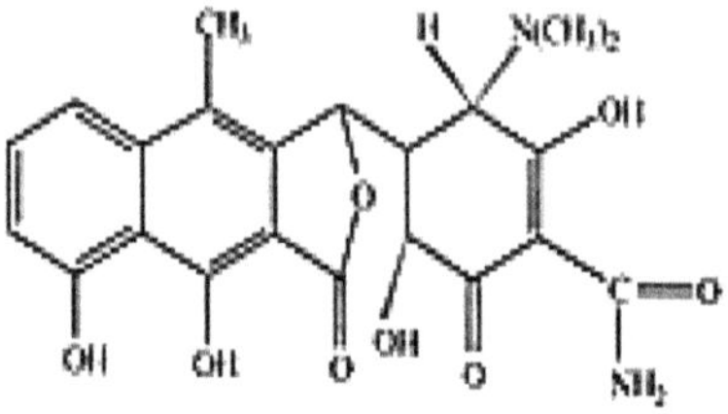

β-Apo-OTC

(The above structures have been copied from the Ph. D. thesis of the main author, drawn by stencils in 1988)

- Oxytetracycline is the second to be discovered having four rings.
- The molecule is not stable in acidic medium.
- The molecule is 'amphoteric' (having acidic and basic functions at one time).
- Position 4 is occupied by dimethyl amino group and is basic in character.
- Position 2 is the carbox-amido group.
- Change of cabox-amido group at position 2, may reduce the activity and increases the toxicity.
- Biological activity of the molecule is mainly due to position 4.
- Position 6 is occupied by hydroxyl group in the back of the ring and methyl group in front of the ring. This hydroxyl group at position 6 is responsible for about 50% degradation of the molecule.

- Positions 1-3 and 10-12 are acidic in character.
- Position 5 is occupied by hydroxyl group and it is believed that there is a strong chemical bonding between position 4 and 5. Due to this believed bonding, the rate of epimerization of the molecule is drastically less.
- Position 4 is responsible for epimerization.

i. Replacing one or both the methyl groups at position 4, biological activity is lost completely.
ii. Change at position 7, the biological activity does not change but change in spectrum takes place with wide range of activity.

Pharmacological uses
Oxytetracycline possesses some level of bacteriostatic activity against almost all medically relevant aerobic and anaerobic bacterial genera, both gram +ive and gram -ive bacteria, used to treat infections caused by the chest infection, pneumonia, and the genital infections. It is also used to treat acne, chronic bronchitis.

Metabolism:
Oxytetracycline works by blocking the ability to make proteins, biological half- life 6-8 hours and excreted through renal system. Given orally, topical.

Adverse effects:
As above

Synthesis of Oxytetracycline 1

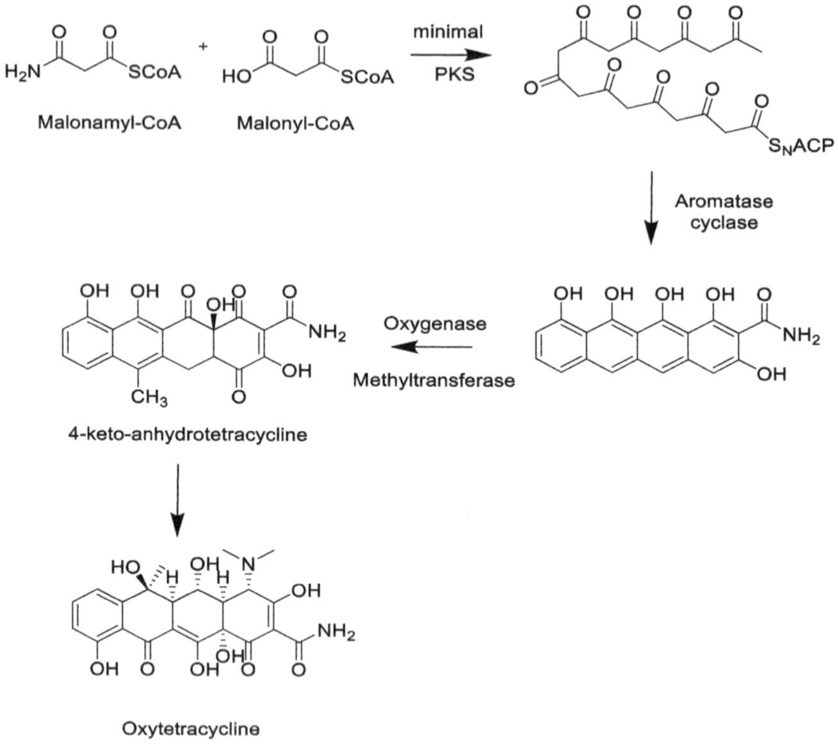

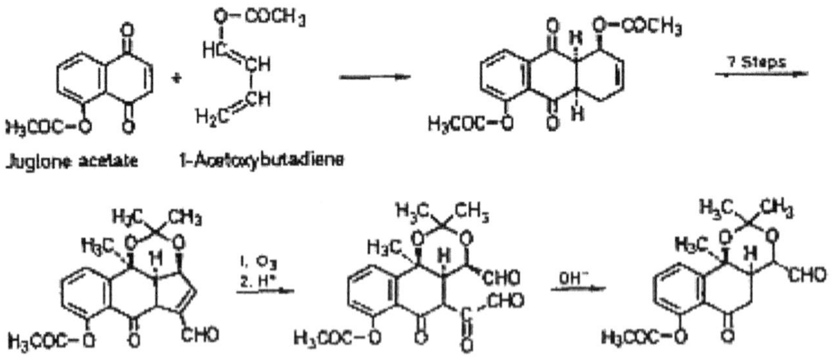

Malonamyl-CoA   Malonyl-CoA

minimal
PKS

Aromatase
cyclase

4-keto-anhydrotetracycline

Oxygenase

Methyltransferase

Oxytetracycline

Juglone acetate   1-Acetoxybutadiene

7 Steps

1, O$_3$
2. H$^+$

OH$^-$

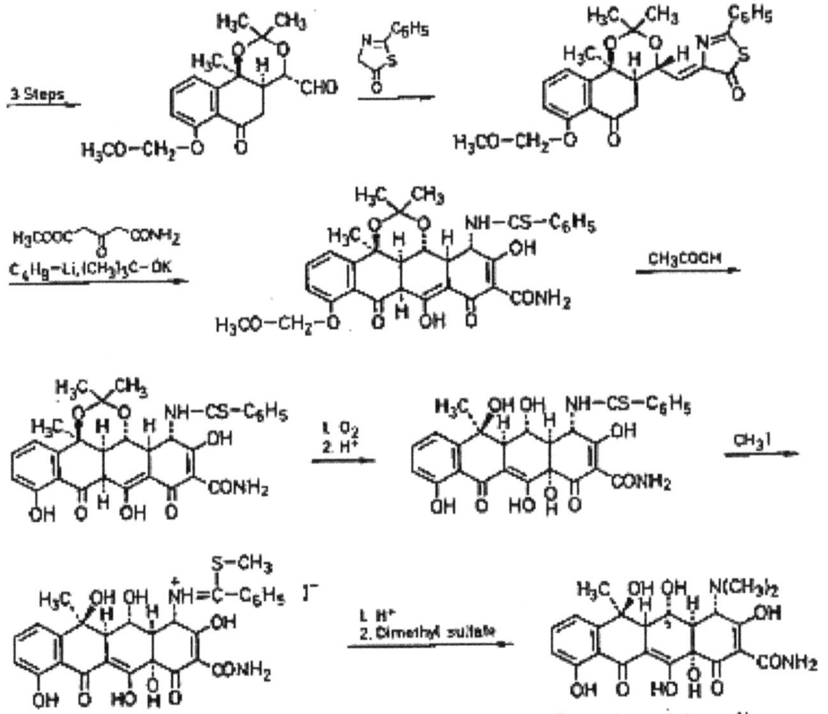

Racemic oxytetracycline

(The above structures have been copied from the Ph. D. thesis of the main author, drawn by stencils in 1988)

TETRACYCLINE

$C_{22}H_{24}N_2O_8$
Molar mass
444.44g/mol

Chemistry

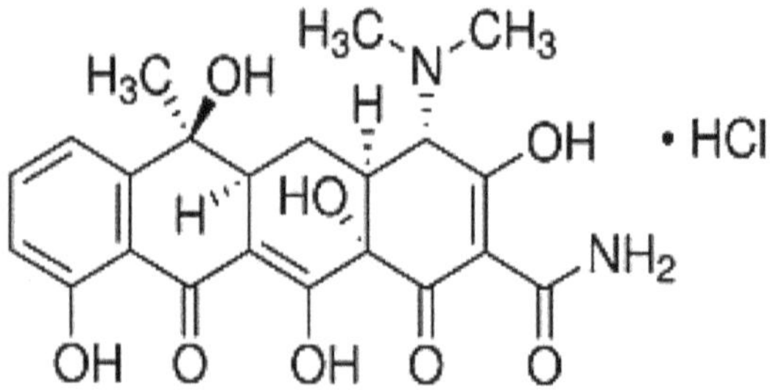

(The above structure has been copied from the Ph. D. thesis of the main author, drawn with stencils in 1988)

Chemistry of Tetracycline

Tetracycline (TC) was first prepared by the catalytic reduction of Chlortetracycline. TC has also been reported to be produced by many strains of Streptomyces aureofaciens, Streptomyces avellanus, streptomyces feofaciens, Streptomyces alboflavus and many others. Among the tetracycline group of antibiotics, TC is most widely used in therapeutics.TC undergoes epimerization at position C-4 resulting in the formation of 4-epitetracycline (ETC). Due to the presence of a hydroxyl group at C-6, acid degradation takes place resulting in the formation of anhydro-tetracycline (ATC) which also undergoes epimerization at -4, resulting in the formation of 4-epianhydrotetracycline (EATC).

This degradation product can also be formed by acid degradation of ETC. Another related compound, 2-acetyl-2-decarboxamidote tetracycline (ADTC) was described by Miller et al. for the purity control of TC is supposed to separate TC, ETC, EATC, ATC and ADTC as shown in the figure below:

314

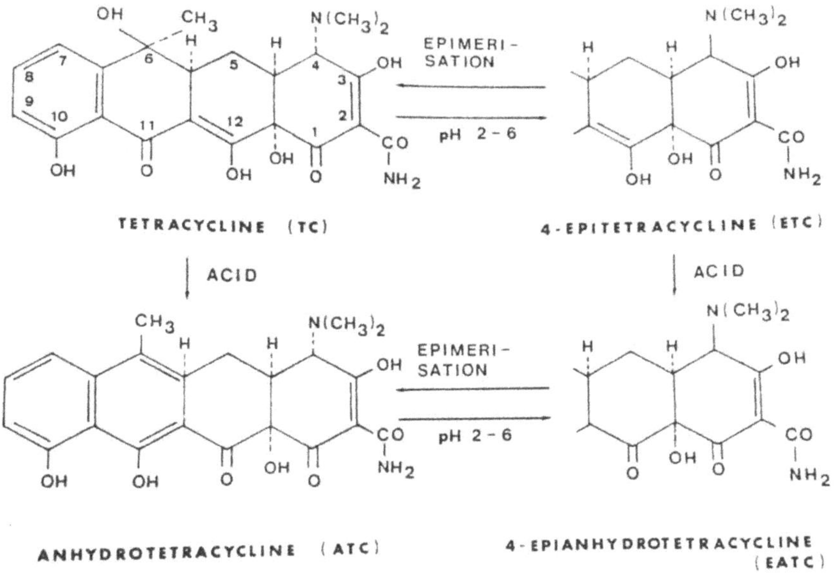

TETRACYCLINE (TC)

4-EPITETRACYCLINE (ETC)

ANHYDROTETRACYCLINE (ATC)

4-EPIANHYDROTETRACYCLINE (EATC)

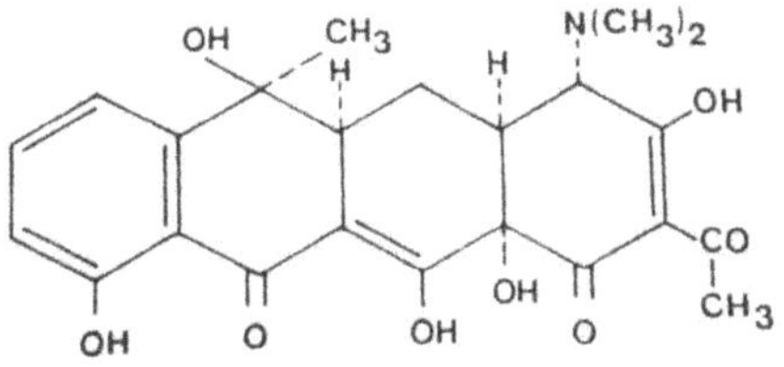

2-ACETYL-2-DECARBOXAMIDOTETRACYCLINE (ADTC)

(The above structures have been copied from the Ph. D. thesis of the main author, drawn with stencils in 1988)

Structure activity relationship (SAR) of TC

- Tetracycline is a group of antibiotics having four rings.
- The molecule is not stable in acidic medium.
- The molecule is 'amphoteric' (having acidic and basic functions at one time).
- Position 4 is occupied by dimethyl amino group and is basic in character.
- Position 2 is the carbox-amido group.

- Change of carbox-amido group at position 2, may reduce the activity and increases the toxicity.
- Biological activity of the molecule is completely due to position 4.
- Position 6 is occupied by hydroxyl group in the back of the ring and methyl group in front of the ring. This hydroxyl group at position 6 is responsible for about 50% degradation of the molecule.
- Positions 1-3 and 10-12 are acidic in character.
- Position 4 is responsible for epimerization.
- Replacing one or both the methyl groups at position 4, biological activity is completely lost.
- Change at position 7, the biological activity does not change but change in spectrum takes place with wide range of activity.

Pharmacological uses
- Tetracycline inhibits protein synthesis by blocking the attachment.
- Tetracycline binds to the 30S subunit of microbial ribosomes. Thus, it prevents introduction of new amino acids to the nascent peptide chain. The action is usually inhibitory and reversible upon withdrawal of the drug.
- Cells are less vulnerable to the effect of tetracyclines, despite the fact that tetracycline binds to the small ribosomal subunit of both prokaryotes and eukaryotes (30S and 40S, respectively) cells.
- Tetracycline is one of the compounds works by blocking the synthesis of protein by the bacteria.
- Originally, Tetracycline possesses some level of bacteriostatic activity against almost all medically relevant aerobic and anaerobic bacterial general.

Metabolism
Bioavailability: 75% (oral)
Metabolism: not metabolized

Biological half- life: 8–11 hours, 57–108 hours (kidney impairment)
Excretion: 60% renal, feces
ROA: Oral

Synthesis of Tetracycline

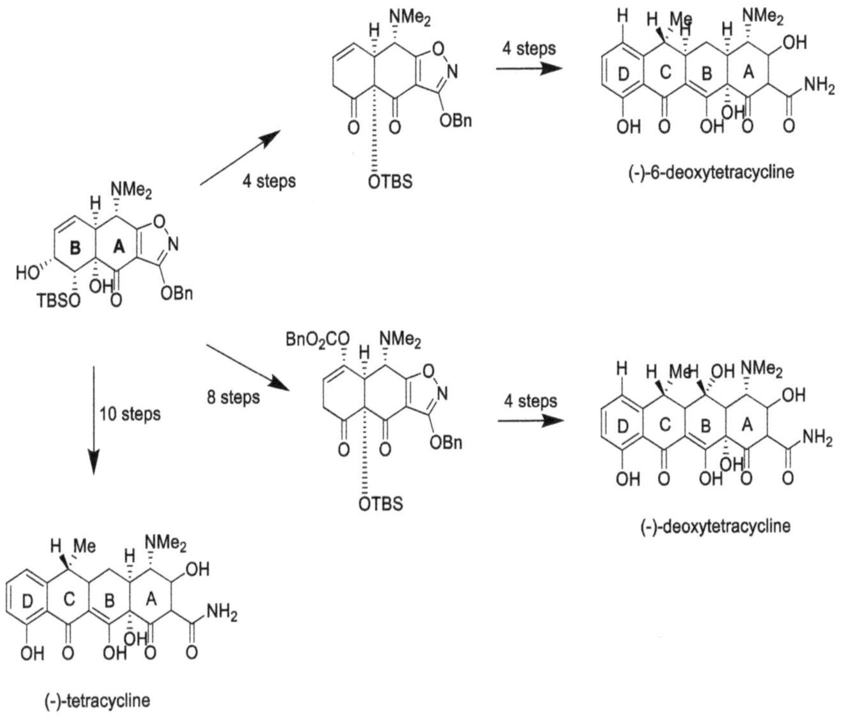

(-)-6-deoxytetracycline

(-)-deoxytetracycline

(-)-tetracycline

Adverse effects

As above

DOXYCYCLINE HYCLATE

$$C_{22}H_{24}N_2O_8$$
Molar mass
444.43 g/mol

Chemistry

317

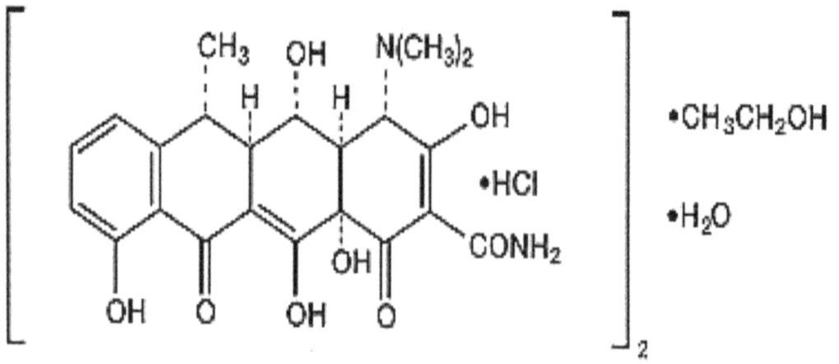

(The above structure has been copied from the Ph. D. thesis of the main author, drawn with stencils in 1988)

Chemistry of Doxycycline

Doxycycline (DOX) was first prepared from oxytetracycline (OTC). Different pathways of DOX synthesis were described by Blackwood et al. as shown in the figure below. Metacycline MTC) is an intermediate product and 6-epidoxycycline (6-EDOX) is much less active byproduct. Therefore MTC, 6-EDOX and to a smaller extent OTC can be present as impurities. DOX not easily epimerises and does not show acid degradation as already explained above. This means that unlike OTC, tetracycline (TC) and chlortetracycline (CTC), DOX must not be analysed for anhydro-derivatives. 6-EDOX can also epimerize to 4, 6-epidoxycycline (4,6-EDOX). Therefore, a good analytical method for the purity control is supposed to separate OTC, 4,6-BDOX, 4-EDOX, MTC, 6-EDOX and DOX.

Structure activity relationship (SAR)

❖ Doxycycline is the antibiotic having four rings.
❖ It is the safest and long- acting compound (one dose for 24 hours).
❖ This molecule is more stable than other tetracyclines.
❖ The molecule is not stable in acidic medium.
❖ The molecule is 'amphoteric' (having acidic and basic functions at one time).
❖ Position 4 is occupied by dimethyl amino group and is basic in character.

318

❖ Position 2 is the carbox-amido group.

❖ Change of cabox-amido group at position 2, may reduce the activity and increases the toxicity.

❖ Biological activity of the molecule is mainly due to position 4.

❖ The methyl group is in front of the ring at position 6 and **No hydroxyl group** exists at position 6 (as in case of chlortetracycline, tetracycline and oxytetracycline). Due to this reason **no degradation of the molecule takes place.**

❖ Positions 1-3 and 10-12 are acidic in character.

❖ Position 5 is occupied by hydroxyl group and it is believed that there is a strong chemical bonding between position 4 and 5. Due to this believed bonding, the rate of degradation of the molecule is about **5% only** as in case of oxytetracycline.

❖ Position 4 is responsible for epimerization.

❖ By replacing one or both the methyl groups at position 4, biological activity is lost completely.

❖ Change at position 7, the biological activity does not change but change in spectrum takes place with wide range of activity.

Pharmacological uses

• Doxycycline is the safest and long -acting compound among tetracycline group of antibiotics.

• It is used in the treatment of number of types of infections.

• In addition to the general indications for all members of the group.

• Doxycycline is frequently used to treat chronic infections.

• In some countries, doxycycline is considered a first-line treatment.

• It is also useful for the treatment of malaria when used with quinine for the prevention of malaria.

• Doxycycline has been shown to improve lung functions in patients with stable symptoms.

• Both doxycycline and minocycline have shown effectiveness in asthma due to immune suppressing effects.

Metabolism

Bioavailability: 100%

Metabolism: In liver

Protein binding: 90%

Biological half- life: 15-25 hours

Excretion: Renal 40%

ROA: Oral, I.V.

Adverse effects

Common side effects include, nausea, vomiting, a red rash.

If used during pregnancy or in young children may result in permanent problems with the teeth changing their color.

Doxycycline becomes dangerous past its expiration date.

Contraindication

As above

Synthesis of Doxycycline

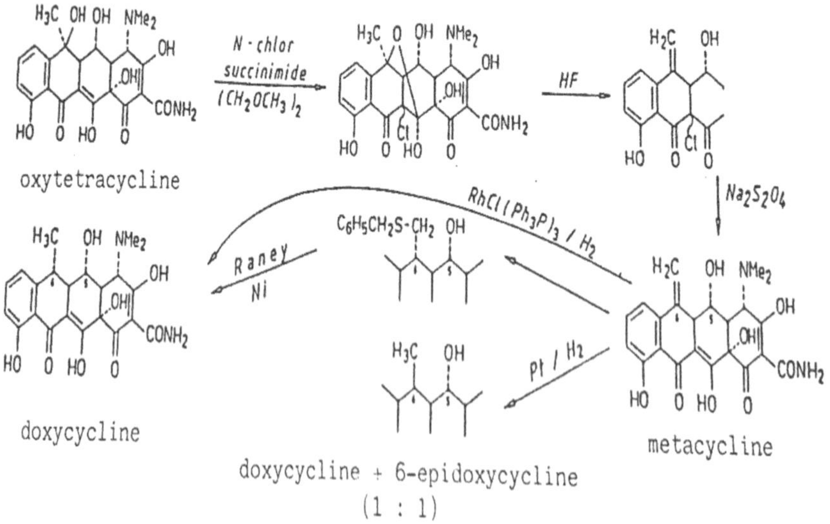

oxytetracycline

doxycycline

doxycycline + 6-epidoxycycline
(1 : 1)

metacycline

**(The above structures have been copied from the Ph. D.
thesis of the main author, drawn with stencils in 1988)**

MINOCYCLINE

$$C_{23}H_{27}N_3O_7$$
Molar mass
457.483

Chemistry

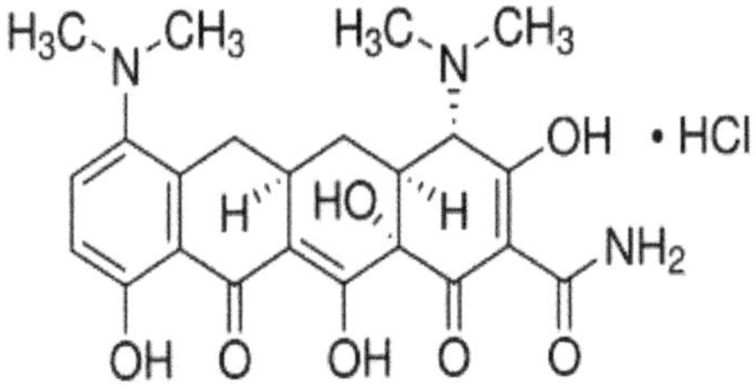

**(The above structure has been copied from the Ph. D.
thesis of the main author, drawn with stencils in 1988)**

Structure activity relationship (SAR) od DOX:

☐ Minocycline is a broader spectrum than the other members of the group.
☐ It is not a naturally occurring antibiotic but was synthesized semi-synthetically from natural tetracycline antibiotic.
☐ It is an antibiotic to inhibit the growth of bacteria, classified as a long-acting type.
☐ It is the safest and long- acting compound (one dose for 24 hours).
☐ This molecule is more stable than other tetracyclines. The molecule is not stable in acidic medium.
☐ The molecule is 'amphoteric' (having acidic and basic functions at one time).

- Position 4 is occupied by dimethyl amino group and is basic in character.
- Position 2 is the carbox-amido group.
- Change of cabox-amido group at position 2, may reduce the activity and increases the toxicity.
- Biological activity of the molecule is mainly due to position 4.
- The methyl group is in front of the ring at position 6 and No hydroxyl group exists at position 6 (as in case of chlortetracycline, tetracycline and oxytetracycline). Due to this reason no degradation of the molecule takes place.
- Position 1-3 and 10-12 are acidic in character.
- Position 5 is occupied by hydroxyl group and it is believed that there is a strong chemical bonding between position 4 and 5. Due to this believed bonding, the rate of degradation of the molecule is about **5% only** as in case of oxytetracycline.
- Position 4 is responsible for epimerization.
- By replacing one or both the methyl groups at position 4, biological activity is lost completely.
- Change at position 7, the biological activity does not change but change in spectrum takes place with wide range of activity.

Metabolism

Minocycline is a relatively poor tetracycline-class antibiotic choice for urinary pathogens sensitive to this antibiotic class, as its solubility in water and levels in the urine are less than all other tetracyclines.

Minocycline is metabolized by the liver and has poor urinary excretion.

Bioavailability: 100%
Metabolism: In liver
Protein binding: 90%
Biological half- life :11-22 hours
Excretion: Mostly through feces and rest through renal
ROA: Oral, I.V., topical

Pharmacological uses

Minocycline is the most lipid-soluble of the tetracycline-class antibiotics, giving it the greatest penetration into the prostate and brain, but also in the greatest amount of CNS.

Recent research has found a tentative benefit from minocycline in schizophrenia.

Adverse effects: As above

Synthesis of Minocycline

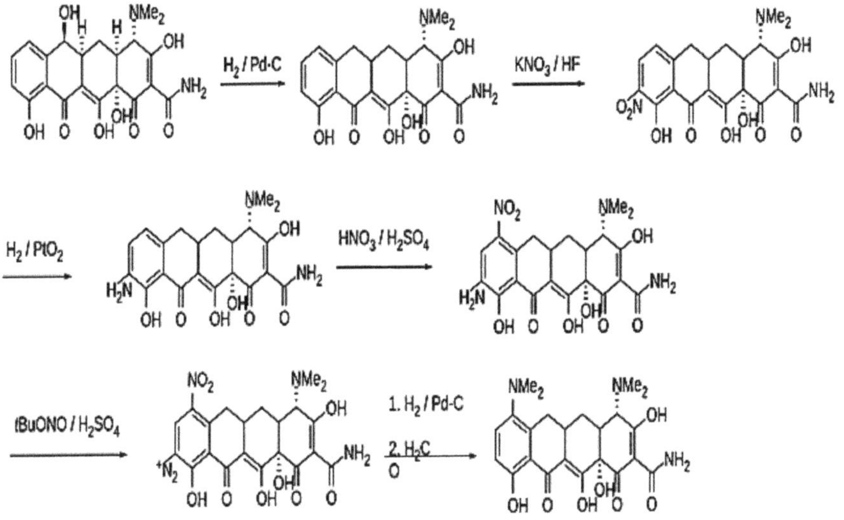

(**The above structures have been copied from the Ph. D. thesis of the main author, drawn with stencils in 1988)**

METACYCLINE / METHACYCLINE

$$C_{22}H_{22}N_2O_8$$
Molar mass
442.42 g/mol

Chemistry

It is used in the industrial synthesis of doxycycline hyclate.

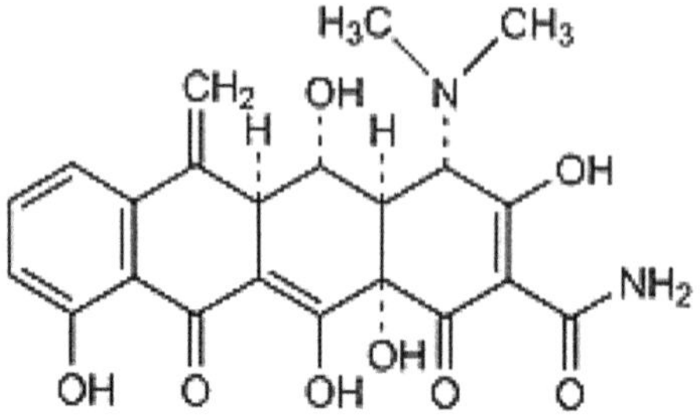

(The above structure has been copied from the Ph. D. thesis of the main author, drawn with stencils in 1988)

Structure activity relationship (SAR) of MTC
As mentioned above

Synthesis of Metacycline

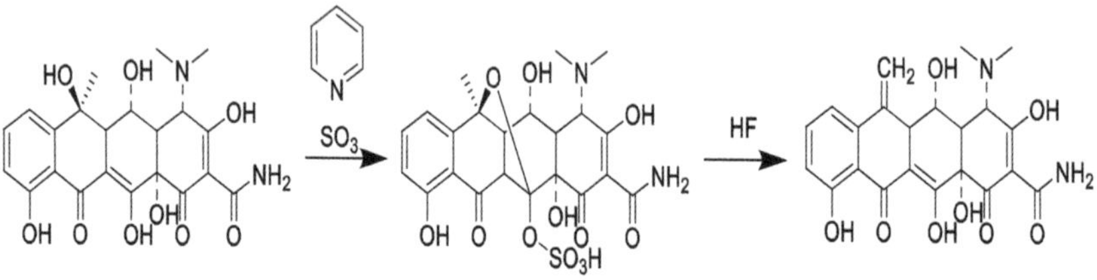

DEMECLOCYCLINE
(DECLOMYCIN)

$$C_{21}H_{21}ClN_2O_8$$
Molar mass
464.85 g/mol

Chemistry

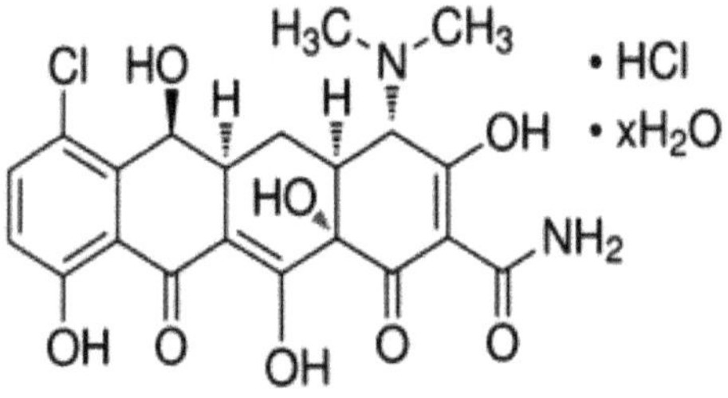

(The above structure has been copied from the Ph. D. thesis of the main author, drawn with stencils in 1988)

CHAPTER 7

POLYPEPTIDE ANTIBIOTICS

7.1 Polypeptide antibiotics in general

Active against Gram-positive bacteria
Tyrocidins A-D (Tyrocidin) (cyclic decapeptides) Gramicidins A-C (Gramicidin) Bacitracins A, A1, B, B1, B2, C, D, E, F, G, and X. (Bacitracin)
Active against Gram-negative bacteria
Polymyxins B, B1, B2, E, M (Polymyxin) (cyclic non-ribosomal polypeptide)
Active against Gram-positive bacteria
Capreomycin (antiphlogistic antibiotic), Viomycin (tuberactinomycin family), Amphomycin, Mikamycins (macrolide antibiotics), (ostreogrycins, streptogramins, vernamycins, pristilinamycins, virginiamycins, staphylomycins.)
Active against staphylococcal bacteria
Vancomycin, Ristocetins

7.2 Active Against Gram-Positive Bacteria

TYROCIDIN

$C_{66}H_{87}N_{13}O_{13}$
Molar mass
1270.47628

Chemistry

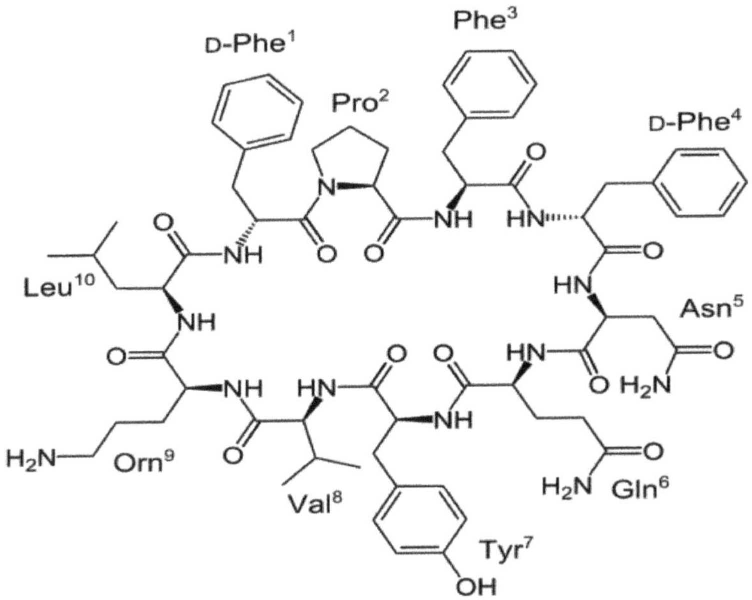

(The above structure has been copied from the Ph. D. thesis of the main author, drawn with stencils in 1988)

A	Tyrocidine A DPhe-Pro-Phe-Dphe-Asn-Gln-Tyr-Val-Orn-Leu		
B	Amino acid position		
Tyrocidine	3	4	7
A	L-Phe	D-Phe	L-Tyr
B	L-Trp	D-Phe	L-Tyr
C	L-Trp	D-Trp	L-Tyr
D	L-Trp	D-Trp	L-Trp

Pharmacology

Tyrocidine appears to perturb the lipid bilayer of a microbe's inner membrane by permeating the lipid phase of the membrane. The exact affinity and location of tyrocidine within the phospholipid bilayer is not yet known.

Tyrocidine A, 46

**(The above structure has been copied from the Ph. D.
thesis of the main author, drawn with stencils in 1988)**

GRAMICIDIN

$$C_{99}H_{140}N_{20}O_{17}$$
Molar mass
1882.332 g·mol^{-1}

Chemistry of Gramicidin C

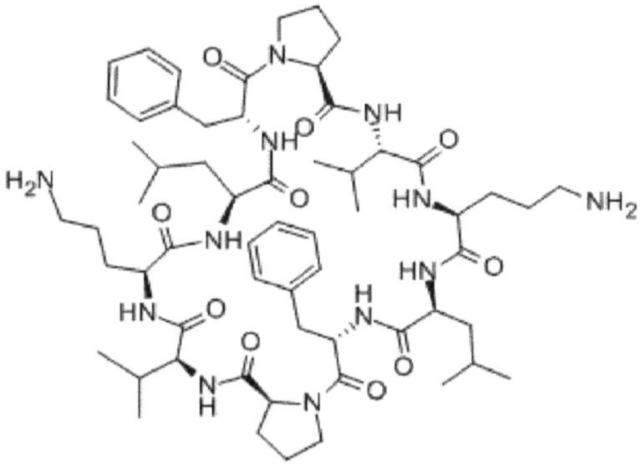

**(The above structure has been copied from the Ph. D.
thesis of the main author, drawn with stencils in 1988)**

Structure activity relationship (SAR)

- Gramicidin A, B and C are non-ribosomal peptides thus they have no genes.
- They consist of 15 L- and D-amino acids. Their amino acid sequence is:
- L-X-Gly-L-Ala-D-Leu-L-Ala-D-Val-L-Val-D-Val-L-Trp-D-Leu-L-Y-D-Leu-L-Trp-D-Leu-L-Trp.
- In natural gramicidin mixes of A, B and C, about 5% of the total gramicidin are isoleucine isoforms.

- Gramicidin form helices. The alternating pattern of D- and L-amino acids is important for the formation of these structures. Helices occur most often as head-to-head.
- Gramicidin can also form antiparallel or parallel double helices, especially in organic solvents. Dimers are long enough to span cellular lipid bilayers.
- Gramicidin mixture is a crystalline solid. Its solubility in water is minimal, 6 mg/l.

Pharmacological uses

Gramicidin work as antibiotics against gram -ive bacteria but not well against gram-negative ones. Gramicidin is used in medicine for sore throat and in topical medicines to treat infected wounds. Gramicidin is also used in for bacterial eye infections. Used to treat eye infections of animals, like horses. Gramicidin is not used internally be toxic to the liver, kidney.

Synthesis of Gramicidin

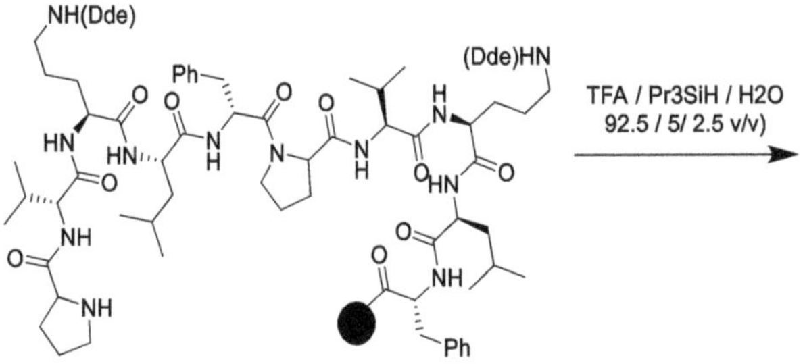

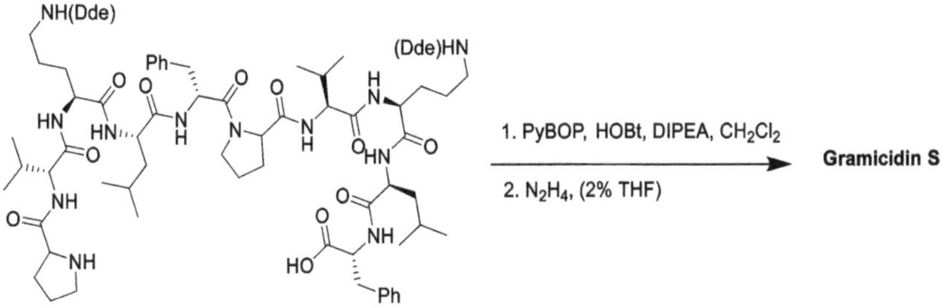

BACITRACIN

$C_{66}H_{103}N_{17}O_{16}S$
Molar mass
1422.69 g/mol g·mol−1

BACITRACIN

$$C_{66}H_{10}3N_{17}O_{16}S$$
Molar mass
1422.69 g/mol g·mol−1

Chemistry

Bacitracin is composed of a mixture of related compounds with
varying degrees of antibacterial activity. Notable fractions include
bacitracin A, A1, B, B1, B2, C, D, E, F, G, and X.

Bacitracin A has been found to have the most antibacterial activity.
Bacitracin B1 and B2 have similar potencies and are approximately
90% as active as bacitracin A.

331

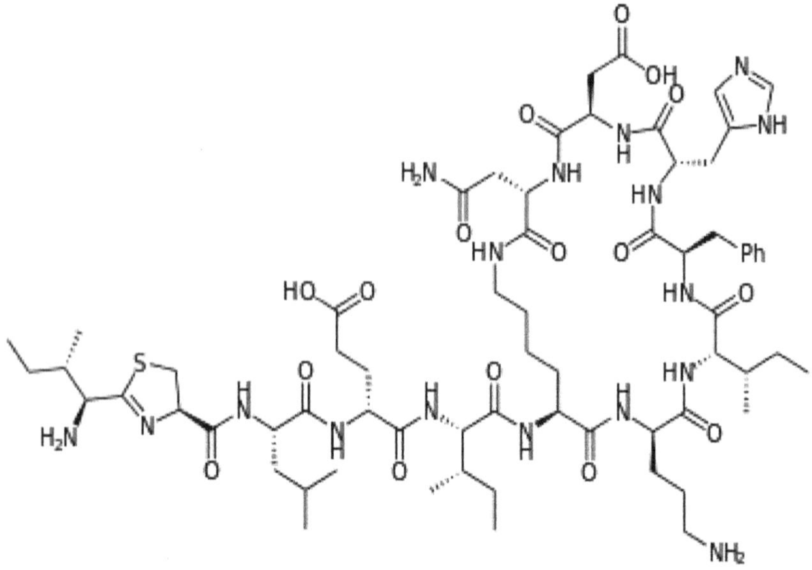

(The above structure has been copied from the Ph. D. thesis of the main author, drawn with stencils in 1988)

Pharmacology

Bacitracin is used in human medicine but though use in animals. As bacitracin zinc salt, in combination with other topical antibiotics "triple antibiotic ointment". It is used for topical treatment of a variety of localized skin and eye infections, as well as for the prevention of wound.

Adverse side effects

As above

7.3   Active Against Gram-Negative Bacteria

POLYMYXIN

Chemistry

Polymyxin B1 and E

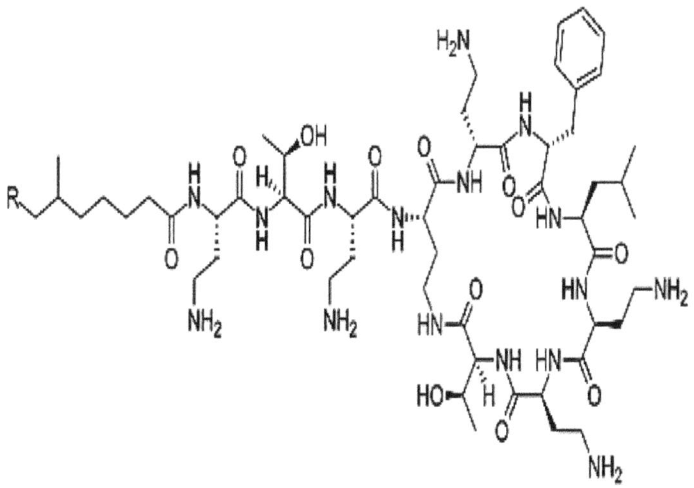

**(The above structure has been copied from the Ph. D.
thesis of the main author, drawn with stencils in 1988)**

Polymyxin B R=H is polymyxin B1, R=CH3 is polymyxin B2)

333

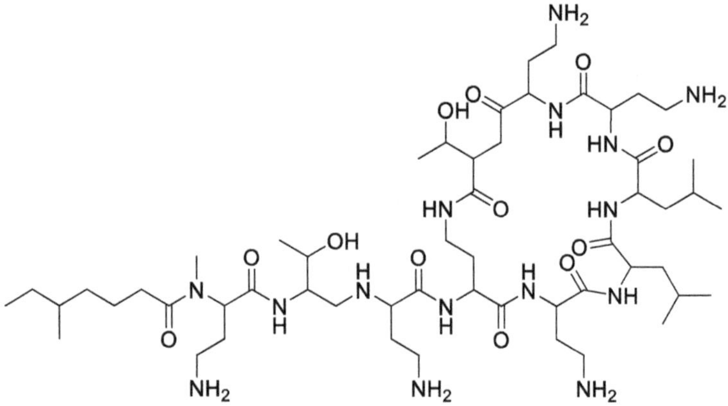

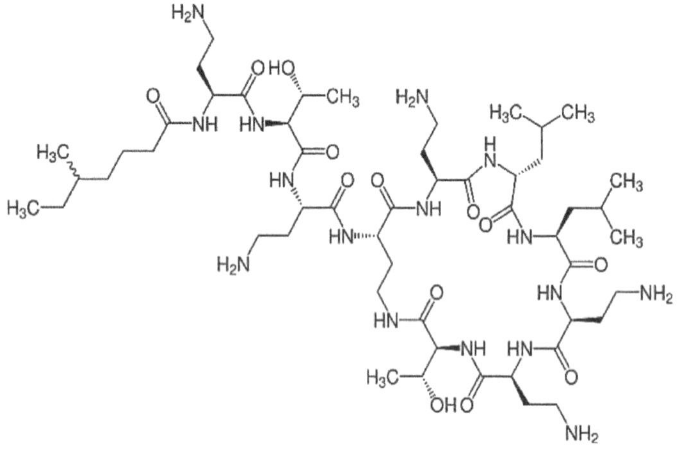

Polymyxin B and E are "Colistin"

(The above structure has been copied from the Ph. D. thesis of the main author, drawn with stencils in 1988)

Pharmacology

- Polymyxins have less effect on gram +ive organisms and are sometimes combined with other agents to broaden the effective spectrum.

- They are also used externally as a cream or drops to treat swimmer's ear and as a component to treat and prevent skin infections.
- Gram-negative bacteria can develop resistance to polymyxins through various modifications.

CHAPTER 8

ANTIBIOTICS DERIVED FROM SUGARS

8.1   General list of antibiotics derived from sugars.

1.	Streptomycin
2.	Dihydrostreptomycin
3.	Neomycins
4.	Paromomycins
5.	Kanamycins
6.	Gentamycin
7.	Sisomicin
8.	Netilmicin
9.	Tobramycin
10.	Dibekacin
11.	Amikacin
12.	Pentisomicin
13.	Spectinomycin

8.1.1   Chemistry of antibiotics of amino sugars

The components of streptomycin: streptidine (aglycone), streptose, and L-glucosamine

The isolation of a new antibiotic in crude form from two cultures of Streptomyces griseus. The substance, streptomycin, had low toxicity and was active against Gram-negative bacteria. This observation was especially encouraging since penicillin and the sulfonamide drugs are chiefly effective against Gram-positive bacteria and there was a real need for a drug to treat Gram-negative microbial infections.

Chemistry in general of Streptomycin

Pure streptomycin is a relatively stable, colorless, water soluble base. It forms tribasic acids and has no characteristic absorption in the ultraviolet. The streptomycin molecule consists of three independent units joined by glycosidic bonds. Degradation studies were naturally directed at a determination of the properties and structure of each of these moieties. The glycosidic linkage between streptidine and streptose is the more labile of the two bonds. When methylstreptobiosaminide dimethyl acetal was treated with acid under more rigorous conditions, the glycosidic bond was hydrolysed and a product was obtained which gave a phenylosazone and a phenylosotriazole having melting points corresponding to those of D-glucose derivatives. The oxidation of the nitrogen-containing carbohydrate from the hydrolysis gave an N-methyl-L-glucosaminic acid. These data indicated that the amino sugar was N-methyl-L-glucosamine.

Chemistry of Streptidine

The presence of monosubstituted guanidino groups in the antibiotic, suggested by the positive Sakaguchi reaction, was confirmed by the stepwise alkaline hydrolysis of the streptidine moiety to strepturea and streptamine. Guanidine was also isolated from degradation mixtures.

Chemical structure of streptomycin

a) **N-Methyl – L- Glucosamine**
b) **Streptidine**
c) **Streptose**

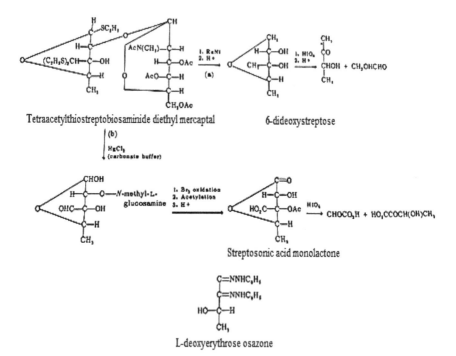

(a)

(b)   (c)

(The above structure has been copied from the Ph. D. thesis of the main author, drawn with stencils in 1988)

Chemistry of Streptose

Tetraacetylthiostreptobiosaminide diethyl mercaptal

6-dideoxystreptose

N-methyl-L-glucosamine

Streptosonic acid monolactone

L-deoxyerythrose osazone

(The above structure has been copied from the Ph. D. thesis of the main author, drawn with stencils in 1988)

8.2 Pharmacological uses and adverse effects of streptomycin in general

Streptomycin and dihydrostreptomycin are absorbed equally well following injection. The potency of streptomycin is expressed in terms of the equivalent weight of the free Base. The antibiotic is not absorbed from the gastrointestinal tract and is consequently not given by the oral route unless a specific local effect is desired. In such instance streptomycin is generally combined with other antimicrobial agents. Streptomycin is excreted in the urine at a much slower rate than penicillin. The injection of 0.5 g. of the sulfate will provide therapeutic concentrations in the serum lasting for about 12 hours. 50-60% may be recovered in the urine in 24 hours.

Note that the carbons numbered with ring atom numbers 1', 2', 3', etc.) refer to the sugar **(streptose)** ring attached to the C4 position of the aminocyclitol systems. It is a general feature of aminoglycosides that the atoms of the ring attached to the C4 position are numbered 1', 2', 3', etc. The same question may be asked about the linkage between **L-glucosamine** and streptose: how it can be made specifically between C2'-OH of **streptose** and the anomeric position of L-glucosamine (C1'').

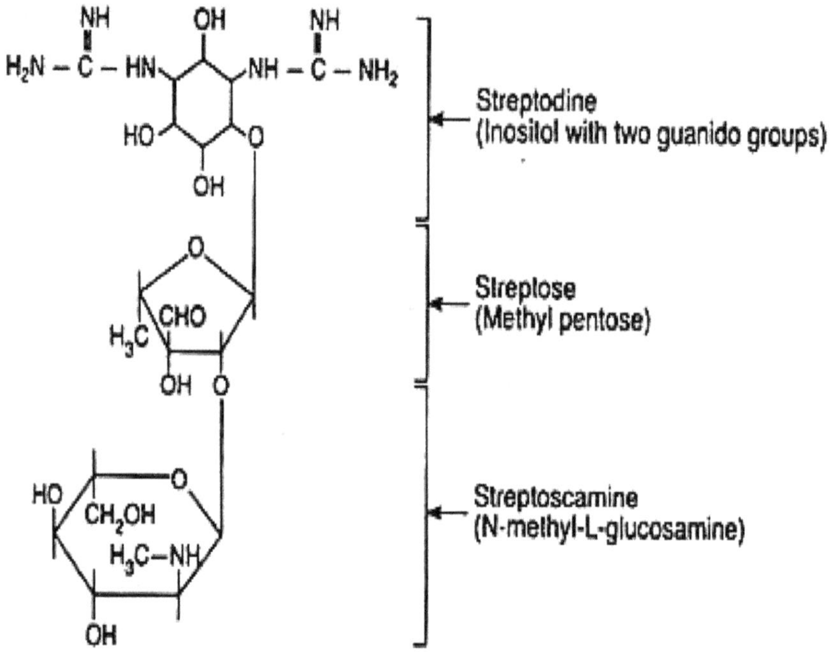

(The above structure has been copied from the Ph. D. thesis of the main author, drawn with stencils in 1988)

The aminoglycosides can be categorized into related groups based upon the glycosidic linkages of the cyclic amino-sugar components to the central aminocyclitol ring: the 4,5-disubstituted group includes neomycin and paromomycin; the 4,6-disubstituted group includes the kanamycins, gentamicins and tobramycin; while the original aminoglycoside, streptomycin, has a six-membered monosubstituted aminocyclitol ring.

Streptamine   2-deoxystreptamine   Streptidine

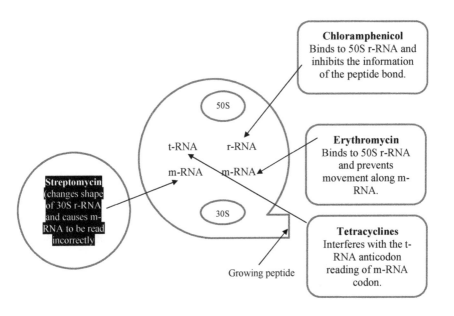

Inhibition of protein synthesis by Antibiotics

8.3 Properties of individual important compounds of antibiotics derived from sugars

STREPTOMYCIN

$C_{21}H_{39}N_7O_{12}$
Molar mass
581.574 g/mol g·mol−1

Chemistry

Streptomycin was discovered in 1943 from soil discovery of streptomycin, the first antibiotic active against tuberculosis". It consists of three components linked glycosidically (by ether bonds):

(i) Streptidine (inositol with two guanido groups)
(ii) Streptose (methyl pentose)
(iii) Streptoscamine (N-methyl-L-glycosamine)

Both guanido groups of streptidine are essential for the antibiotic activity and removal of one group reduces antibiotic activity upto 90%.

(iv) By doing so, the streptomycin causes a structural change which interferes with the recognition site of codon-anticodon interaction resulting in misreading of the genetic message carried by messenger RNA (mRNA).

Structure activity relationship

❏ Avtivity largely depends upon the hydrogen ion concentration of the medium and its composition and biologically active more in alkaline state.
❏ In acid medium, activity is decreased.
❏ Treated with hydroxylamine, phenylhydrazine, there is a complete loss of activity.
❏ The presence of D- mannose sugar, makes the drug less active.
❏ Catalytic hydration gives dihydrostreptomycin, with less activity but is more stable.
❏ Streptidine unit has no biological activity.
❏ Introduction of cysteine molecule, results in a deactivation.
❏ The reduction of aldehydic group to primary alcohol in dihydrostreptomycin, does not abolish biological activity.

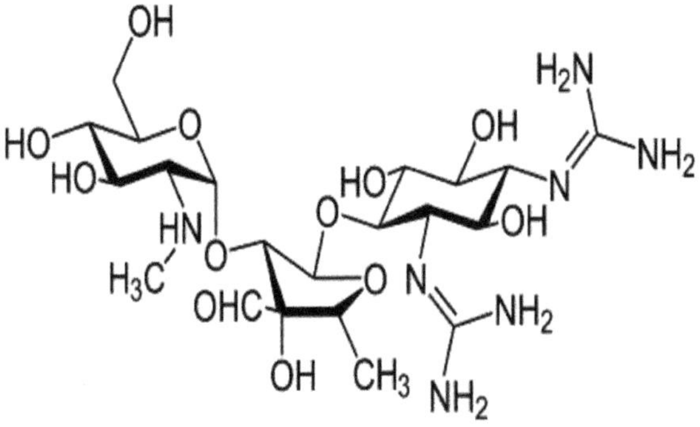

**(The above structure has been copied from the Ph. D.
thesis of the main author, drawn with stencils in 1988)**

Pharmacology

For active tuberculosis it is often given together with INH, rifamycin
and pyrazinamide. It is not the first line treatment, except in
medically under-served populations where the cost of more expensive
treatments is prohibitive. It may be useful in cases where resistance
to other drugs is identified. Streptomycin also is used as a pesticide,
to combat the growth of bacteria beyond human applications.

Metabolism

Bioavailability	84% to 88% i.m. (est.) 0% by mouth
Elimination half life	5-6 hours
Metabolism	Kidneys

Common side effects
Common side effects include, vomiting, numbness of the face, fever,
and rash.

Biosynthesis of Streptomycin

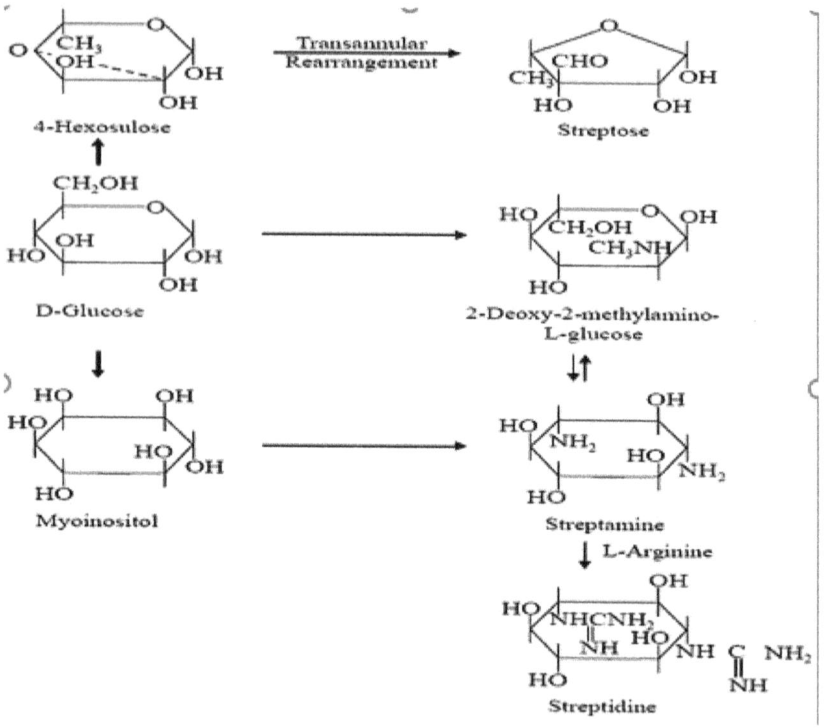

(The above structures have been copied from the Ph. D. thesis of the main author, drawn with stencils in 1988)

DIHYDROSTREPTOMYCIN

$$C_{21}H_{41}N_7O_{12}$$
Molar mass
583.59 g/mol g·mol−1

Chemistry

Dihydrostreptomycin is a derivative of streptomycin that has a bactericidal effect.

It is a semisynthetic aminoglycoside antibiotic used in the treatment of tuberculosis.

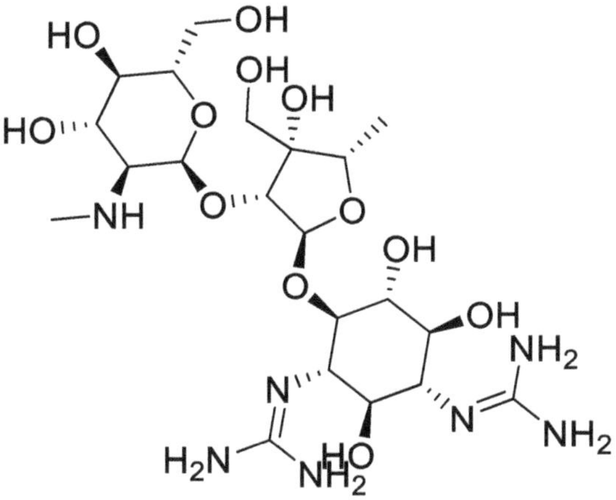

NEOMYCIN

$C_{23}H_{46}N_{6}O_{13}$
Molar mass
614.650 g·mol^{-1}

Chemistry

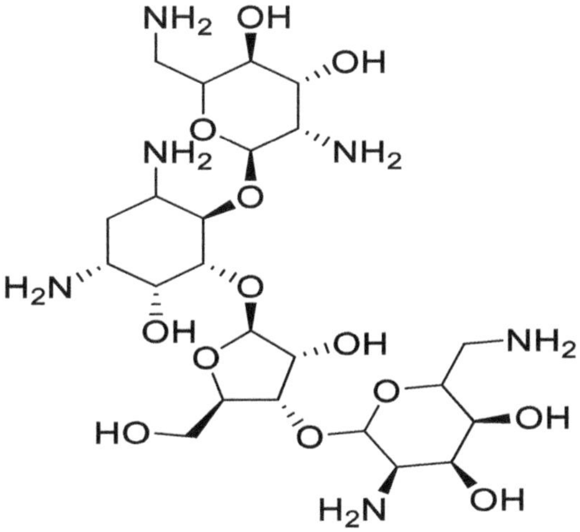

(The above structure has been copied from the Ph. D. thesis of the main author, drawn with stencils in 1988)

Neomycin belongs to aminoglycoside class of antibiotics that contain two or more amino sugars connected by glycosidic bonds. It is a basic compound that is most active with an alkaline reaction.

Pharmacology
Neomycin is typically used as a topical preparation, such as Neosporin (neomycin/polymyxin B/bacitracin). Neomycin has good activity against Gram-positive and Gram-negative bacteria but is very ototoxic. Its use is thus restricted to oral treatment of intestinal infections.

Metabolism
Enterobacter cloacae: >16μg/ml
Escherichia coli: 1μg/ml
Proteus vulgaris: 0.25μg/ml

Bioavailability	-
Elimination half life	2-3 hours
Metabolism	-

Common side effects
As above

PAROMOMYCIN

$C_{23}H_{47}N_5O_{18}S$
Molar mass
615.629 g/mol g·mol^{-1}

Chemistry

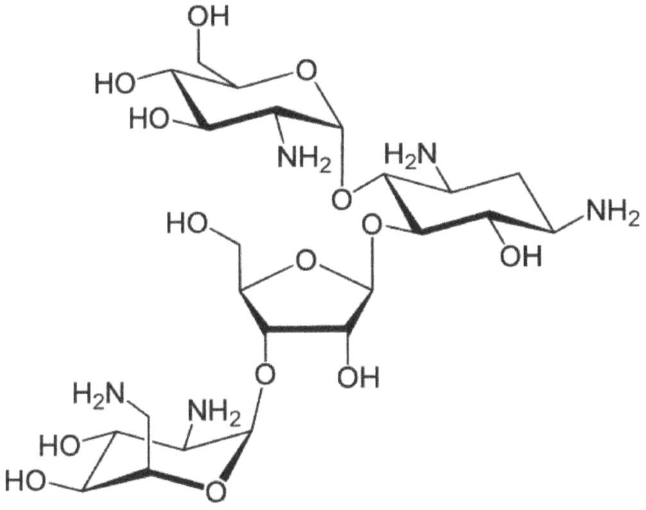

(The above structure has been copied from the Ph. D. thesis of the main author, drawn with stencils in 1988)

Pharmacology

Paromomycin is used to treat a number of parasitic infections. It is a first line treatment for amebiasis or giardiasis. It is generally a second line treatment option, is an effective treatment for ulcerative cutaneous leishmaniasis, according to the results of a phase-3, randomized, double-blind, parallel group–controlled trial.

Pharmacokinetics

GI absorption is poor. Any obstructions or factors which impair GI motility may increase the absorption of the drug from the digestive tract. Almost 100% of the oral dose is eliminated unchanged via feces. Any absorbed drug will be excreted in urine.

Common side effects

As above

KANAMYCIN

$$C_{18}H_{36}N_4O_{11}$$
Molar mass
484.499 g·mol⁻¹

Chemistry

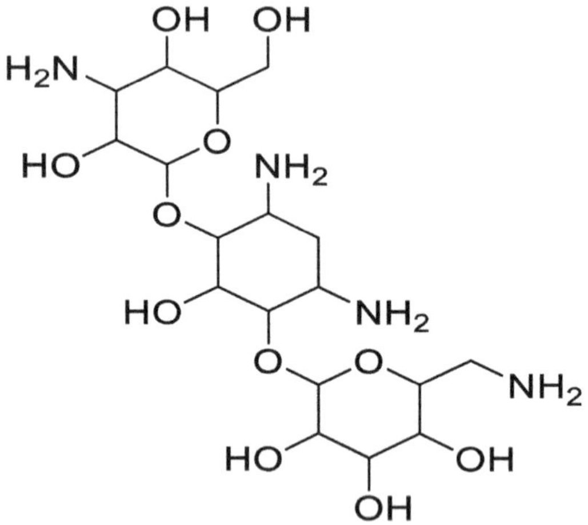

Pharmacology
Kanamycin is indicated for short term treatment of bacterial infections caused by one or more of the pathogens species (both indole-positive and indole-negative). In cases of serious infection when the causative organism is unknown.

Metabolism

Bioavailability	very low after by mouth
Elimination half life	2 hours 30 minutes
Excretion	Urine (as unchanged drug)

Common side effects
Gastrointestinal effects, Myasthenia gravis, Blurring of vision, Neuromuscular blockade,
Malabsorption syndrome.

GENTAMYCIN

$$C_{21}H_{43}N_5O_7$$
Molar mass
477.596 g/mol g·mol^{-1}

Chemistry

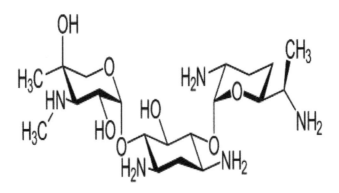

(The above structure has been copied from the Ph. D.
thesis of the main author, drawn with stencils in 1988)

Pharmacology
Gentamicin used to treat several types of infections. It can be given i.v.

Metabolism

Bioavailability	limited bioavailability by mouth
Elimination half life	2 hours
Excretion	Kidneys

Common side effects
Nephrotoxicity and ototoxity.

Contraindications
Gentamicin should not be used if a person has a history of other serious toxic reaction to gentamicin.

Synthesis of Gentamycin

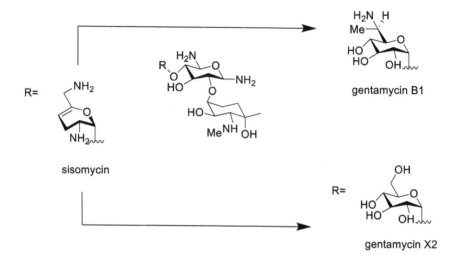

R= sisomycin

gentamycin B1

R= gentamycin X2

TOBRAMYCIN

$C_{18}H_{37}N_5O_9$
Molar mass
467.515 g/mol g·mol⁻¹

Chemistry

**(The above structure has been copied from the Ph. D.
thesis of the main author, drawn with stencils in 1988)**

Pharmacology
Like all aminoglycosides, tobramycin does not pass the GIT so given i.v. in the muscle. The nebulized formulation is indicated in the treatment of chronic infections.

Metabolism
Protein binding < 30%

Common side effects
Like other aminoglycosides, tobramycin can cause otitis.

AMIKACIN

$$C_{22}H_{43}N_5O_{13}$$
Molar mass
585.603 g/mol g·mol^{-1}

Chemistry

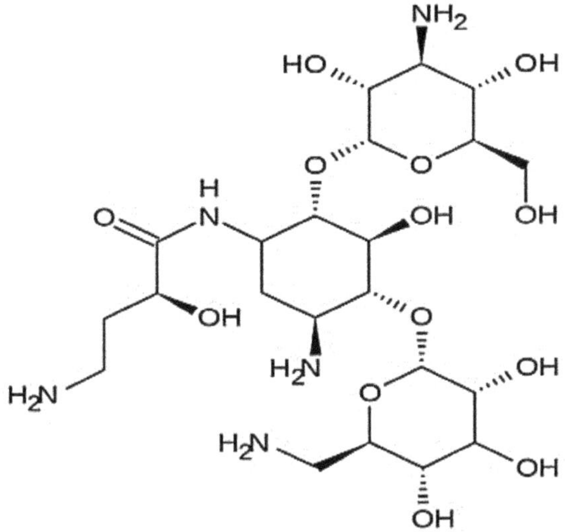

(The above structure has been copied from the Ph. D. thesis of the main author, drawn with stencils in 1988)

351

Pharmacology

Amikacin is most often used for treating severe infections with aerobic bacteria, Bone and joint infections.

Pharmacokinetics

Bioavailability	>90%
Protein binding	0–11%
Metabolism	Mostly unmetabolized
Elimination half life	2–3 hours
Excretion	Kidneys

Common side effects

Amikacin, like other can cause otitis, balance problems.

SPECTINOMYCIN

$$C_{14}H_{24}N_2O_7$$
Molar mass
332.35 g/mol g·mol^{-1}

Chemistry

Spectinomycin was discovered in 1961.

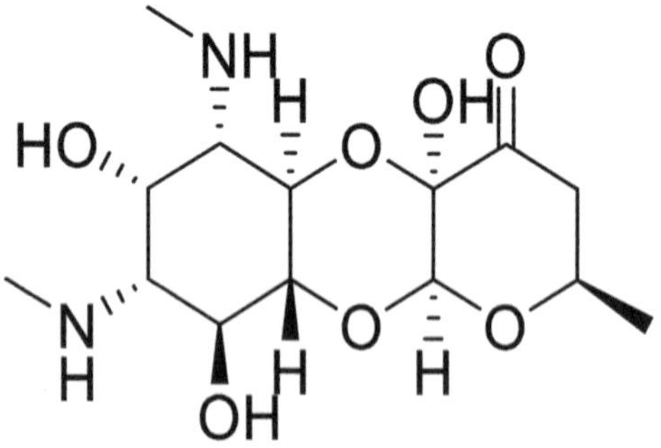

Pharmacology

Spectinomycin is given especially in patients who are allergic to penicillin.

Common side effects

Common side effects include pain at the area of injection, rash, nausea, fever and trouble sleeping.

CHAPTER 9

ANTIBIOTICS DERIVED FROM ACETATES AND PROPIONATE

1.	Tetracycline group of antibiotics *(discussed already in Chapter 6)*
2.	Griseofulvin
3.	Fusidic acid

9.1 Properties of individual important compounds of antibiotics derived from acetates or propionates

GRISEOFULVIN

$$C_{17}H_{17}ClO_6$$
Molar mass
352.766 g·mol^{-1}

Chemistry

Griseofulvin was discovered in 1939 from a mold.

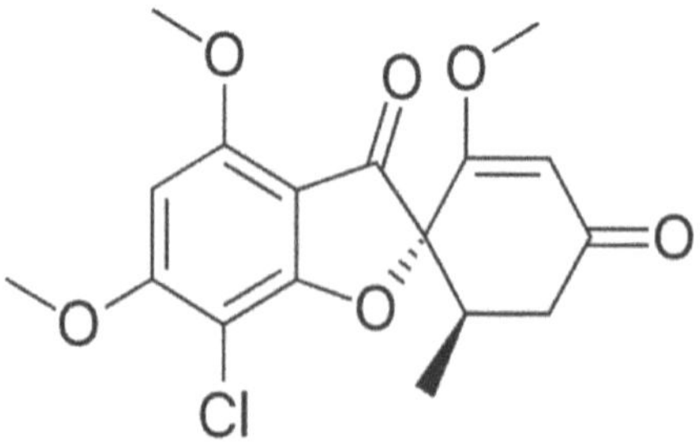

(The above structure has been copied from the Ph. D. thesis of the main author, drawn with stencils in 1988)

Pharmacology

Griseofulvin is used orally only for dermic use.

Common side effects

Confusion, Diarrhea, Dizziness, Fatigue, Headache, impairment of liver enzymatic activity Itching, Nausea, Skin rashes, Swelling and Upper abdominal pain.

Synthesis of Griseofulvin

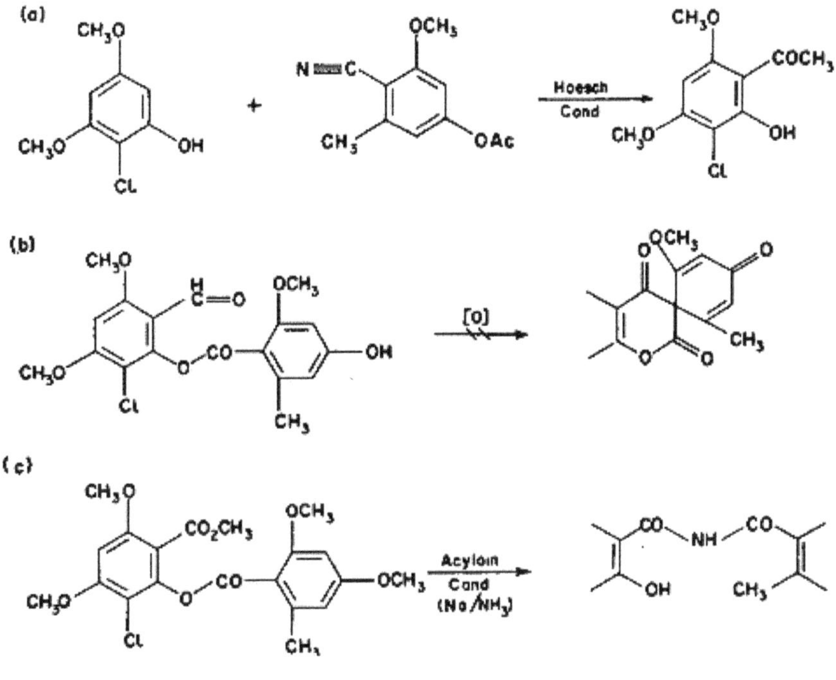

(The above structures have been copied from the Ph. D. thesis of the main author, drawn with stencils in 1988)

FUSIDIC ACID

$$C_{31}H_{48}O_6$$
Molar mass
516.709 g·mol^{-1}

Chemistry

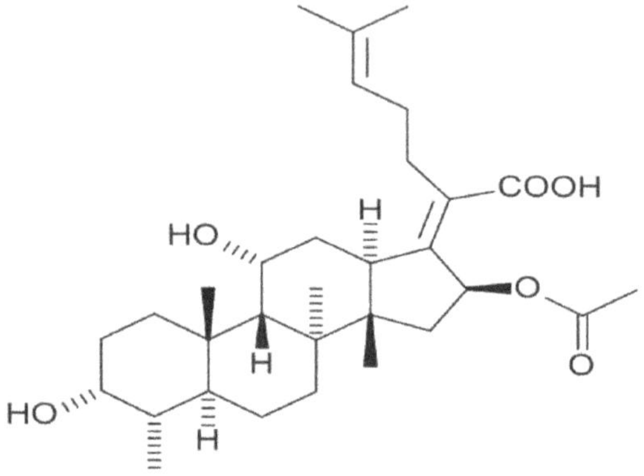

(The above structure has been copied from the Ph. D. thesis of the main author, drawn with stencils in 1988)

Pharmacology

Fusidic acid is effective primarily on gram +ive bacteria. Topical fusidic acid is occasionally used as a treatment for for acne, fusidic acid is often partially effective at improving acne symptoms.

Pharmacokinetics

Bioavailability	91% oral bioavailability
Protein binding	97-99%
Elimunation half life	Approximately 5-6 hours

Common side effects

Fucidin occasionally cause liver upsets, which can produce jaundice (yellowing of the skin and the whites of the eyes).

356

Contraindications

There is inadequate evidence of safety in human pregnancy.

Interactions

Fusidic acid should not be used with quinolone antibiotics with which they are antagonistic.

Synthesis of Fusidic acid

CHAPTER 10

MACROLIDE ANTIBIOTICS

10.1 List of macrolide antibiotics (old)

1.	Erythromycin
2.	Oleandomycin
3.	Carbomycin
4.	Spiramycins
5.	Leucomycins *(kitasamycins)*
6.	Avermactins

Newer macrolide antibiotics
(azalids)

1.	Azithromycin
2.	Clarithromycin
3.	Fidaxomicin

10.2 Chemistry of macrolides antibiotics

The macrolides are a class of that consist of a large ring to which one or more de-oxysugar, usually cladinose and desosamine may be attached. These antibiotics are so designated because of the presence of a macrocyclic lactone ring. They are predominantly active against gram-positive bacteria and include erythromycin, carbomycin, spiramycin and leucomycins (kitasamycins). Further rosaramicin, with higher activity than erythromycin aoagins gram – negative pathogens as well against *Mycoplasma* and *Chlamydia*, shows promising therapeutic efficacy in the treatment of bacterial prostatitis. Avermactins possess potent activity against nematodes.

Approved macrolide antibiotics:

Erythromycin, Clarithromycin, Azithromycin and Fidaxomicin.

Non-approved macrolide antibiotics:

Carbomycin A, Josamycin, Kitasamycin, Oleeandomycin, Midecamycin / Midecamycin Acetate, Solithromycin, Spiramycin, Troleandomycin, Tylosine, Telithromycin and Roxithromycin.

Ketolides
Are a class of antibiotics that are structurally related to the macrolides. They are used to treat respiratory tract infections caused by macrolide-resistant bacteria. Ketolides are especially effective, as they have two ribosomal binding sites (Telithromycin).

Fluoroketolides
Fluoroketolides are a class of antibiotics that are structurally related to the ketolides. The fluoroketolides have three ribosomal interaction sites (Solithromycin).

General interactions of macrolides
Macrolides should not be taken with colchicine as it may lead to colchicine toxicity. Symptoms of colchicine toxicity include gastrointestinal upset, fever, myalgia, pancytopenia, and organ failure. Macrolide therapy still produces substantial anti-inflammatory results.

10.3 Properties of individual important compounds of macrolide antibiotics

ERYTHROMYCIN

$$C_{37}H_{67}NO_{13}$$
Molar mass
733.937 g·mol^{-1}

Chemistry

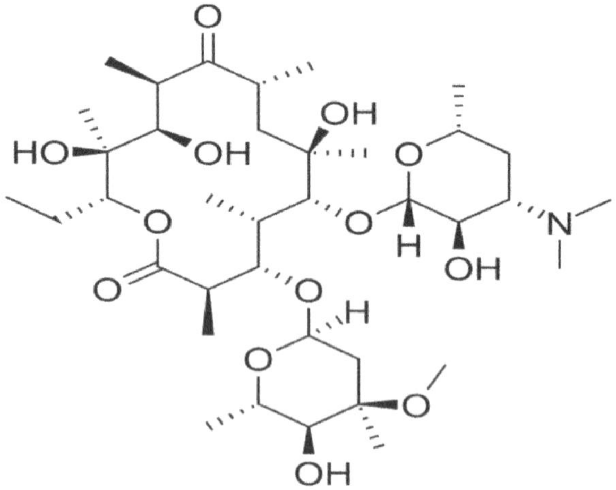

(The above structure has been copied from the Ph. D. thesis of the main author, drawn with stencils in 1988)

Structure activity relationship

❑ Dimethyl amino group plays vital role in the biological activity of erythromycin.

❑ Substitution of one N- methyl group by hydrogen, ethyl, propyl, isobutyl deprives the biological activity.

❑ When hydrogen concentration is raised, the activity of erythromycin increases.

❑ The presence of sodium chloride and semicarbazone has no effect on the molecules's biological activity.

❑ The sugar residues are essential for antibacterial activity.

360

Degradation of Erythromycin

$$H_3C-CH_2-CH-\underset{\underset{\overset{|}{CH_3}}{|}}{C}-\underset{\overset{|}{H}}{C}-\underset{\overset{|}{H}}{C}-\overset{\overset{\overset{O}{\|}}{}}{C}-\underset{\overset{|}{H}}{\overset{CH_3}{C}}-CH_2-\underset{\underset{desosaminyl}{OH}}{\overset{CH_3}{C}}-\underset{\overset{|}{H}}{\overset{H}{C}}-\underset{\overset{|}{O}}{C}-\underset{\underset{cladinosyl}{\overset{|}{O}}}{\overset{CH_3}{\overset{|}{C}}}-CH_3$$

Erythromycin

↓ Sodium borohydride

Dihydroerythromycin

↓ MeOH-HCl

5-O-desosaminyldihydroerythronolide

↓ 2N HCl

$$H_3C-CH_2-CH-\underset{\underset{\overset{|}{CH_3}}{|}}{C}-\underset{\overset{|}{H}}{C}-\underset{\overset{|}{H}}{C}-\overset{\overset{\overset{O}{\|}}{}}{C}-\underset{\overset{|}{H}}{\overset{CH_3}{C}}-CH_2-\underset{\underset{desosaminyl}{OH}}{\overset{CH_3}{C}}-\underset{\overset{|}{H}}{\overset{H}{C}}-\underset{\overset{|}{O}}{C}-\underset{\underset{cladinosyl}{\overset{|}{O}}}{\overset{CH_3}{\overset{|}{C}}}-CH_3 \cdots C=O$$

Dihydroerythronolide

↓ OH⁻
   IO₄⁻

$$\overset{\overset{O}{\|}}{CH}-\underset{\overset{|}{H}}{C}-\underset{\overset{|}{OH}}{\overset{CH_3}{C}}-\underset{\overset{|}{H}}{\overset{H}{C}}-\overset{CH_3}{C}-CO_2\overset{}{CH}COCH_3 \quad (C_2H_5)$$

$$\overset{\overset{O}{\|}}{CH}-\underset{\overset{|}{CH_3}}{C}-\underset{\overset{|}{OH}}{\overset{H}{C}}-\underset{\overset{|}{H}}{\overset{H}{C}}-\overset{CH_3}{C}-CH_2COCH_3$$

Pharmacokinetics

Bioavailability	30 – 65%
Protein binding	90%
Metabolism	Liver, 2-15% excreted unchanged
Elimination half-life	1.5 hours
Excretion	Bile

Common side effects

Include abdominal cramps, vomiting, and diarrhea, may include liver problems, appears to be safe to use during pregnancy.

Conversion of Erythromycin to Roxithromycin

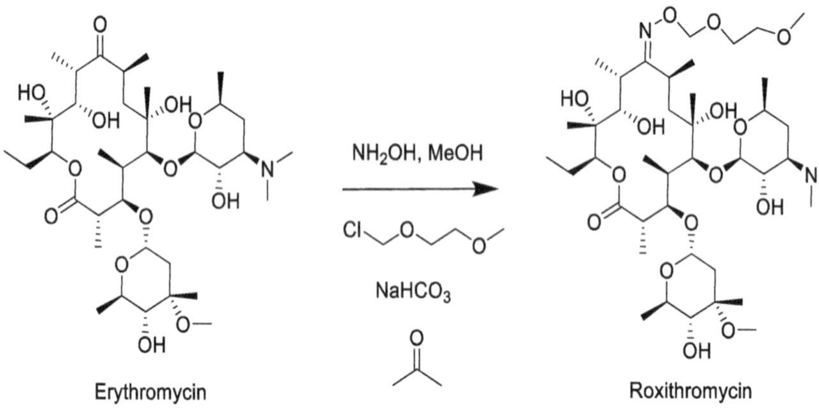

Erythromycin

NH₂OH, MeOH

Roxithromycin

NaHCO₃

Synthesis of Erythromycin (condensed)

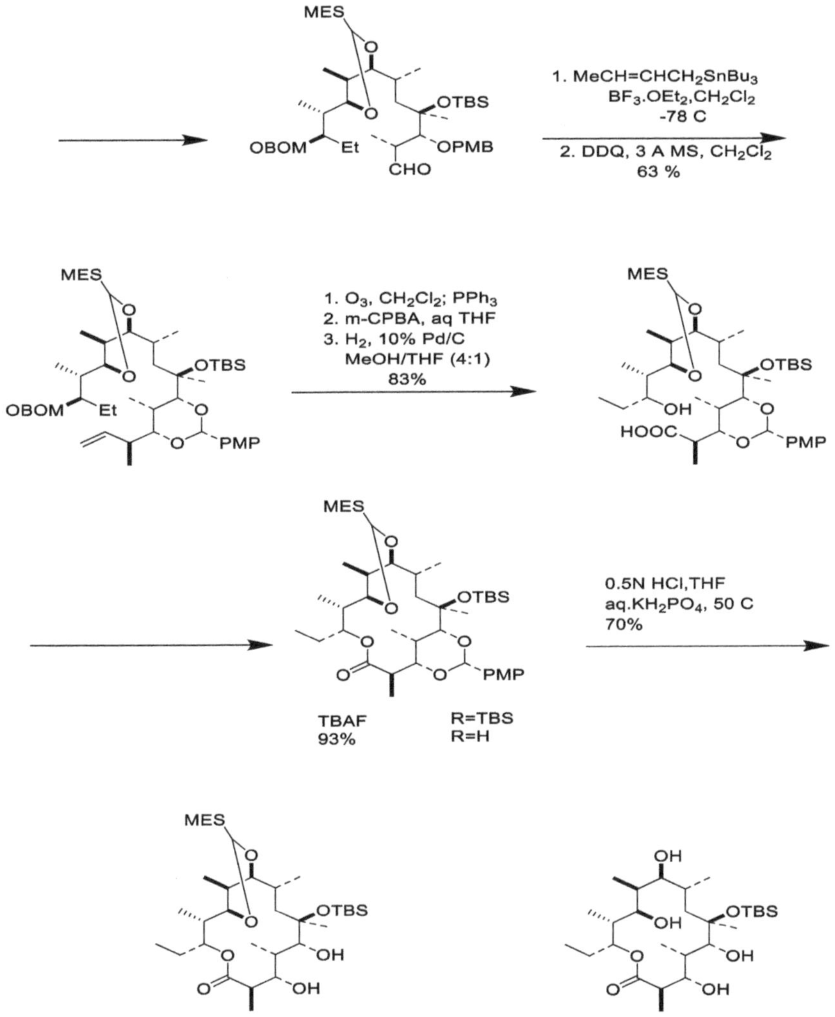
MES
OTBS
OBOM
Et
OPMB
CHO
1. MeCH=CHCH2SnBu3
BF3.OEt2,CH2Cl2
-78 C
2. DDQ, 3 A MS, CH2Cl2
63 %
PMP
1. O3, CH2Cl2; PPh3
2. m-CPBA, aq THF
3. H2, 10% Pd/C
MeOH/THF (4:1)
83%
OH
HOOC
0.5N HCl,THF
aq.KH2PO4, 50 C
70%
TBAF
93%
R=TBS
R=H

OLEANDOMYCIN

$C_{35}H_{61}NO_{12}$

Molar mass

687.858 g/mol g·mol⁻

Chemistry

Pharmacology

Oleandomycin can be employed to inhibit the activities of bacteria responsible for causing infections in the upper respiratory tract much like Erythromycin can.

Mechanism of Action

AZITHROMYCIN

$$C_{38}H_{72}N_2O_{12}$$
Molar mass
748.996 g/mol g·mol⁻

Chemistry

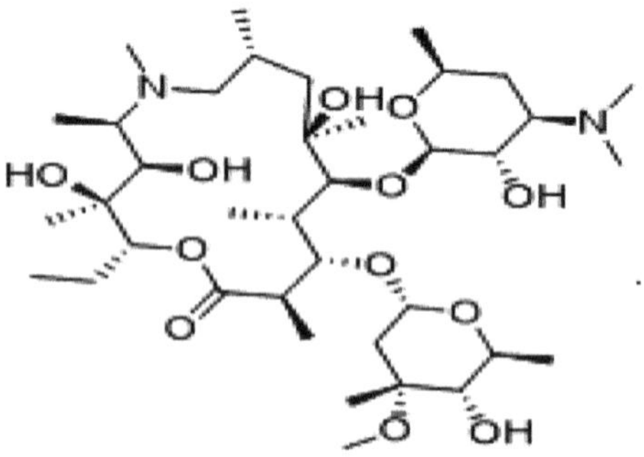

Synthesis of Azithromycin

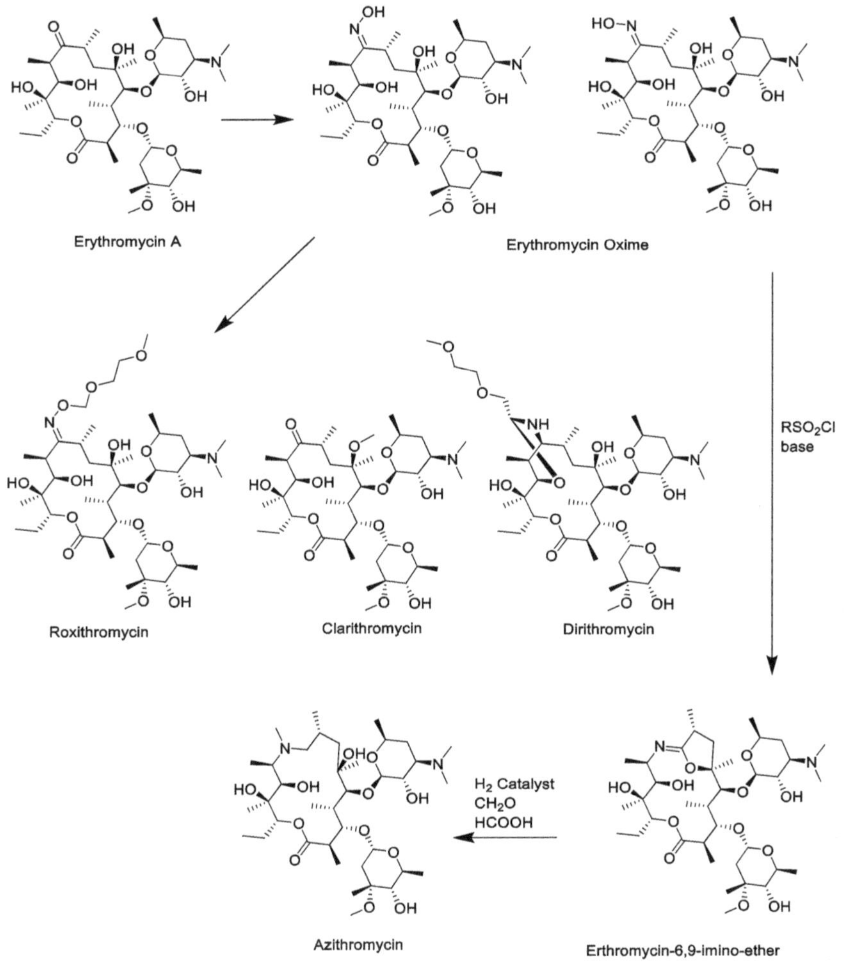

Erythromycin A

Erythromycin Oxime

RSO$_2$Cl
base

Roxithromycin

Clarithromycin

Dirithromycin

H$_2$ Catalyst
CH$_2$O
HCOOH

Azithromycin

Erthromycin-6,9-imino-ether

CLARITHROMYCIN

C$_{38}$H$_{69}$NO$_{13}$
Molar mass
747.953 g/mol g·mol^{-1}

Chemistry

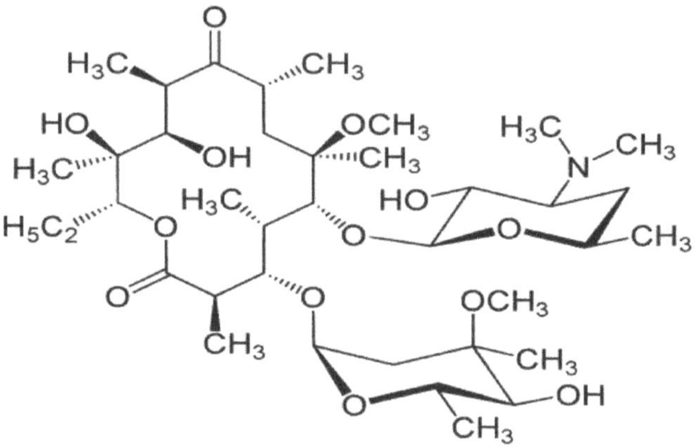

(The above structure has been copied from the Ph. D. thesis of the main author, drawn with stencils in 1988)

Pharmacology

Clarithromycin is primarily used to treat number of bacterial infections and as an alternative to penicillin, is effective against upper and lower respiratory tract infections, skin and soft tissue infections and helicobacter pylori infections associated with duodenal ulcers.

Pharmacokinetics

Unlike erythromycin, clarithromycin is acid-stable, so can be taken orally without having to be protected from gastric acids. It is readily absorbed and diffuses into most tissues. Due to the high concentration in phagocytes, clarithromycin is actively transported to the site of infection.

Common side effects

Common side effects include nausea, vomiting, headaches, and diarrhea. Liver problems have been reported.

Contraindications

Clarithromycin should not be taken by people who are allergic to other macrolides or inactive ingredients in the tablets, including microcrystalline cellulose, croscarmelose sodium, and magnesium stearate.

Synthesis of Clarithromycin

Erythromycin

2,3'-O-benzyloxycarbonyl Erythromycin

Methylation is carried out at 6-OH group of the 2,3'-O-benzyloxycarbonyl Erythromycin using methyl iodide in a suitable base solvent.

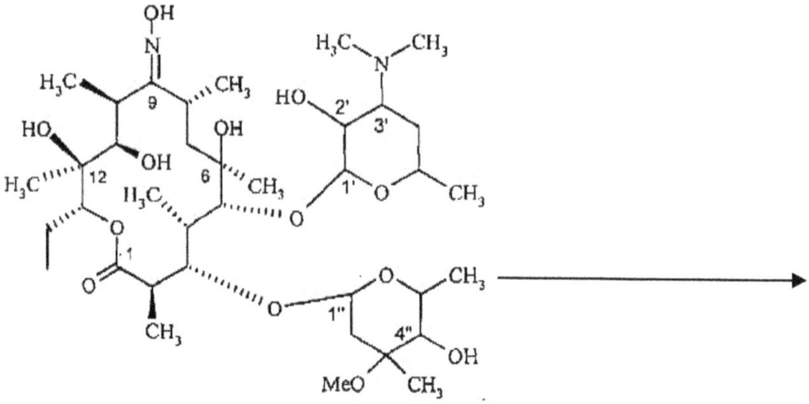

Erythromycin-9-Oxime

2,3'-O-benzyloxycarbonyl Erythromycin is removed by hydrogenolysis and the subjected to reductive methylation in presence of excess formaldehyde.

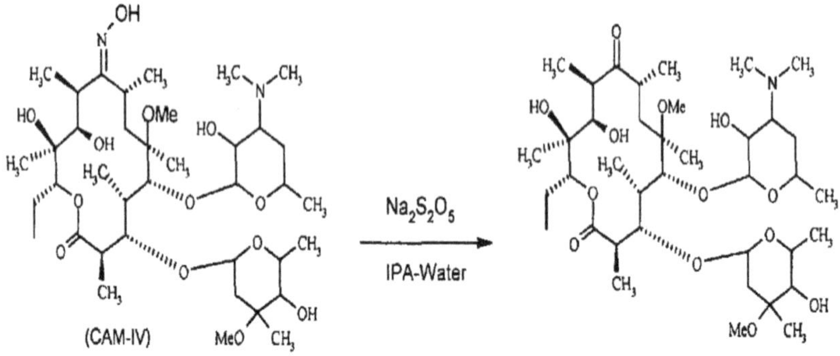

Clarithromycin-9 oxime   Clarithromycin

The above structures have been copied from the Ph. D. thesis of the main author, drawn with stencils in 1988)

Clarithromycin-9 oxime is treated with sodium metabisulphite in isopropyl alcohol (IPA) and water (1:1) v/v, 6-8 hours reflux condensation at 80 ° C to get Clarithromycin.

FIDAXOMICIN

$C_{52}H_{74}Cl_2O_{18}$
Molar mass
1058.04 g/mol g·mol^{-1}

Chemistry

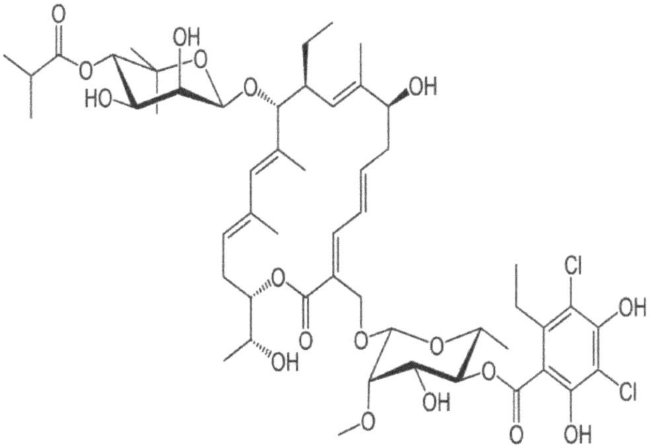

**(The above structure has been copied from the Ph. D.
thesis of the main author, drawn with stencils in 1988)**

Pharmacology
It is currently one of the most expensive antibiotics approved for use.

Pharmacokinetics

Bioavailability	Minimal systemic absorption
Elimination half-life	11.7 ± 4.80 hours
Excretion	Urine (<1%), faeces (92%)

Common side effects
As above

CARBOMYCIN

$C_{42}H_{67}NO_{16}$
Molar mass
841.97848

Chemistry

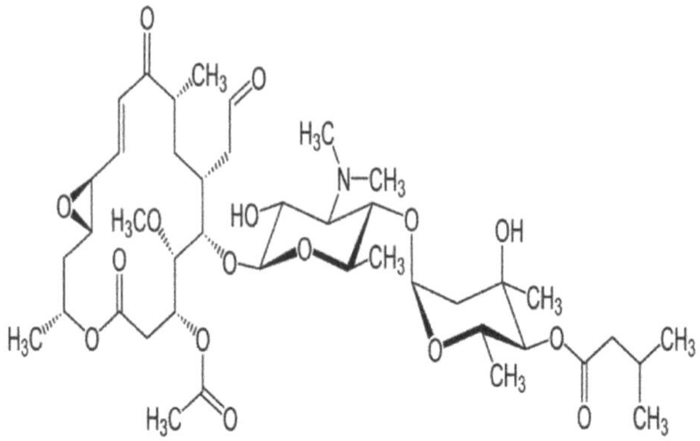

(The above structure has been copied from the Ph. D. thesis of the main author, drawn with stencils in 1988)

Pharmacology
Active in inhibiting the growth of gram +ive bacteria.

CHAPTER 11

POLYENE ANTIBIOTICS

11.1 List of polyene antibiotics

1.	Natamycin *(pimaricin)*
2.	Nystatin
3.	Amphotericin B
4.	Hachimycin *(trichomycin)*
5.	Candicidin
6.	Pecilocin *(variotin)*
7.	Fumagillin

11.2 Properties of individual important compounds of polyene antibiotics

NYSTATIN

$C_{47}H_{75}NO_{17}$
Molar mass
926.09 g·mol^{-1}

Chemistry

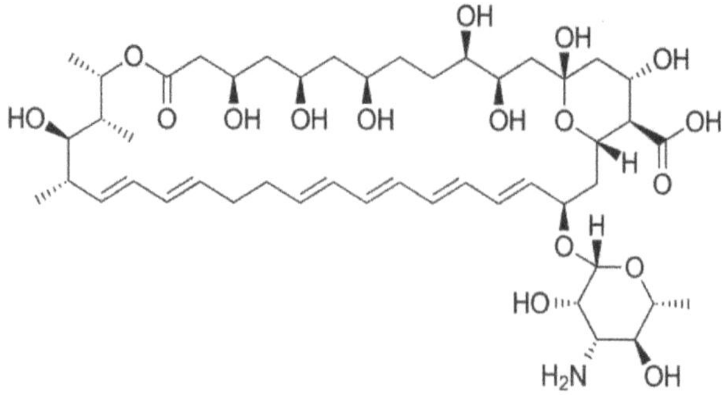

The above structure has been copied from the Ph. D. thesis of the main author, drawn with stencils)

These chiefly antimycitic antibiotics owe their name to the presence of several conjugated double bonds. Classical drugs of this group are used for the local treatment of infections. Further polyene antibiotics are used orally against amoebisis.

Pharmacology
Oral nystatin is used in the treatment for fungal infection.
In certain cases, nystatin has been used to prevent the spread of mold on objects.

Pharmacokinetics

Bioavailability	0% on oral ingestion
Metabolism	None (not extensively absorbed)
Elimination half life	Dependent upon GI transit time
Excretion	100% fecal

Common side effects
Bitter taste and nausea are more common than most other adverse effects. Diarrhea, abdominal pain. Rarely, tachycardia, bronchospasm, facial swelling, muscle aches.

AMPHOTERICIN B

$$C_{47}H_{73}NO_{17}$$
Molar mass
924.091 g·mol^{-1}

Chemistry
It is a subgroup of the macrolide antibiotics and exhibits similar structural elements.

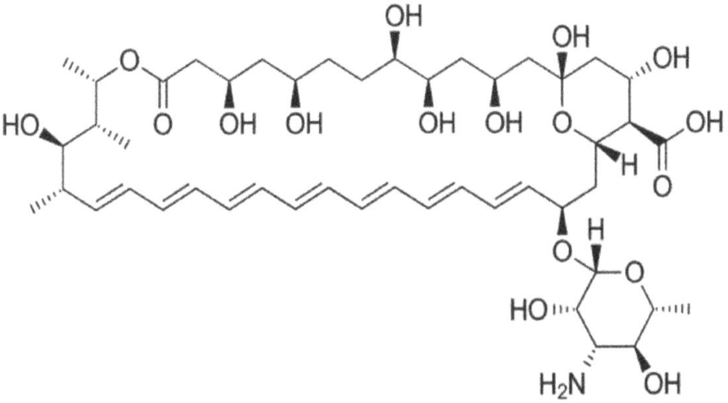

The above structure has been copied from the Ph. D. thesis of the main author, drawn with stencils)

Pharmacology
Amphotericin B is an antifungal medication and leishmaniasis. It is considered first line therapy for invasive mucomycosis infections, cryptococcal meningitis, and certain aspergillus and candidal infections.

Pharmacokinetics

Bioavailability	100% I.V.
Metabolism	Kidneys 40% in urine and biliary
Elimination half life	Initial phase 24 hours
	Second phase about 15 days
Excretion	40% in urine and biliary

Common side effects

High fever, shaking chills, hypotension, anorexia, nausea, vomiting, headache, dyspnea, tachypnea, drowsiness and generalized weakness. In addition, electrolyte imbalances such as hypokalemia and hypomagnesemia are also common. It appears to be relatively safe in pregnancy.

FUMAGILLIN

$$C_{26}H_{34}O_7$$
Molar mass
458.54 g/mol g·mol^{-1}

Chemistry

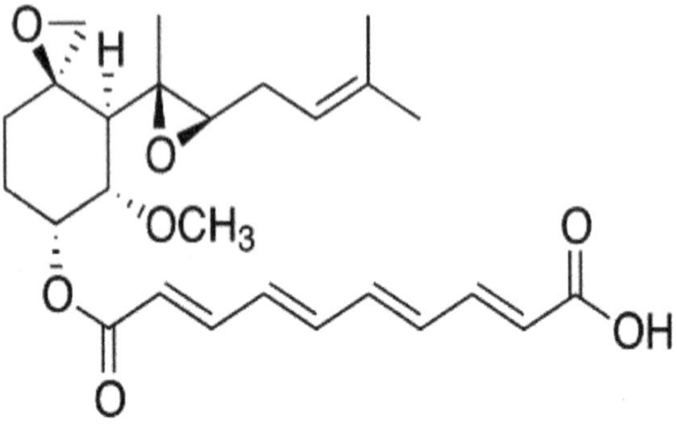

The above structure has been copied from the Ph. D. thesis of the main author, drawn with stencils)

Pharmacology

It was originally used against microsporidian parasites infections.

374

CHAPTER 12

MACROCYCLIC ANTIBIOTICS

12.1 List of macrocyclic antibiotics

(RIFAMYCINS)

1.	Rifamycin B
2.	Rifampin *(rifampicin)*
3.	Rifamycin SV
4.	Rifamide

12.2 Properties of individual important macrocyclic antibiotics

RIFAMYCIN

$$C_{37}H_{47}NO_{12}$$
Molar mass
697.778 g·mol−1

Chemistry

Rifamycins comprise a group of macrocyclic antibiotics which are predominantly effective against gram- positive organisms. They contain a chromophoric naphthohydroquinone system which is spanned by a long aliphatic bridge and hence belongs to the group of ansa compounds. The various compounds of this group differ in structure of their hydroquinone moieties. The most important id rifampin with less intestinal absorption have to given parentrally.

Structure activity relationship

❖ The aq. Solution of rifamycin on aeration gives rifamycin S. This convertion is carried through the formation of rifamycin O, which is hydrolysed to rifamycin S, having a quinone ring. The biological activity of rifamycin in vivo and vitro is much stronger than that of the parent compound.

❖ When rifamycin S is reduced, it produces rifamycin SV. When the quinone group is reduced to quinol group, is much active physiologically than rifamycin S.

❖ Rifamycin B can be oxidized to rifamycin O, which shows epioxide linkage and it has been found to have same antibacterial activity as rifamycin.

Pharmacology

Rifamycin have been used for the treatment of HIV-related tuberculosis.

Biosynthesis of Rifamycin

The first information on the rifamycin came from studies using the stable isotope Carbon-13 and to establish the origin of the carbon skeleton. The general scheme of biosynthesis starts with the uncommon starting unit, 3-amino-5-hydroxybenzoic acid (AHBA), via type I polyketide pathway (PKS I) in which chain extension is performed using 2 acetate and 8 propionate units.

Synthesis of Rifamycin

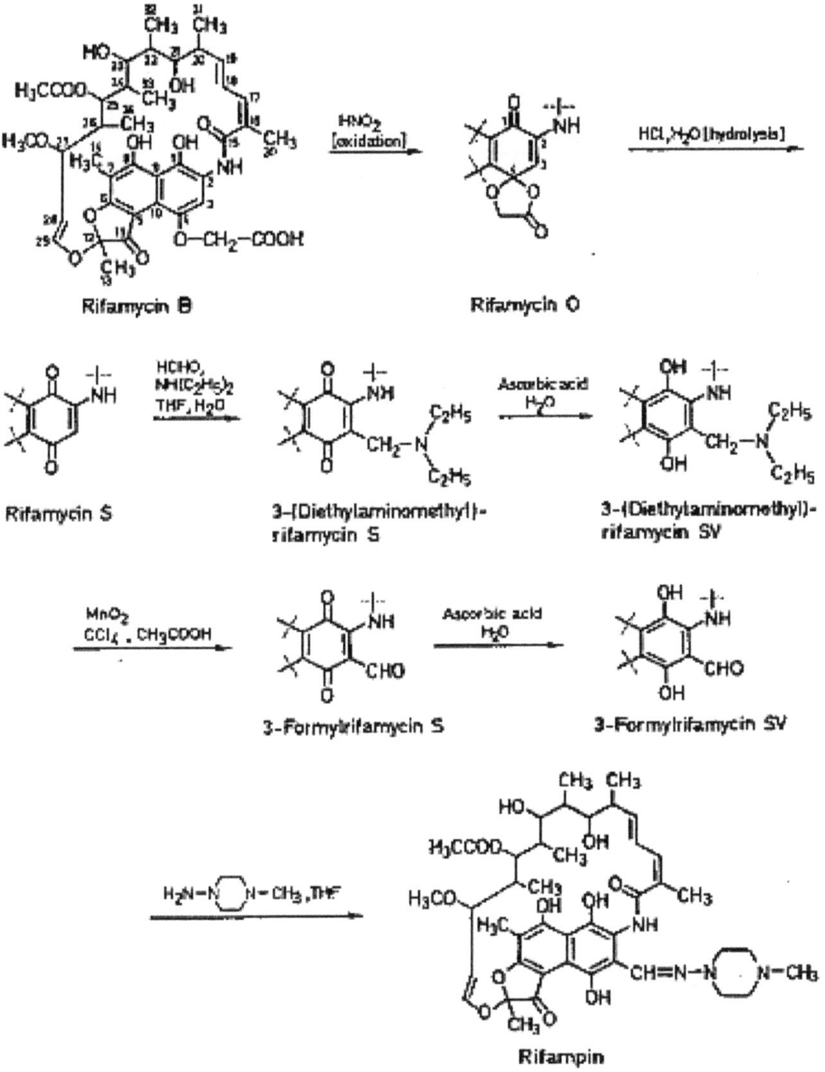
HNO2 [oxidation]
HCl, H2O [hydrolysis]
Rifamycin B
Rifamycin O
HCHO, NH(C2H5)2 THF, H2O
Ascorbic acid H2O
Rifamycin S
3-(Diethylaminomethyl)-rifamycin S
3-(Diethylaminomethyl)-rifamycin SV
MnO2 CCl4, CH3COOH
Ascorbic acid H2O
3-Formylrifamycin S
3-Formylrifamycin SV
THF
Rifampin

(The above structure has been copied from the Ph. D. thesis of the main author, drawn with stencils in 1988)

CHAPTER 13

ANTIBIOTICS FROM VARIOUS OTHER STRUCTURES

13.1 List of antibiotics with other various structures

1.	Vancomycin *(tricyclic glycosylated nonribosomal peptide)*
2.	Ristocetin
3.	Lincomycin *(lincosamide antibiotic)*
4.	Clindamycin
5.	Fosfomycin
6.	Novobiocin *(aminocoumarin antibiotic)*
7.	Puromycin *(aminonucleoside antibiotic)*

13.2 Properties of individual important antibiotics with various structures

VANCOMYCIN

$$C_{66}H_{75}Cl_2N_9O_{24}$$
Molar mass
1449.3 g.mol^{-1} g·mol^{-1}

Chemistry

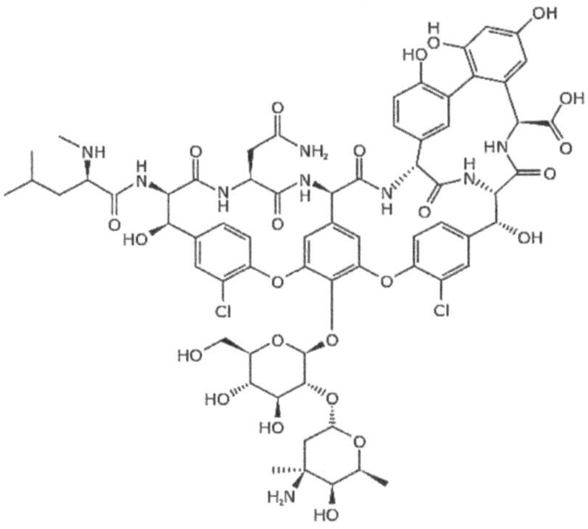

**The above structure has been copied from the Ph. D.
thesis of the main author, drawn with stencils in 1988)**

Pharmacology

Treatment of serious infections caused by susceptible organisms
resistant to penicillin (methicillin-resistant S. aureus. For treatment
of infections caused by Gram-positive microorganisms in patients
with serious allergies to beta-lactam antimicrobials. Vancomycin is
considered a last resort medication for the treatment of sepsis and
lower respiratory tract, skin, and bone infections.

Pharmacokinetics

Bioavailability	Negligible (by mouth)
Metabolism	Excreted unchanged
Elimination half life	4 - 6 hours (adults)
	6 - 10 days adults with impaired renal function
Excretion	Urine (IV), feces (by mouth)

Adverse effects

Local pain, which may be severe. Vancomycin has traditionally been considered a nephrotoxic and ototoxic drug.

RISTOCETIN

$$C_{94}H_{108}N_8O_{44}$$
Molar mass
2053.89052

Chemistry

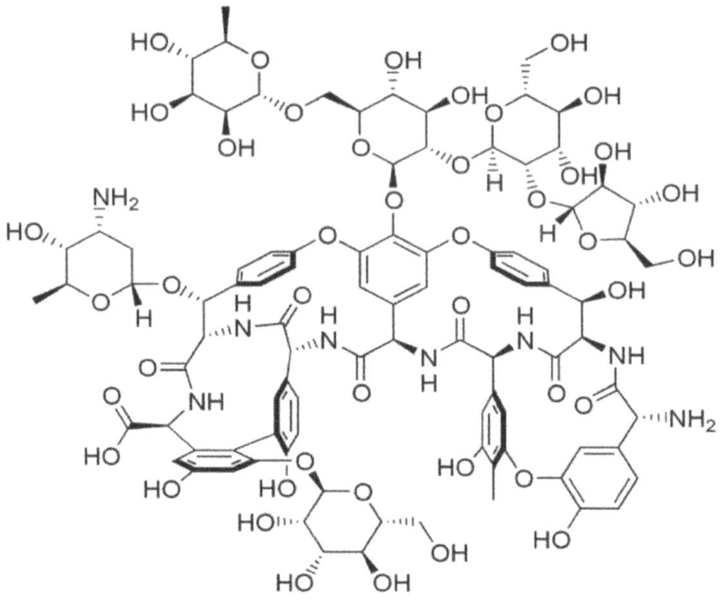

(The above structure has been copied from the Ph. D. thesis of the main author, drawn with stencils in 1988)

Pharmacology
Ristocetin is an antibiotic no longer used clinically.

LINCOMYCIN

$C_{18}H_{34}N_2O_6S$
Molar mass
406.54 g·mol^{-1}

Chemistry

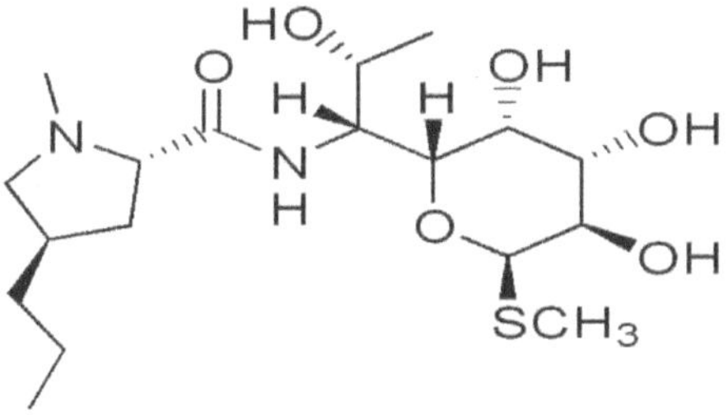

**(The above structure has been copied from the Ph. D.
thesis of the main author, drawn with stencils in 1988)**

Pharmacology

Lincomycin is a narrow spectrum antibiotic with activity against Gram-positive bacteria.

Pharmacokinetics

I.V., I.M.

Bioavailability	N/A
Metabolism	
Elimination half life	5.4 ± 1.0 h after IM or IV administration
Excretion	Renal and biliary

CLINDAMYCIN

$C_{18}H_{33}ClN_2O_5S$
Mola mass
424.98 g/mol g·mol−1

Chemistry

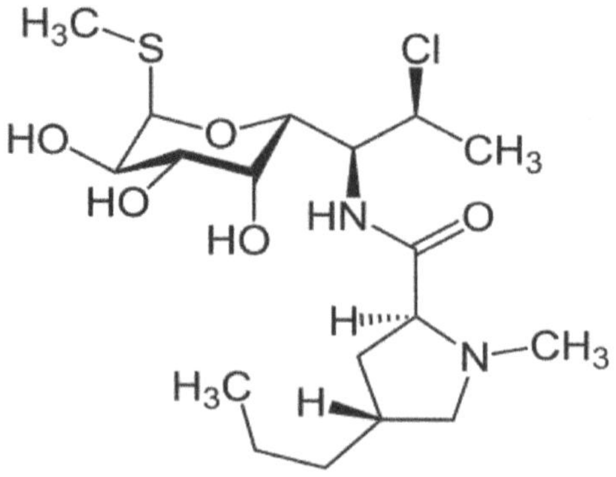

(The above structure has been copied from the Ph. D. thesis of the main author, drawn with stencils in 1988)

Pharmacology
Clindamycin is effective in treating malaria.

Pharmacokinetics

Bioavailability	90% (by mouth) –5% (topical)
Protein binding	95%
Metabolism	Hepatic
Elimination half life	2-3 hours
Excretion	Biliary and renal

Adverse effects
Include: diarrhea, pain, dryness, burning, itching, scaliness, or peeling of skin.

FOSFOMYCIN

$C_3H_7O_4P$
Molar mass
138.059 g/mol g·mol^{-1}

Chemistry

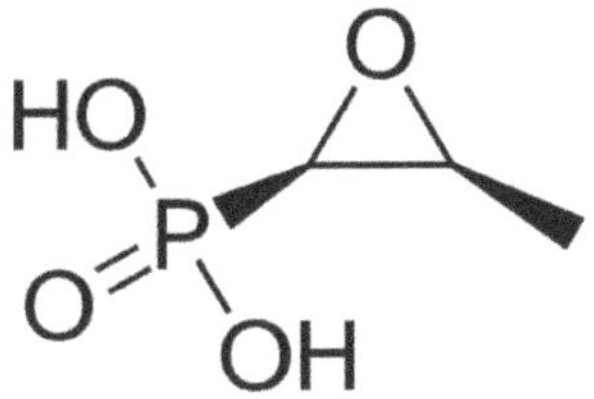

(The above structure has been copied from the Ph. D. thesis of the main author, drawn with stencils in 1988)

Pharmacology

Fosfomycin has broad antibacterial activity against both Gram-positive and Gram-negative pathogens.

Pharmacokinetics

Bioavailability	30–37% (by mouth
Protein binding	N/A
Metabolism	N/A
Elimination half life	5-7 hours
Excretion	Kidney and feacal

NOVOBIOCIN
(albamycin or cathomycin)

$$C3_1H_{36}N_2O_{11}$$
Molar mass
612.624 g·mol−1

Chemistry:

Novobiocin is an aminocoumarin. Novobiocin may be divided up into three fragments:

 ➢ a benzoic acid derivative

➤ a coumarin residue
➤ the sugar novobiose

Novobiocin, also known as albamycin or cathomycin, is produced by the actinomycete, which has been identified as a subjective synonym for S. spheroides. Other aminocoumarin antibiotics include:

- clorobiocin
- coumermycin A1

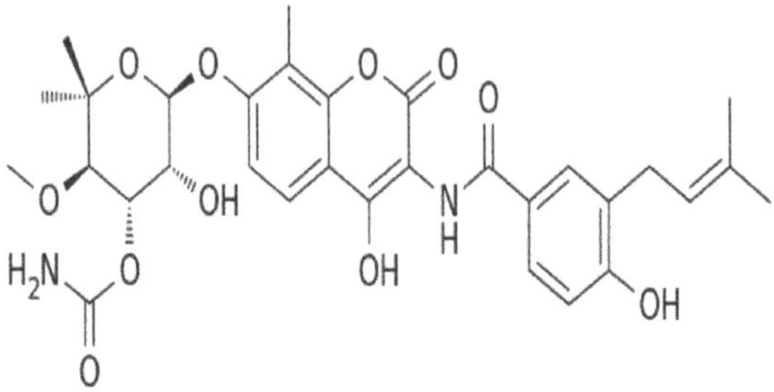

(The above structure has been copied from the Ph. D. thesis of the main author, drawn with stencils in 1988)

Structure–activity relationship
In structure activity relationship it was found that removal of the carbomoyl group located on the novobiose sugar leads to a dramatic decrease in inhibitory activity of novobiocin.

Pharmacology
It is active against to differentiate it from the other coagulase-negative which is resistant to novobiocin, in culture.

Pharmacokinetics

Bioavailability	Negligible oral bioavailability
Metabolism	Excreted unchanged
Elimination half life	6 hours
Excretion	Renal

PUROMYCIN

$$C_{22}H_{29}N_7O_5$$
Molar mass
471.50956 g/mol^{-1}

Chemistry

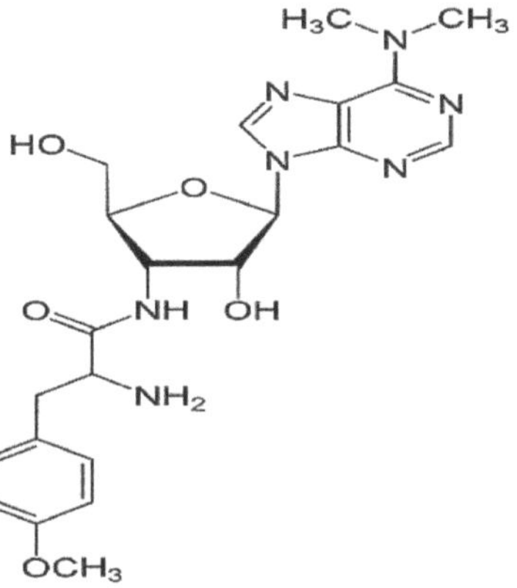

**(The above structure has been copied from the Ph. D.
thesis of the main author, drawn with stencils in 1988)**

Pharmacology
Puromycin is selective for various infections.

CHAPTER 14

SYNTHETIC QUINOLONE GROUP OF ANTIBIOTICS (MACROCYCLIC)

14.1 General chemistry of Quinolone antibiotics (macrocyclic)

The quinolones synthetic antibacterial agents, a naphthyridine derivative introduced for the treatment of urinary tract infections. Isosteric heterocyclic groupings in this class included:

o   the quinolines (nortoxacin, ciprotloxacin, and lomefloxacin),
o   the naphthyridine (nalidixic acid and enoxacin),
o   the cinnolines (cinoxacin).

Structure-activity studies have shown that the 1,4-dihydro-4-oxo-3-pyridine carboxylic acid moiety is essential for antibacterial activity. The pyridine system must be annulated with an aromatic ring. Isosteric replacements of Nitrogen for carbon atoms at positions 2 (cinnolines), 5 (1,5-napthyridines), 6 (1.6-naphthyridines), and 8 (1.8-naphthyridines) are consistent with retained antibacterial activity. Introduction of substituents at position 2 greatly reduces or abolishes activity, positions 5, 6, 7 (especially), and 8 of the annulated ring systems may be substituted to good effect.

Formation of Chelate

The quinolones may form chelates with metal ions such as Ca*, Mg, Zn*, Fe, and Bi. The stoichiometry of the chelate formed will depend on a variety of factors, such as the relative concentrations of chelating agent (quinolone) and metal ion present.

14.2 List of quinolone antibiotics

FIRST GENERATION
Oxolinic acid, Rosoxin
Structurally related drugs but not formally 4-quinolon include:
Cinoxacin, Nalidixic acid, Piromidic acid, Pepimidic acid

SECOND GENERATION
Second generation is sub-divided in class 1 and class 2
Ciprofloxacin, Fleroxacin, Lomefloxacin, Nadifloxacin, Norfloxacin, Ofloxacin, Pefloxacin, Rufloxacin
Structurally related drug but not formally 4-quinolon include: Enoxacin

THIRD GENERATION
Unlike the first and second generation, the third generation is active against *streptococci*.
Balofloxacin, Grepafloxacin, Levofloxacin, Pazufloxacin, Sparfloxacin, Temafloxacin
Structurally related third generation drug but not formally 4-quinolons include: Tosufloxacin

---

FOURTH GENERATION

This generation **FLUROQUINOLONES** unlike 1-3 generations, act at DNA gyrase and topoisomerase IV. This dual action slows the development of resistance.

Clinafloxacin, Gatifloxacin, Moxifloxacin, Sitafloxacin, Prulifloxacin, Besifloxacin, Delafloxacin

Structurally related fourth generation drug but not formally 4-quinolons include:
Ozenoxacin

Two structurally related fourth generation drugs but not formally 4-quinolons include:

Gemifloxacin, Trovafloxacin

VETERINARY COMPOUNDS

Flumequine (first generation), Danofloxacin, Difloxacin, Enrofloxacin, Ibafloxacin, Marbofloxacin, Orbifloxacin, Sarafloxacin

---

14.3 General chemistry of quinolone antibiotics

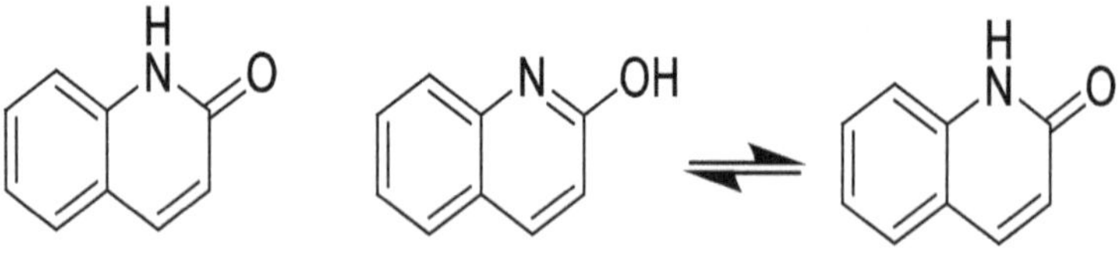

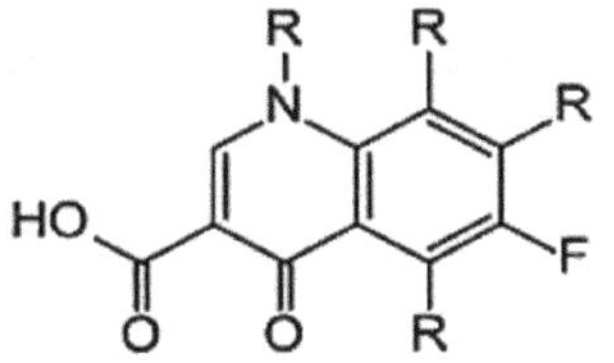

General structure of quinolone antibiotics
R = is / may be alkyl or phenyl
F = is fluorine (it is fluoroquinolones)

(The above structure has been copied from the Ph. D.
thesis of the main author, drawn with stencils in 1988)

A quinolone antibiotic is any member of a large group of broad -spectrum bactericides that share a bicyclic core structure related to the compound 4 - quinolone. They are used in human and veterinary medicine to treat bacterial infections. Nearly all quinolone antibiotics in modern use are fluoroquinolones.

1,8 – naphthyridine
1,8 - diazanaphthalene

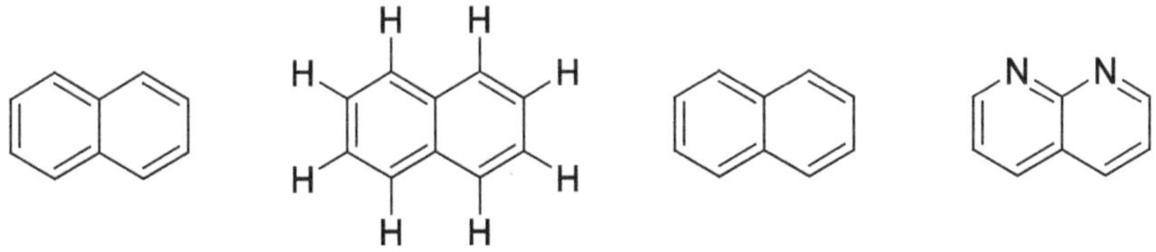

Topoisomerase inhibitor / inhibit DNA replication

First generation
Nalidixic acid

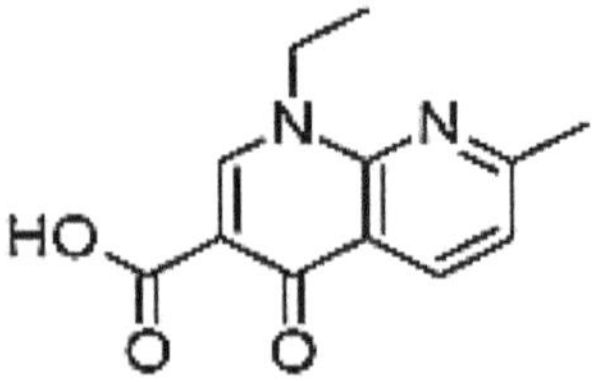

Second generation
Ciprofloxacin

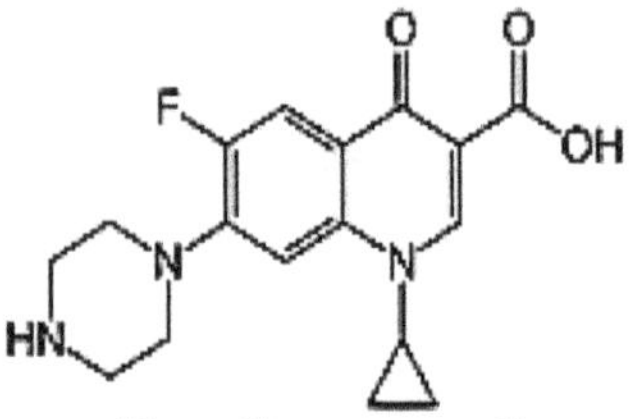

Third generation
Levofloxacin, oral, i.v., eyedrops

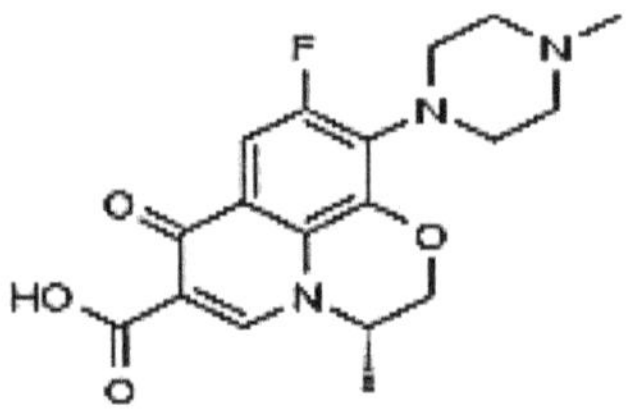

Fourth generation
Moxifloxacin, oral, i.v., eyedrops

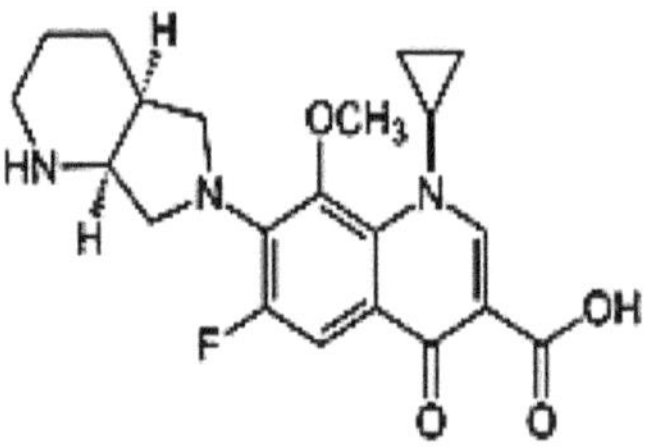

(The above structures have been copied from the Ph. D. thesis of the main author, drawn with stencils in 1988)

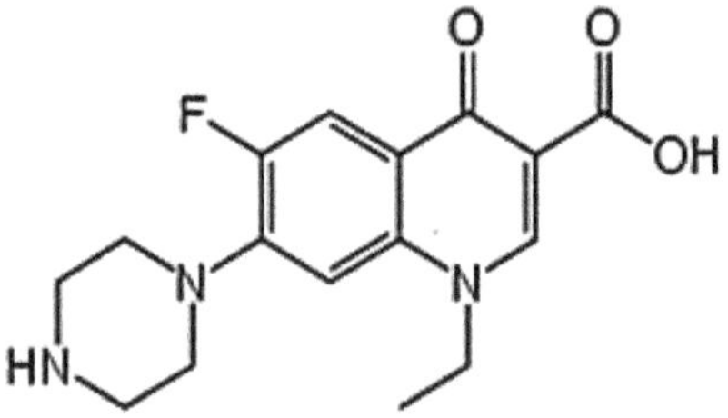

Structure of Norfloxacin

Pharmacokinetic properties of some fluoroquinolone

Type of Fluoroquinolone drug	Half-life (h)	Oral bioavailability (%)	Peak serum concentration (mcg/ml)	Oral dose (mg)	Primary route of excretion

390

Ciprofloxacin	3-5	70	2.4	500	Renal
Gatifloxacin	8	98	3.4	400	Renal
Gemifloxacin	8	70	1.6	320	Renal and non-renal
Levofloxacin	5-7	95	5.7	500	Renal
Lomefloxacin	8	95	2.8	400	Renal
Moxifloxacin	9-10	>85	3.1	400	Non-renal
Norfloxacin	3.5-5	80	1.5	400	Renal
Ofloxacin	5-7	95	2.9	400	Renal

14.4 Properties of individual important compound from quinolone group of antibiotics

FIRST GENERATION	Nalidixic acid
SECOND GENERATION (Flouroquinolone)	Norfloxacin Ciprofloxacin Ofloxacin Enoxacin Lomefloxacin Rufloxacin
THIRD GENERATION	Levofloxacin
FOURTH GENERATION	Moxifloxacin

NALIDIXIC ACID

$$C_{12}H_{12}N_2O_3$$
Molar mass
232.235 g/mol g·mol−1

Chemistry

Nalidixic acid is the first of the synthetic quinolone. In a technical sense, it is a naphthyridone, not a quinolone: its ring structure contains two nitrogen atoms, unlike quinoline, which has a single nitrogen atom. Synthetic quinolone antibiotics were discovered in the 1960.

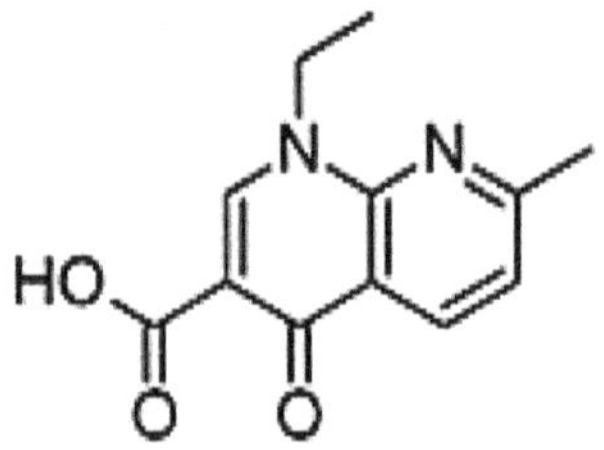

(The above structure has been copied from the Ph. D. thesis of the main author, drawn with stencils in 1988)

Pharmacology
Nalidixic acid is effective primarily against gram-negative bacteria, In higher concentrations, it is bactericidal, meaning that it kills bacteria instead of merely inhibiting their growth. Oral administration.

Pharmacokinetics

Protein binding	90%
Metabolism	Partially hepatic
Elimination half life	6-7 hours, longer in renal impairment

Common side effects
Common adverse effects include rash, itchy skin, blurred or double vision, halos around lights, changes in color vision, nausea, vomiting and diarrhea. Convulsions and hyperglycemia.

Synthesis of nalidixic acid

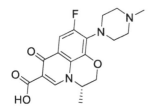

(The above structures have been copied from the Ph. D. thesis of the main author, drawn with stencils in 1988)

Nalidixic acid

Ciprofloxacin

Levofloxacin

Moxifloxacin

CIPROFLOXACIN
(Fluoroquinolone)

$$C_{17}H_{18}FN_3O_3$$
Molar mass
331.346 g/mol g·mol⁻¹

Chemistry

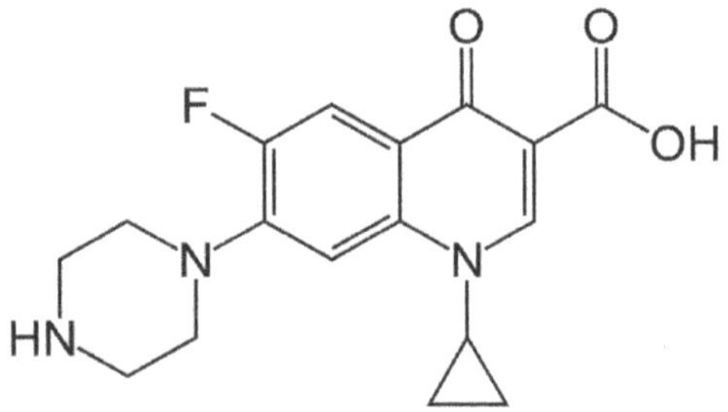

(The above structure has been copied from the Ph. D. thesis of the main author, drawn with stencils in 1988)

Pharmacology
Ciprofloxacin is the most widely used of the second-generation quinolones, to treat a wide variety of infections, including infections of bones and joints. Ciprofloxacin only treats bacterial infections; it does not treat viral infections for certain uses including acute sinusitis, lower respiratory tract infections.

Pharmacokinetics
Penetration into the central nervous system is relatively modest, with cerebrospinal fluid levels normally less than 10% of peak serum concentrations. The serum half-life of ciprofloxacin is about 4–6 hours, with 50-70% of an administered dose being excreted in the urine as unmetabolized drug.

Bioavailability	70%
Protein binding	30%
Metabolism	Liver
Elimination half life	3-5 hours
Excretion	Kidneys

Common side effects

Adverse effects can involve the tendons, muscles, joints, nerves, and the central nervous system.

Interactions

Ciprofloxacin interacts with certain foods and several other drugs leading to undesirable increases or decreases in the serum levels or distribution of one or both drugs.

(a)TEA, toluene (b) Cyclopropylamine, (c) Potassium carbonate + DMF, (d) piperazine

Synthesis of Ciprofloxacin

(a) TEA, (b) piperazine), (c)H_2, (d) HNO_3 +HCl, (e) HNO_3 + $CaCl_2$, (f) Raney nickle

OFLOXACIN
(Fluoroquinolone)

$$C_{18}H_{20}FN_3O_4$$
Molar mass
361.368 g/mol g·mol^{-1}

Chemistry

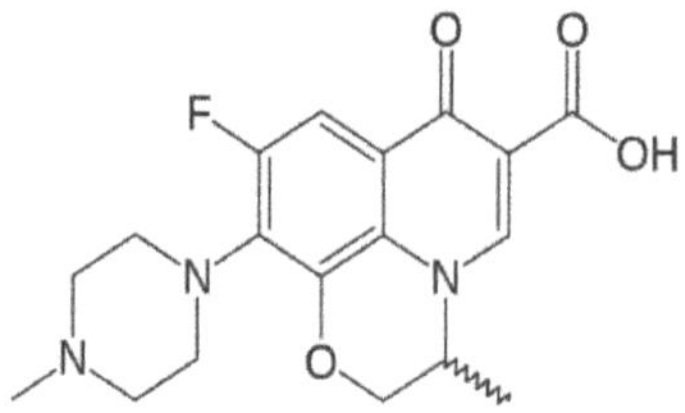

(The above structure has been copied from the Ph. D. thesis of the main author, drawn with stencils in 1988)

Pharmacology
Uncomplicated skin and skin structure infections. Mixed Infections. Acute, uncomplicated urethral and cervical gonorrhea.

Pharmacokinetics
The ofloxacin in the tablet form is roughly 98% following oral administration, reaching maximum serum concentrations within one to two hours.

Between 65% and 80% of an administered oral dose of ofloxacin is excreted unchanged via the kidneys within 48 hours of dosing. Therefore, elimination is mainly by renal excretion.

Bioavailability	85-95%
Protein binding	32%
Metabolism	Liver
Elimination half life	8-9 hours
Excretion	Kidneys

Common side effects
The concomitant administration of a nonsteroidal anti-inflammatory drug with a quinolone, may increase the risk of central nervous system stimulation and convulsive seizures.

Contraindications

Ofloxacin is now considered to be for the treatment of certain sexually transmitted diseases.

ENOXACIN
(Fluoroquinolone)

$C_{15}H_{17}FN_4O_3$
Molar mass
320.319 g/mol g·mol−1

Chemistry

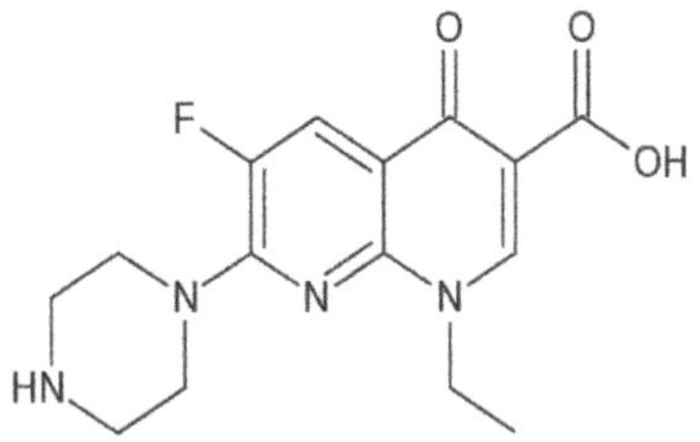

(The above structure has been copied from the Ph. D. thesis of the main author, drawn with stencils in 1988)

Pharmacology

Enoxacin is an oral broad-spectrum, articularly GIT including infectious diarrhea.

Pharmacokinetics

The serum elimination half-life, in subjects with normal renal function, is approximately 6 hours. Approximately 60% of an orally administered dose is excreted in the urine as unchanged drug within 24 hours. A small amount of a dose of drug administered is excreted in the bile.

Common side effects

Enoxacin, like other fluoroquinolones, is known to trigger seizers.

397

Interactions

Co-administration with these substances can lead to therapeutic failure of the antibiotic due to decreased absorption by the intestinal tract.

LOMEFLOXACIN
(Fluoroquinolone)

$C_{17}H_{19}F_2N_3O_3$
Molar mass
351.348 g/mol g·mol^{-1}

Chemistry

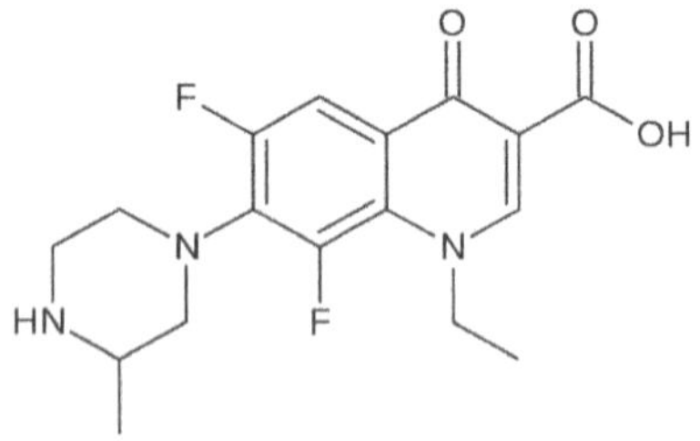

(The above structure has been copied from the Ph. D. thesis of the main author, drawn with stencils in 1988)

Pharmacology
is used to treat infections to prevent urinary tract infections.

Pharmacokinetics
protein binding: 10 %, Elimination half- life: 8 hours

RUFLOXACIN
(Fluoroquinolone)

$C_{17}H_{18}FN_3O_3S$
Molar mass
363.406 g/mol g·mol^{-1}

Chemistry

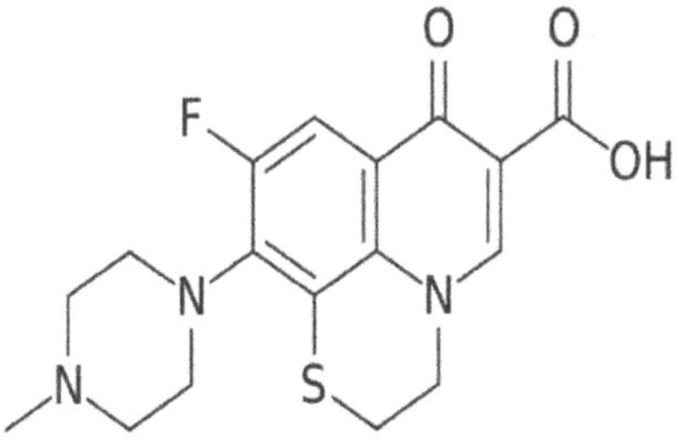

**(The above structure has been copied from the Ph. D.
thesis of the main author, drawn with stencils in 1988)**

Nemonoxacin is a non-fluorinated quinolone antibiotic undergoing
clinical trials. It has the same mechanism of action as fluouroquinolones.
Is more potent than Levofloxacin and moxifloxacin.

NEMONOXACIN

$C_{20}H_{25}N_3O_4$
Molar mass
371.437 g·mol^{-1}

Chemistry
Nemonoxacin is a non-fluorinated.

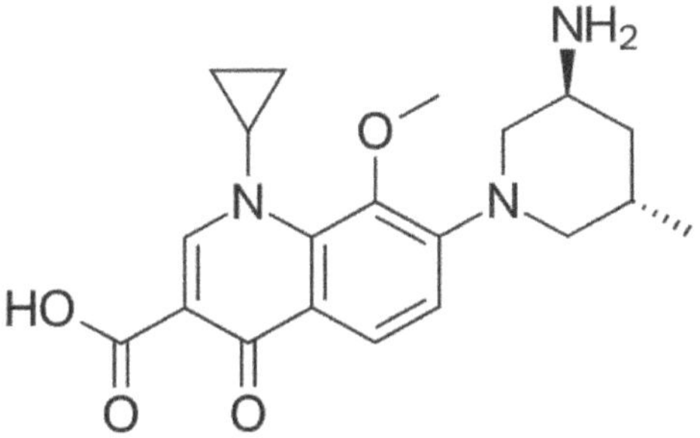

**(The above structure has been copied from the Ph. D.
thesis of the main author, drawn with stencilsin 1988)**

399

Pharmacology

Nemonoxacin has a broad spectrum of activity against gram +ive and gram -ive bacteria and atypical pathogens, including activity against (MRSA) (MIC90 1 g/ml).

CHAPTER 15

ANTINEOPLASIC ANTIBIOTICS
(Cancer or malignant tumor or malignant neoplasm)

15.1 Etiological factors responsible that may develop cancer cell

i. Radiation

- ❖ Ionizing radiation
- ❖ Radioactive elements
- ❖ Ultraviolet radiation

ii. Chemical substances

- ❖ Air pollution
- ❖ Alimentary factors

iii. Iatrogenic chemical factors

- ❖ Drugs
- ❖ Hormones

iv. Personal habits

- ❖ Smoking
- ❖ Alcohol
- ❖ Sex life
- ❖ Circumcision

v. Parasites

vi. Viruses

Teratoma	Tumor made up of several different types of tissue, such as hair, muscle, teeth, or bone or development of new cancer including cells of the body organ tissues. (comprise mesodermal and endodermal elements).
Anticarcinogen	Antitumor, antineoplastics, anti-cancers.
Cytotoxic	Cancer.
Mutation	Is a change in a DNA sequence that can result from DNA copying mistakes made during cell division, exposure to ionizing radiation, exposure to chemicals called mutagens or infection causd by the viruses.
Mutagen	Is a physical or chemical agent that changes the genetic material, usually DNA.
Dermoid	Is composed of only of dermal and epidermal element.
Somatic hypermutation:	is a cellular mechanism by which the immune system adapts to the new foreign elements that confront it.
Metastasis	Secondary cancer originating from parent cancer.
Neoplasm	A neoplasm is a type of abnormal and excessive growth, called neoplasia. The growth of a neoplasm is uncoordinated with that of the normal surrounding tissue, and persists in growing abnormally, even if the original trigger is removed. This abnormal growth usually forms a mass when it may be called a tumor.
Carcinogenesis	also called oncogenesis or tumorigenesis, is the formation of a cancer, whereby normal cells are transformed into cancer cells.

The central role of DNA damage and epigenetic defects in DNA repair genes in carcinogenesis.

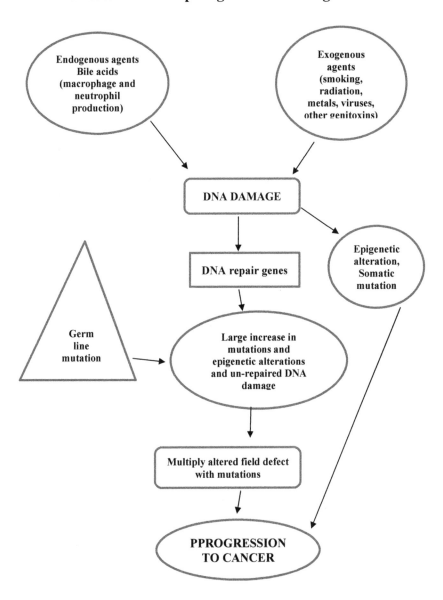

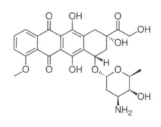

Daunorubicin

Doxirubicin

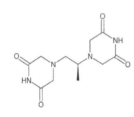

Epirubicin

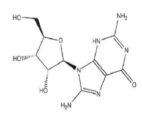

Idarubicin

Dexrazoxane

Trastuzumab

(The above structures have been copied from the Ph. D. thesis of the main author, drawn with stencils in 1988)

Trastuzumab in breast cancer

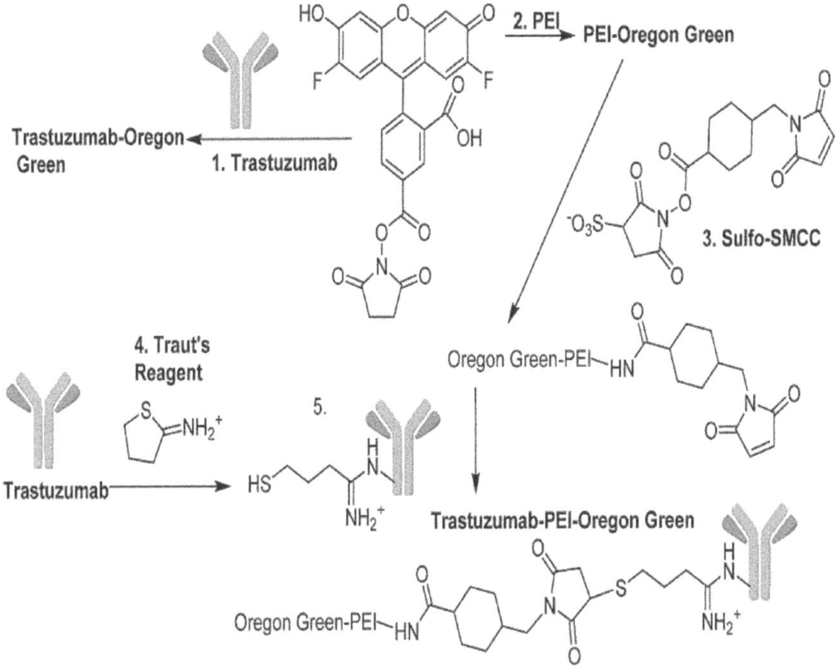

(The above structures have been copied from the Ph. D. thesis of the main author, drawn with stencils in 1988)

This chemicall heterogenous group of antibiotics many therapeutically active compounds. Some of these antibiotics have proved to be active clinivally, used as single or in combination therapy in certain malignant diseases.

Epirubicin

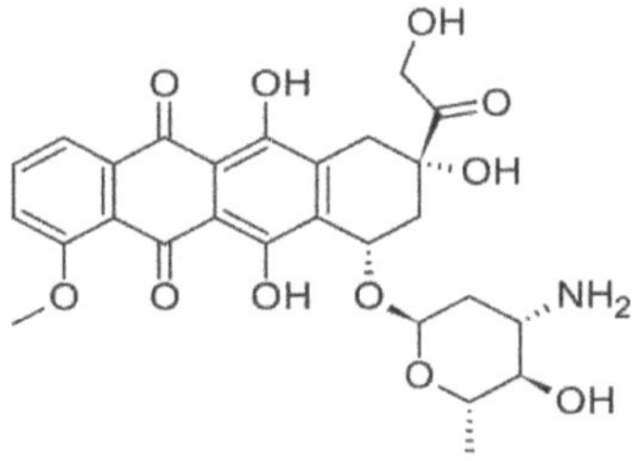

Pirarubicin

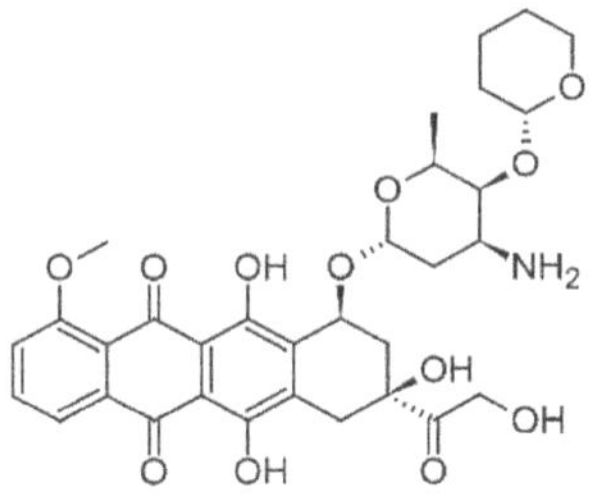

(The above structures have been copied from the Ph. D. thesis of the main author, drawn with stencils)

Nogalamycin   Menogaril

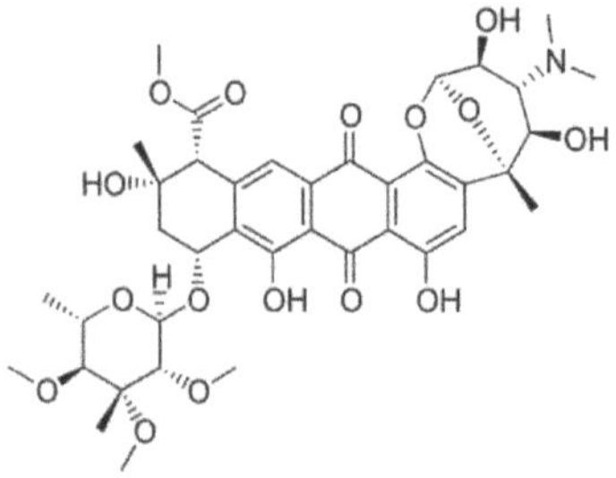

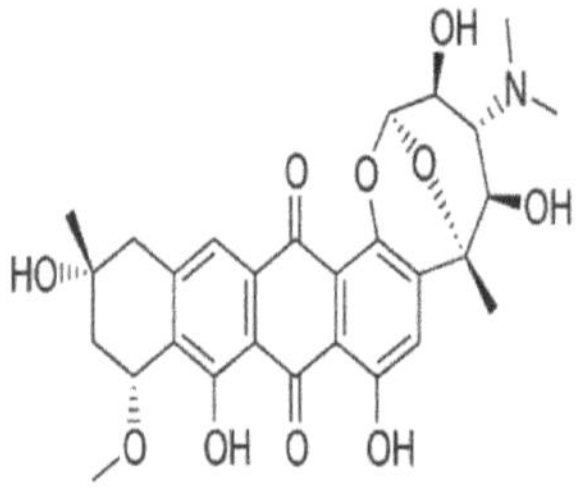

(The above structures have been copied from the Ph. D. thesis of the main author, drawn with stencil in 1988)

❖ Hair loss, Infertility, Teratogenicity, Peripheral neuropathy, Cognitive impairment Tumor lysis syndrome, Organ damage, Limitation of cytotoxic therapy, Resistance of cytotoxic therapy

Mechanism of action in general

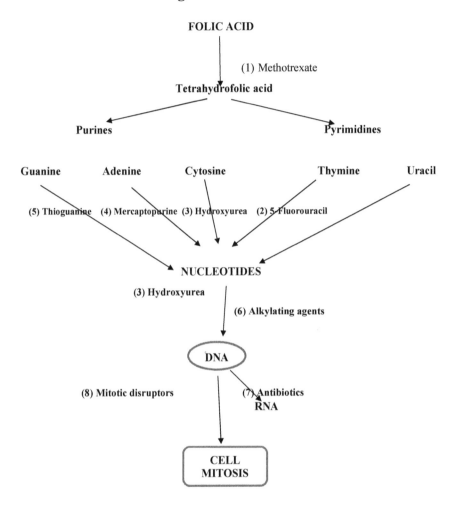

15.2 Classification of chemically heterogenous group of antitumor antibiotics

Antitumor agents are classified by their effects on cell survival as a function of dose. For many drugs, including alkylating agents, cell survival is exponentially related to dose, and a plot of log cell survival against drug concentration gives a straight line. They exert their cytotoxicity regardless of the cell cycle phase and are termed noncell cycle phase-specific, other drugs include antimetabolites and mitotic inhibitors, which act at one phase of the cell cycle (cell cycle phase-specific), show a plateau after an initial low-dose exponential region.

1.	Sarkomycin
2.	L-azaserine
3.	6-diazo-5-oxo-L-norleucine
4.	Mitomycin C
5.	Stretonigrin
6.	Bleomycin
7.	Peplomycin
8.	Streptozocin
9.	Dactinomycin (actinomycin D)
10.	Daunorubicin (daunomycin or rubidomycin)
11.	Doxorubicin (adriamycin)
12.	Aclarubicin (aclacinimycin A)
13.	Mithramycin (aureolic acid)

Some of the above listed antibiotics are very successful clinically as a single agent or in combination with other antitumor agents in malignant diseases.

- Doxorubicin brought about remissions in sarcoma, breast cancer, acute leukemia, neuroblastoma and Wilms tumor. Acrarubicin showed similar effectiveness as doxorubicin but less cardiotoxic. Daunorubicin has shown effectiveness n acute leukemias.
- Dactinomycin in testicular carcinoma.
- Bleomycin and peplomycin in squamous cell carcinomas and testicular carcinoma.

- Mithramycin in testicular embryonal cell carcinoma.
- Stretozocin in islet cell carcinoma of the pancreas.

Anti-tumor drugs are classified as chemotherapeutic agents such as methotrexate, chlorambucin, 6-mercaptopurine, cyclophosphamide, 5-fluorouracil, cytarabine, carmustine, procarbazine, cisplatin, mechlorethamine and doxifluridine. All these drugs mentioned above may be use alone or in combination of antitumor antibiotics.

The vinca alkaloids (vinblastine and vincristine), isolated from a plant (*Cantharanthus roseus or Vinca rosea*) are not antibiotics but falls in a broader definition. These alkaloids display a powerful antimitotic (Antimitotic agents are the compounds that arrest cells multiplication in mitosis) activity by interference with spindle formation including metaphase arrest. Despite their close structural similarity, vinblastine and vincristine differ both in clinical spectrum of activity and toxicity. Vincristine causes less bone marrow depression the vinblastine, but more neuro toxic effects. Vincristine is effective in the treatment of acute lymphoblastic leukemia, lympho sarcoma and neuroblastoma. Vinblastine is used in the treatment of Hodgkin's disease, testicular carcinoma and methotrexate- resistant chriocarcinoma.

15.3 List of important antitumor antibiotics

(commonly used in therapy)

1.	**DACTINOMYCIN** *(Actinomycin D)*
2.	**DAUNORUBICIN** *(Daunomycin)*
3.	**DOXORUBICIN** *(Adriamycin)*
4.	**IDARUBICIN**

5.	ACLARUBICIN (*Aclacinomycin A*)
6.	PIRARUBICIN
7.	ESORUBICIN
8.	EPIRUBACIN
9.	CARUBICIN (*Carminomycin*)
10.	ADREAMYCINOL
11.	DAUNOMYCINOL
12.	NOGALAMYCIN
13.	MENOGARIL
14.	MITHRAMYCIN PLICAMYCIN or MITHRACIN (*Aureolic acid derivatives*)
15.	BLEOMYCIN (A2)
16.	BLEOMYCIN (A5) (*Pingyangmycin*)
17.	MITOMYCIN A1, B1, C1, D1
18.	OLIVOMYCIN (*Chromomycins used in Japan, Variamycins used in Russia*)

15.4 Properties of individual antitumor antibiotics with various structures

DACTINOMYCIN
(*Actinomycin D*)

$C_{62}H_{86}N_{12}O_{16}$
Molar mass
1255.42 g/mol g·mol^{-1}

Chemistry

(actinomycin D) is a crystalline antibiotic composed of a phenoxazone chromophore and two cyclic peptide chains obtained as a product of fermentation by Streptomyces parvulus. The drug intercalates into DNA between adjacent guanine–cytosine base pairs and inhibits DNA-directed RNA synthesis.

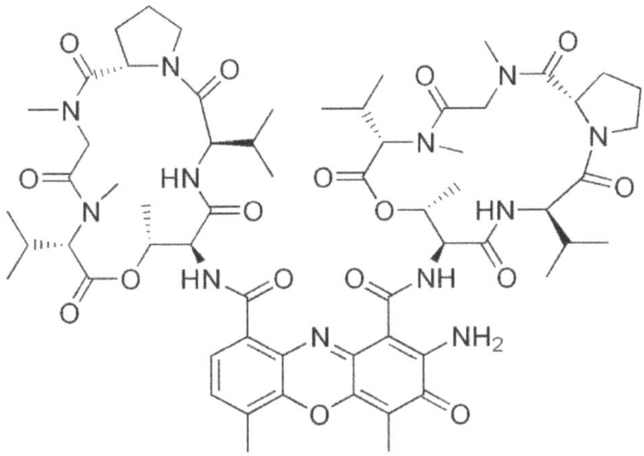

(The above structures have been copied from the Ph. D. thesis of the main author, drawn with stencils in 1988)

Pharmacology
Dactinomycin is used to treat a number of different type of cancers. It is also used in adjunct to radiotherapy.

Pharmacokinetics

Protein binding	5%
Elimination half life	36 hours
Administration	I.V.

DAUNORUBICIN
(Daunomycin)

411

$$C_{27}H_{29}NO_{10}$$
Molar mass
527.52 g/mol
563.99 g/mol (HCl salt) g·mol⁻¹

Chemistry

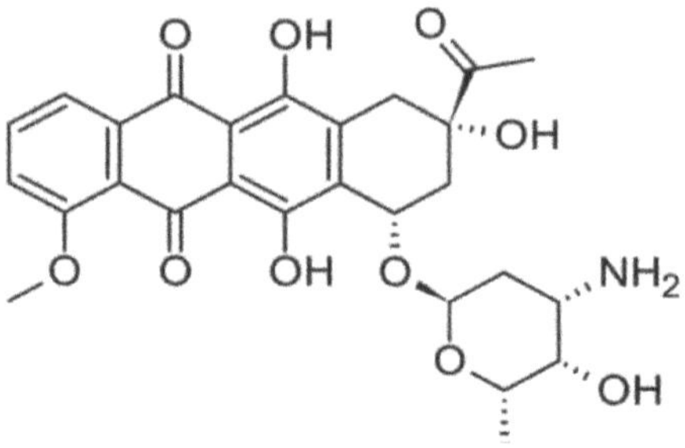

(The above structure has been copied from the Ph. D. thesis of the main author, drawn with stencils in 1988)

Pharmacology

It slows or stops the growth of cancer cells in the body. Treatment is usually performed together with other chemotherapy drugs.

Pharmacokinetics

Protein binding	5%
Metabolism	Liver
Elimination half life	26.7 hours
Excretion	Biliary and urinary
	I.M., I.V., S.C.

Common side effects

Hair loss, vomiting, Inflammation of the inside of the mouth. Severe side effects include cardiac problems.

Synthesis of Daunorubicin 1

Daunorubicin and doxorubicin are efficient agents for cancer treatment. Benzoic acid ester derivatives of daunorubicin were synthesized by nucleophilic esterification of the 14-bromodaunorubicin with the potassium salt of the corresponding benzoic acid, resulting in good yields.

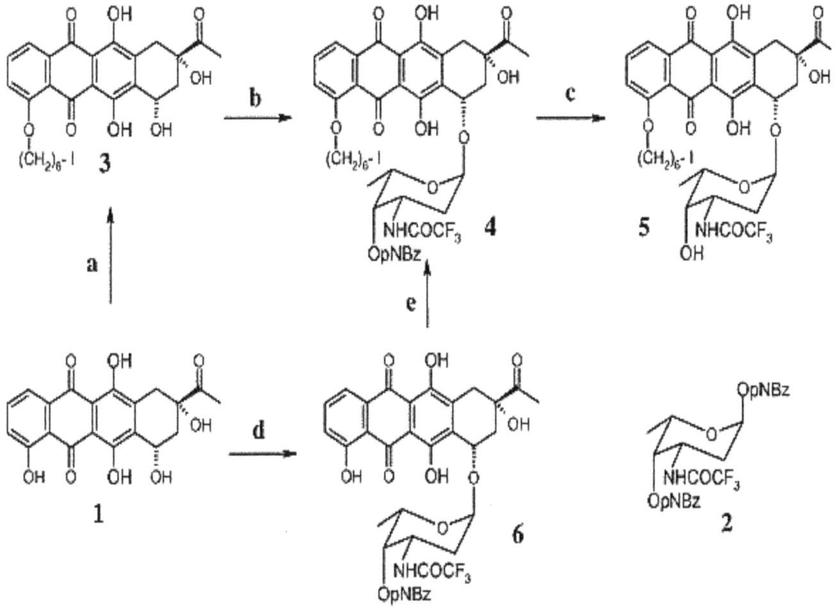

(The above structures have been copied from the Ph. D. thesis of the main author, drawn with stencils in 1988)

413

Synthesis of Daunorubicin 2

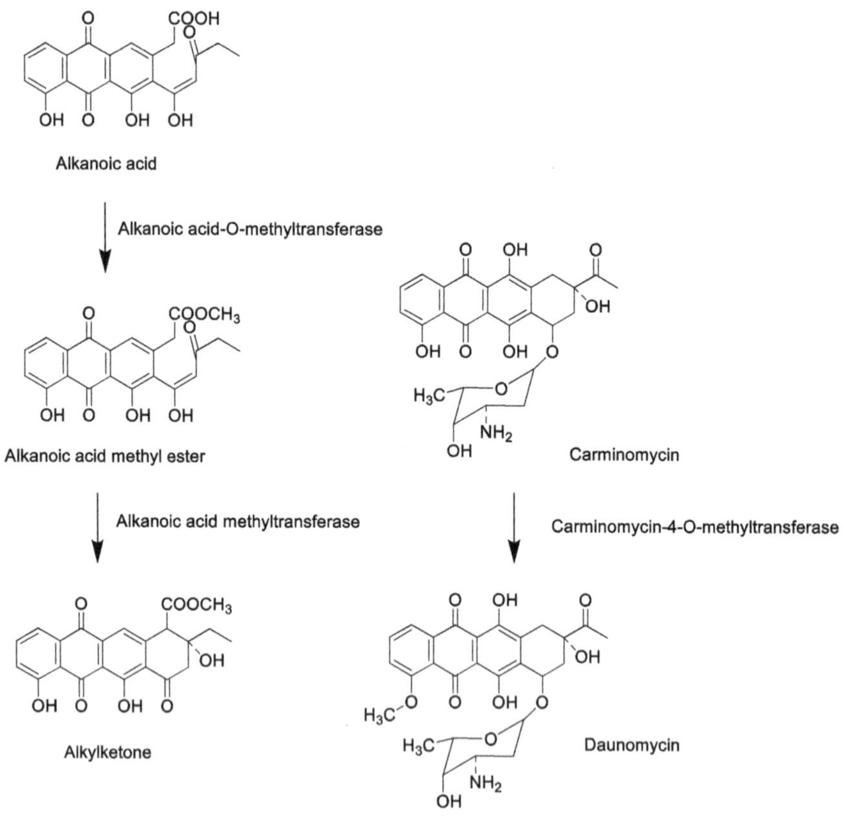

Alkanoic acid

Alkanoic acid-O-methyltransferase

Alkanoic acid methyl ester

Carminomycin

Alkanoic acid methyltransferase

Carminomycin-4-O-methyltransferase

Alkylketone

Daunomycin

DOXORUBICIN
(Adriamycin)

$C_{27}H_{29}NO_{11}$
Molar mass
543.525 g·mol^{-1}

Chemistry

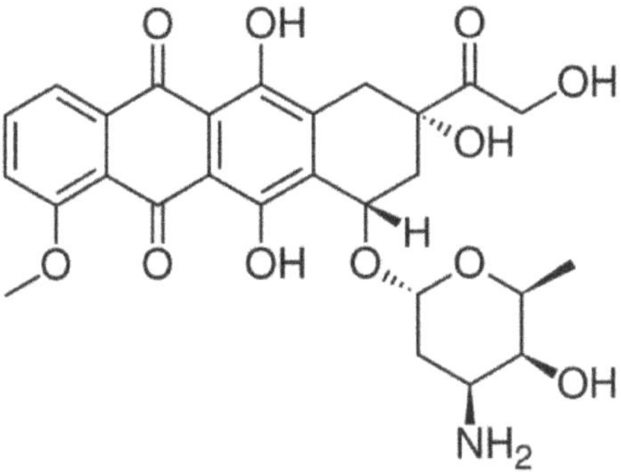

**(The above structure has been copied from the Ph. D.
thesis of the main author, drawn with stencils in 1988)**

Pharmacology

Doxorubicin is commonly used to treat cancers. Commonly used doxorubicin-containing AC (Adriamycin, cyclophosphamide, hydroxydaunorubicin and FAC.

Pharmacokinetics

Protein binding	75%
Bioavailability	5% by mouth
Metabolism	Liver
Elimination half life	3.5 hours
Excretion	Urine 5-10%,
	Faces40-50%
	I.V., Intravesical

Common side effects

Doxorubicin-induced cardiomyopathy typically results in dilated cardiomyopathy, with all four cardiac chambers being enlarged, rash.

Synthesis of Doxorubicin

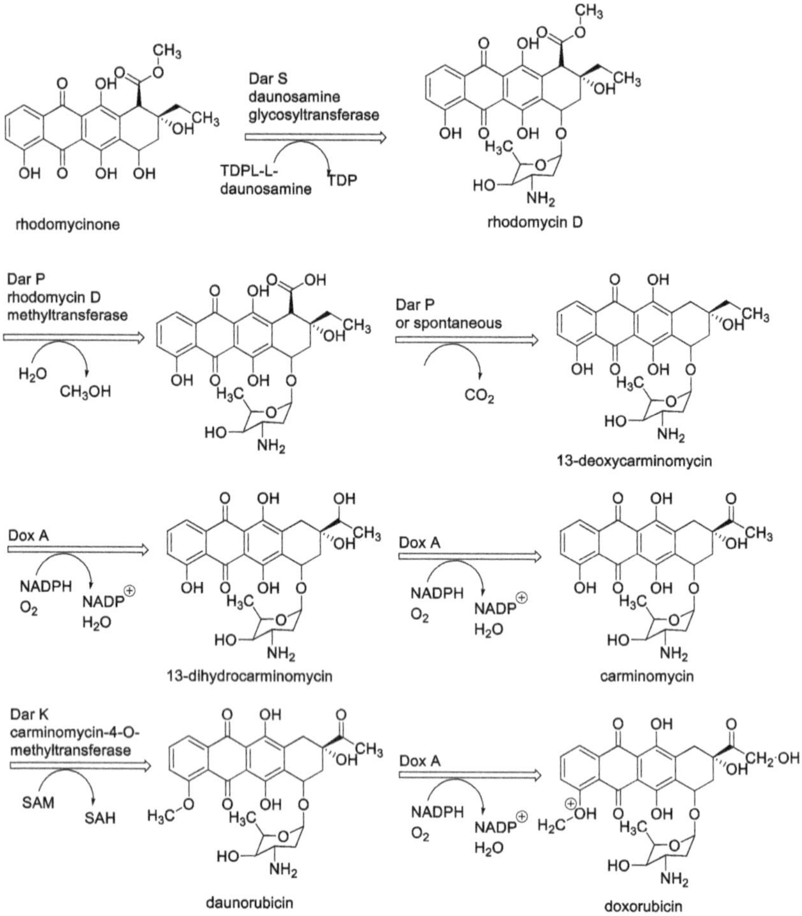

rhodomycinone

Dar S
daunosamine
glycosyltransferase

TDPL-L-
daunosamine → TDP

rhodomycin D

Dar P
rhodomycin D
methyltransferase

H_2O
CH_3OH

Dar P
or spontaneous

CO_2

13-deoxycarminomycin

Dox A

NADPH
O_2 → NADP$^{\oplus}$
H_2O

13-dihydrocarminomycin

Dox A

NADPH
O_2 → NADP$^{\oplus}$
H_2O

carminomycin

Dar K
carminomycin-4-O-
methyltransferase

SAM → SAH

daunorubicin

Dox A

NADPH
O_2 → NADP$^{\oplus}$
H_2O

doxorubicin

IDARUBICIN

$$C_{26}H_{27}NO_9$$
Molar mass
497.494 g/mol g·mol^{-1}

Chemistry

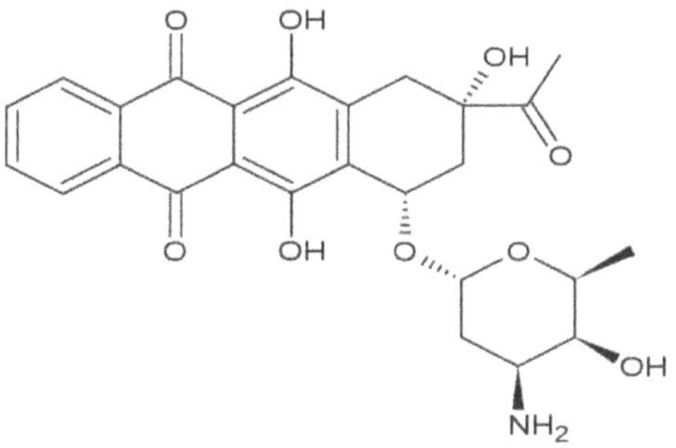

(The above structure has been copied from the Ph. D. thesis of the main author, drawn with stencils in 1988)

Pharmacology

It inserts itself into DNA and prevents DNA unwinding by interfering with the enzyme.

It is used for treatment of in blast crisis.

Pharmacokinetics

Protein binding	97%
Elimination half life	22 hours

Common side effects

Diarrhea, stomach cramps, nausea and vomiting. Contraindicated in pregnancy

ACLARUBICIN
(Aclacinomycin A)

$C_{42}H_{53}NO_{15}$
Molar mass
811.86 g/mol g·mol⁻¹

Aclarubicin or aclacinomycin A is a drug that is used in the cancer treatment.

It is obtained from soil bacteria.

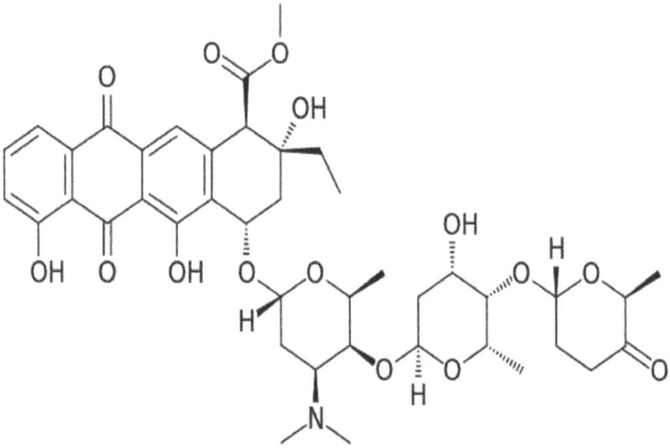

(The above structure has been copied from the Ph. D. thesis of the main author, drawn with stencils in 1988)

Pharmacokinetics

Protein binding	97%
Elimination half life	22 hours
	I.V.

PIRARUBICIN

$C_{32}H_{37}NO_{12}$
Molar mass
627.63 g/mol g·mol^{-1}

Chemistry

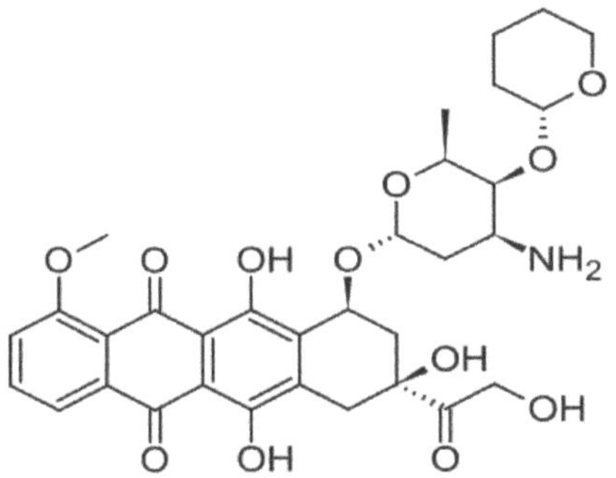

(The above structure has been copied from the Ph. D. thesis of the main author, drawn with stencils in 1988)

CARUBICIN
(Carminomycin)

$C_{26}H_{27}NO_{10}$
Molar mass
513.49 g/mol

Chemistry

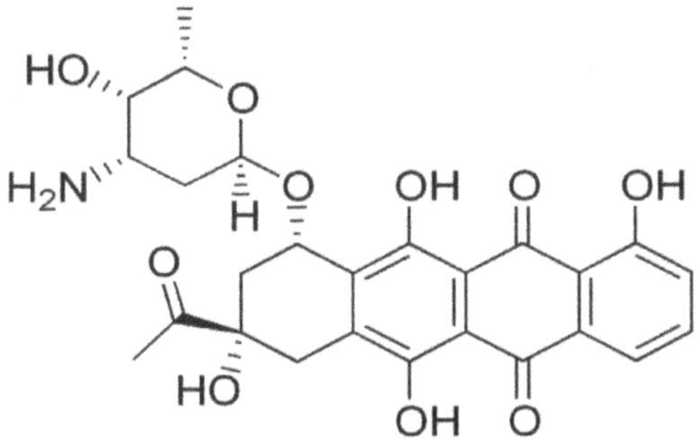

(The above structure has been copied from the Ph. D. thesis of the main author, drawn with stencils in 1988)

419

NOGALAMYCIN

$C_{39}H_{49}NO_{16}$
Molar mass
787.80 g/mol

Chemistry

Nogalamycin is an antibiotic produced by the soil. It has antitumor effects but is also highly cardiotoxic. The less cardiotoxic semisynthetic analog was developed in the 1970s. Currently nogalamycin and menogaril are not used clinically.

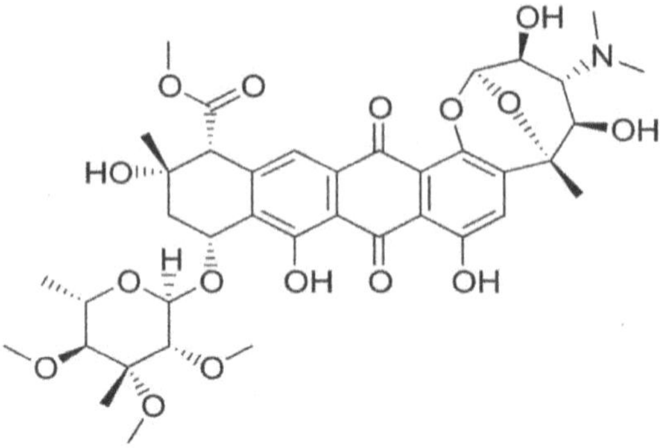

(The above structure has been copied from the Ph. D. thesis of the main author, drawn with stencils in 1988)

MENOGARIL

$C_{28}H_{31}NO_{10}$
Molar mass
541.55 g/mol

Chemistry

Menogaril is was developed in late 1970s. It has even stronger anticancer activity than nogalamycin and has less toxicity than

420

nogalamycin. However, its development for clinical use was cancelled due to only moderate success with relatively high incidence of serious toxicity.

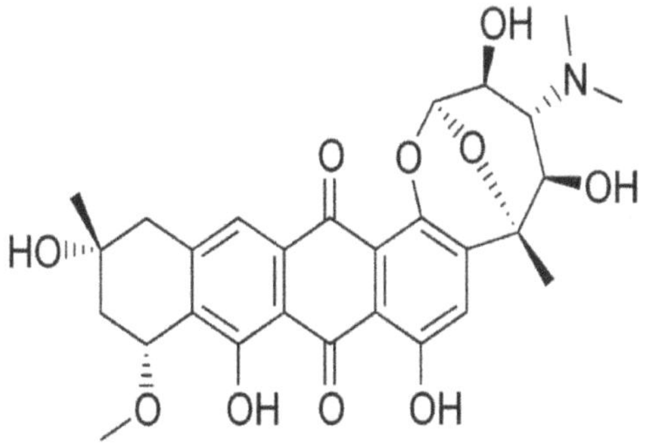

(The above structure has been copied from the Ph. D. thesis of the main author, drawn with stencils in 1988)

MITHRAMYCIN
(Palicamycin, Methracin)
(Aureolic acid derivatives)

$C_{52}H_{76}O_{24}$
Molar mass
1085.15 g/mol g·mol⁻¹

Chemistry

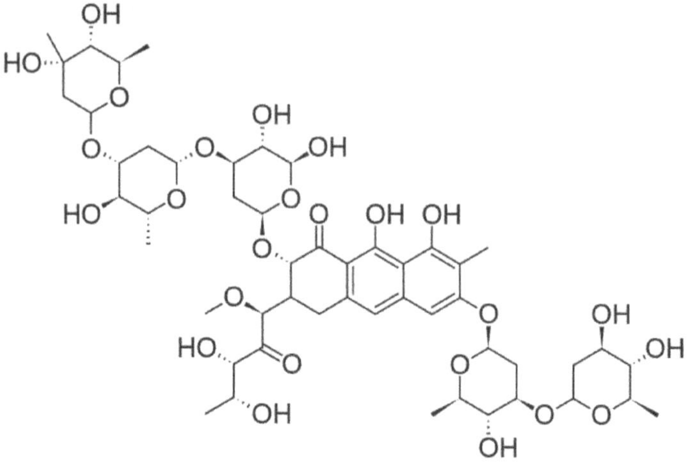

(The above structure has been copied from the Ph. D. thesis of the main author, drawn with stencils in 1988)

Synthesis of Mithramycin

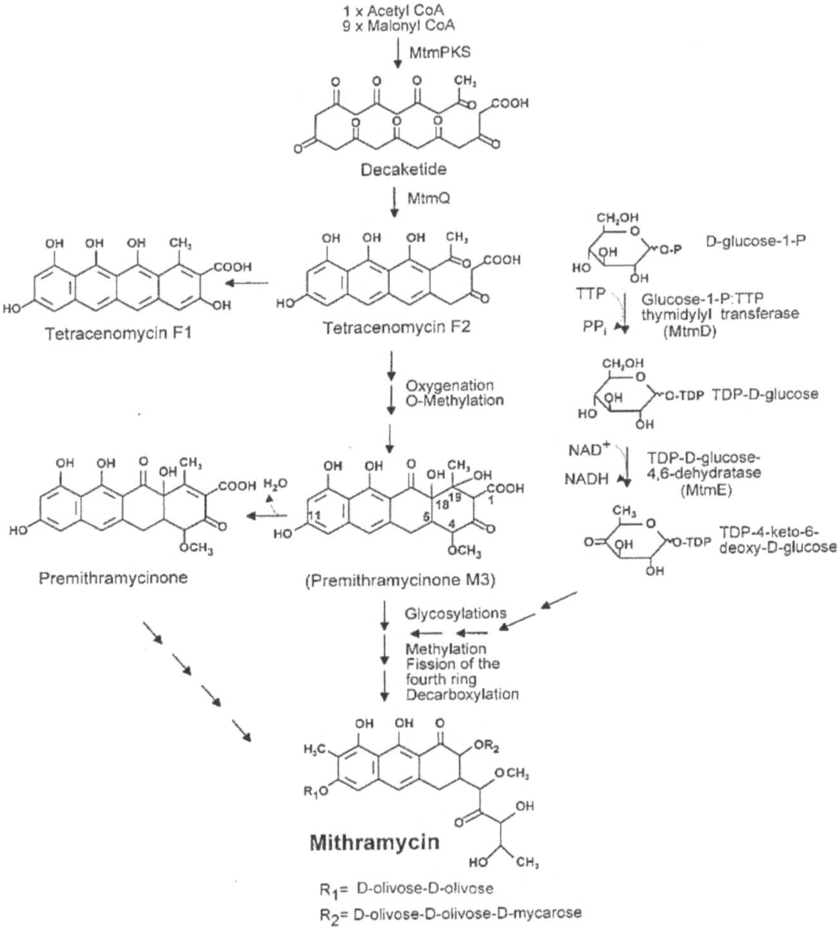

(The above structures ha been copied from the Ph. D. thesis of the main author, drawn with stencils in 1988)

BLEOMYCIN
(Glycopeptide antibiotic)

$$C_{55}H_{84}N_{17}O_{21}S_3$$
Molar mass
1415.551 g·mol^{-1}

Bleomycin was first discovered in 1962 when the Japanese scientist found anticancer activity while screening culture filtrates and published his discovery in 1966.

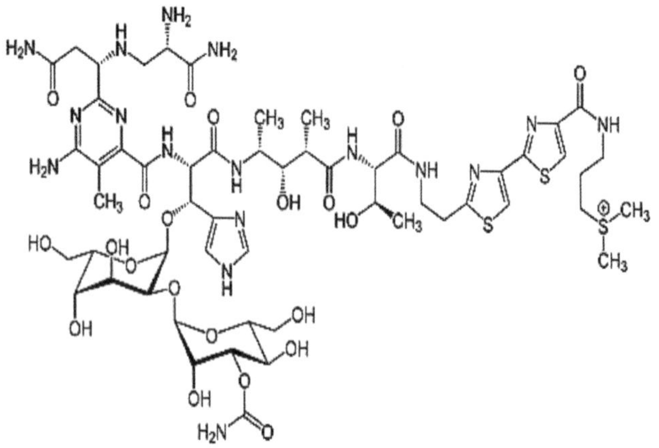

(The above structure has been copied from the Ph. D. thesis of the main author, drawn with stencils in 1988)

Bleomycin is a medication and can be given intravenously, by injection into a muscle or under the skin. It may also be administered inside the chest to help prevent the recurrence due to cancer. Common side effects include weight loss, vomiting, and rash. Bleomycin may cause harm to the baby if used during pregnancy.

Pharmacokinetics

Bioavailability	70% by I.M., 100% by S.C., 45% following intraperitoneal or intrapleural
Elimination half life	2 hours
Excretion	65% through renal

Side effects

The most common are flu-like symptoms and include rash, hair loss, chills, and discoloration of fingers and toes. The most serious complication of bleomycin, occurring upon increasing dosage is impaired lung function. Any previous treatment with bleomycin should therefore always be disclosed to the anesthetist prior to undergoing a procedure.

BLEOMYCIN A2
(Bleomycin)
BLEOMYCIN A5
(Pingyangmycin)

MITOMYCIN A1, B1, C1, D1
MITOMYCIN C

$$C_{15}H_{18}N_4O_5$$
Molar mass
334.332 g·mol−1

Chemistry

The mitomycins are a family of aziridine-containing isolated. They include mitomycin A, mitomycin B, and mitomycin C. When the name mitomycin occurs alone, it usually refers to mitomycin C. Mitomycin C is used as a medicine for treating various disorders associated with the growth and spread of cells. Mitomycin was discovered in the 1950s by Japanese scientists.

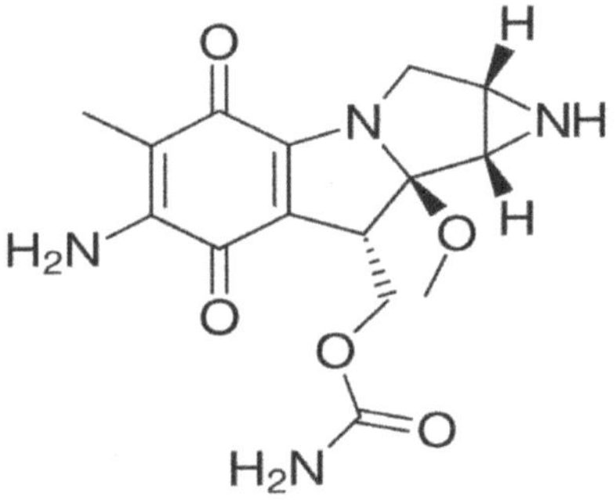

(The above structure has been copied from the Ph. D. thesis of the main author, drawn with stencils in 1988)

425

It is given i.v. to treat upper gastro-intestinal cancers as well as by bladder instillation. It causes delayed toxicity and therefore it is usually administered at 6-weekly intervals. Prolonged use may result in permanent bone-marrow damage. Mitomycin C is used to treat symptoms of wound healing, corneal excimer laser surgery. Mitomycin C has also been used intravenously in several areas.

Pharmacokinetics

Metabolism	Hepatic
Bioavailability	
Elimination half life	8-48 hours
Excretion	
Administration	I.V., topical

Synthesis of Mitomycin (condensed)

426

CHAPTER 16

ANTI-TUBERCLOSTATIC ANTIBIOTICS

16.1 List of anti-tuberclostatics

Rifamycins (macrocyclic antibiotics)	Already discussed under chapter 12.
Streptomycin (amino sugar)	Already discussed under chapter 8.
Capreomycin (antiphlogistic antibiotic)	Already discussed under chapter 7.
Viomycin (tuberactinomycin family)	Already discussed under chapter 7.
Amphomycin (lipopeptide antibiotic)	Already discussed under chapter 7.
Mikamycins (macrolide antibiotics)	Already discussed under chapter 7.
Cycloserine	Under discussion in the running chapter 16.
And many others.	

Active against Gram-positive bacteria	Capreomycin (antiphlogistic antibiotic)
	Viomycin (tuberactinomycin family)
	Amphomycin
	Mikamycins (macrolide antibiotics)
	(ostreogrycins, streptogramins, vernamycins, pristilinamycins, virginiamycins, staphylomycins.)
Active against staphylococcal bacteria	Vancomycin
	Ristocetins

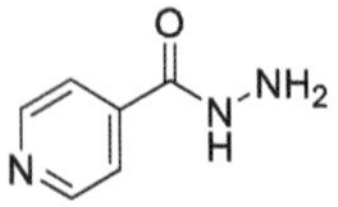

Isoniazid

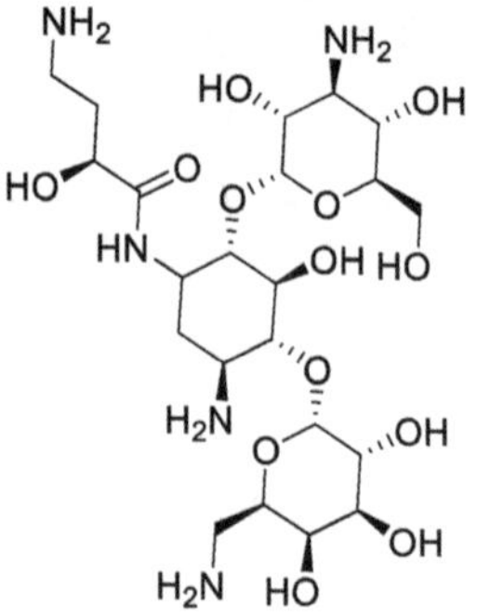

Amikacin

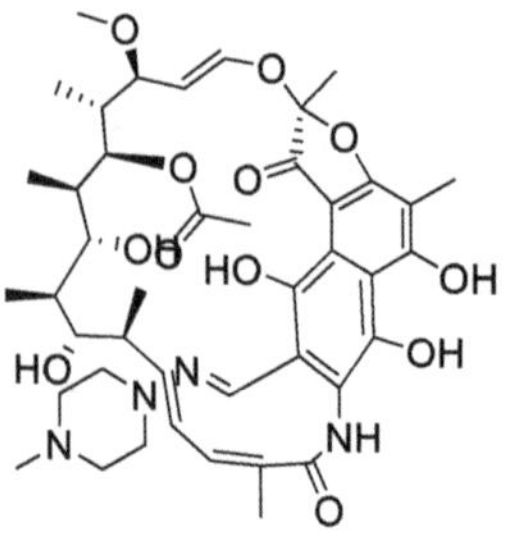

Rifampicin

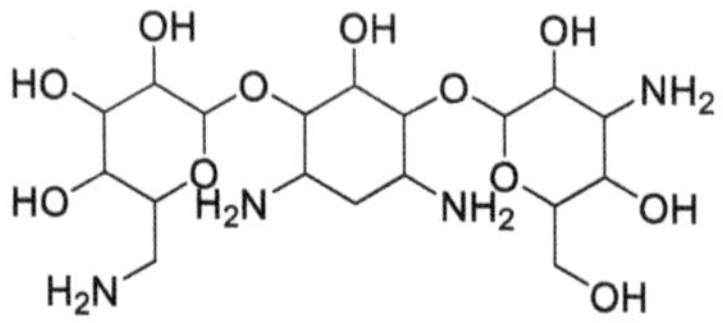

Kanamycin

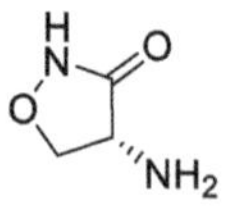

cycloserine

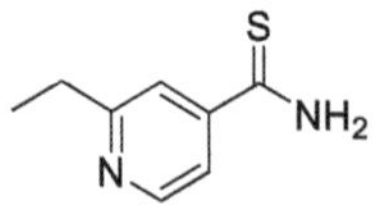

Ethionamide

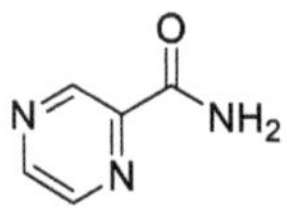

Pyrazinamide

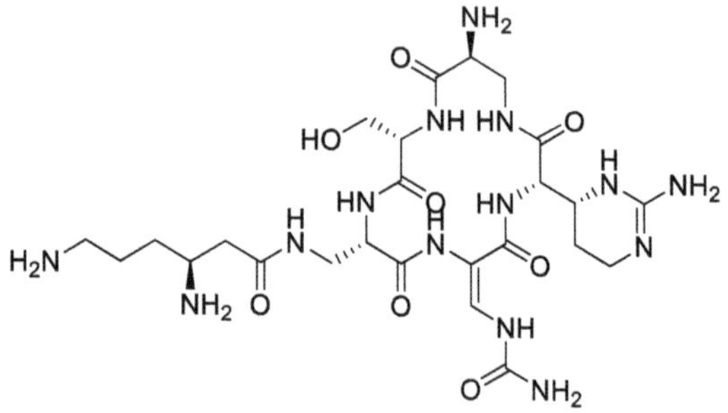

Capreomycin

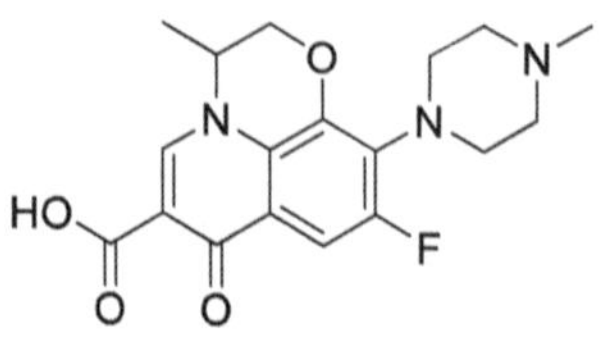

Ofloxacin

16.2 Chemistry of important anti-TB antibiotic drug

(Rifamycin)

The rifamycin are a group of chemically related antibiotics obtained from Streptomyces mediterranei. They belong to a new class of antibiotics called as an mycins that contain a macrocyclic ring bridged across two nonadjacent positions of an aromatic nucleus. The rifamycin and many of their semisynthetic derivatives have a broad spectrum of antimicrobial activity. They are most notably active against gram-positive bacteria and M. tuberculosis. However, they are also active against some gram-negative bacteria and many viruses. Rifampin, a semisynthetic derivative of rifamycin B, was released as an antitubercular agent in the United States in 1971. A second semisynthetic derivative, rifabutin, was approved in 1992 for the treatment of atypical mycobacterial infections.

It may, however, interfere with liver function in some patients and should not be combined with other potentially hepatotoxic drugs, nor employed in patients with impaired hepatic function (e.g., chronic alcoholics). The incidence of hepatotoxicity was significantly higher when rifampin was combined with isoniazid than when they are either agent was combined with ethambutol.

16.3 Active against gram-positive bacteria

CAPREOMYCIN

$$C_{25}H_{44}N_{14}O_8$$
Molar mass
668.706 g/mol g·mol^{-1}

Chemistry

Capreomycin, an antiphlogistic antibiotic which was produced in 1960, and be applied in clinic in 1968. In 1979, capreomycin was used in the area of antituberculosis by inhibiting the growth of mycobacterium tuberculosis.

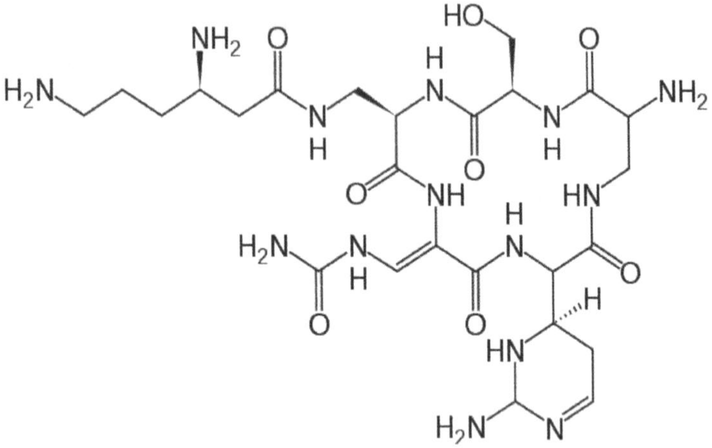

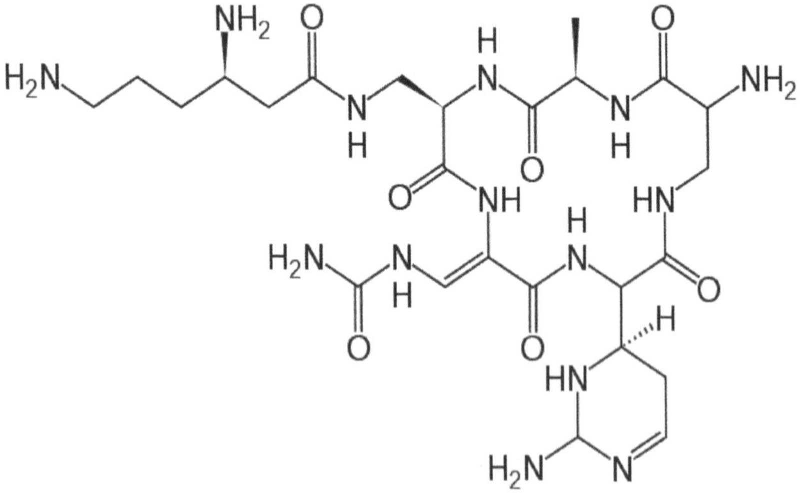

(The above structures have been copied from the Ph. D. thesis of the main author, drawn with stencils in 1988)

430

Pharmacology

Capreomycin is given in combination with others for the treatment.

Adverse side effects

Hematuria, urine output or urinary frequency significantly increased or decreased, loss of appetite or extreme thirst (hypokalemia, renal toxicity). Hearing loss, tinnitus, gait instability, dizziness, dyspnea, lethargy, extreme weakness (neuromuscular blockade, renal toxicity, hypokalemia), nausea or vomiting.

CYCLOSERINE

Chemistry

Saromycin is an antibiotic that has been isolated from the different Streptomyces species: S. orchaceus, S. garyphallus and S. lavandulus. It is stable in alkaline media only.

Pharmacology

Although, cycloserine exhibits antibiotic activity in vitro against a wide variety spectrum of both Gram -ive and Gram +ive organism, its relatively weak potency and frequent toxic reactions limit its use in treating TB.

Synthesis of Cycloserine 1

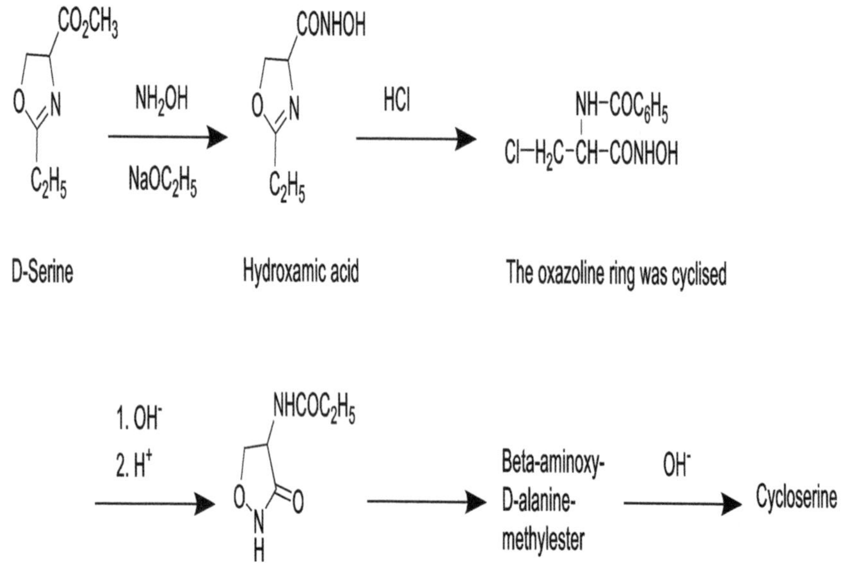
CO2CH3
NH2OH
NaOC2H5
CONHOH
HCl
NH-COC6H5
Cl–H2C-CH-CONHOH
C2H5
D-Serine
Hydroxamic acid
The oxazoline ring was cyclised
1. OH-
2. H+
NHCOC2H5
Beta-aminoxy-
D-alanine-
methylester
OH-
Cycloserine

CAPREOMYCIN

$C_{25}H_{44}N_{14}O_8$
Molar mass
668.706 g/mol g·mol^{-1}

Chemistry

Capreomycin 1A

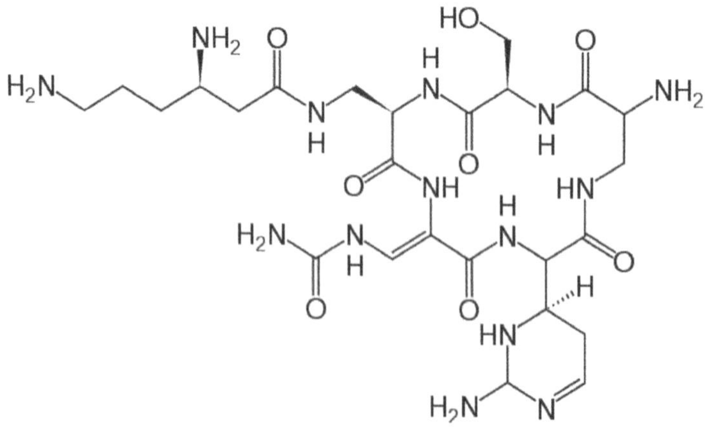

Capreomycin 1B

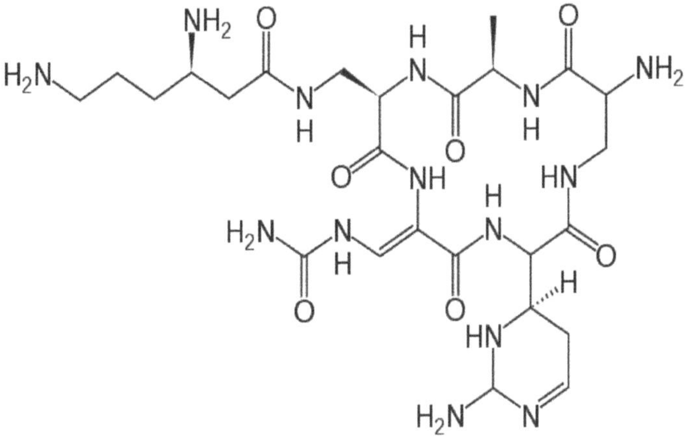

(The above structures have been copied from the Ph. D. thesis of the main author, drawn with stencils in 1988)

Pharmacology

Capreomycin is given in combination with others for the treatment. Other side effects include in the inability to breathe. Capreomycin is commonly grouped with the amino-glycosidic family of medications. It is not recommended with streptomycin.

Adverse side effects

Hematuria, urine output or urinary frequency increased, loss of appetite or extreme thirst (hypokalemia, renal toxicity). Hearing loss, tinnitus, gait instability, dizziness, dyspnea, lethargy, extreme weakness (neuromuscular blockade, renal toxicity, hypokalemia), nausea or vomiting. It may cause kidney or hearing problems in the baby.

VIOMYCIN

$C_{25}H_{43}N_{13}O_{10}$
Molar mass

685.691 g/mol g·mol⁻¹

Chemistry

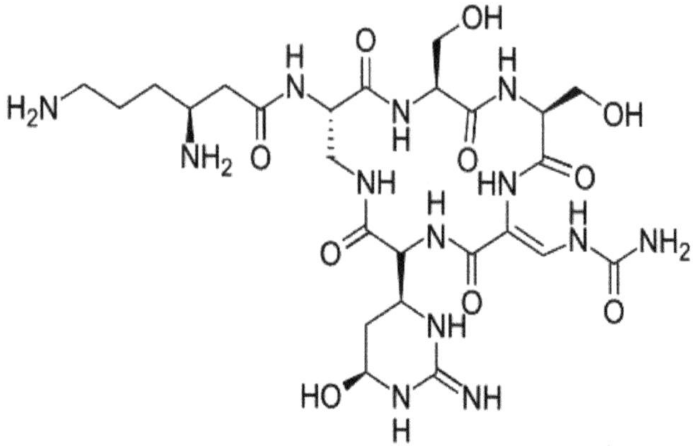

(The above structure has been copied from the Ph. D. thesis of the main author, drawn with stencils in 1988)

AMPHOMYCIN
(lipopeptide)

Streptomyces is a bacterium species from the genus of Streptomyces which has been isolated from soil. Streptomyces can also be produced by fungi.

MIKAMYCINS

Mikamycins are a group of macrolide antibiotics. Mikamycin can refer to pristinamycin IIA.

Mikamycin A; Virginiamycin M1

Mikamycin A

$C_{28}H_{35}N_3O_7$
Molar mass

434

525.602 g·mol^{-1}

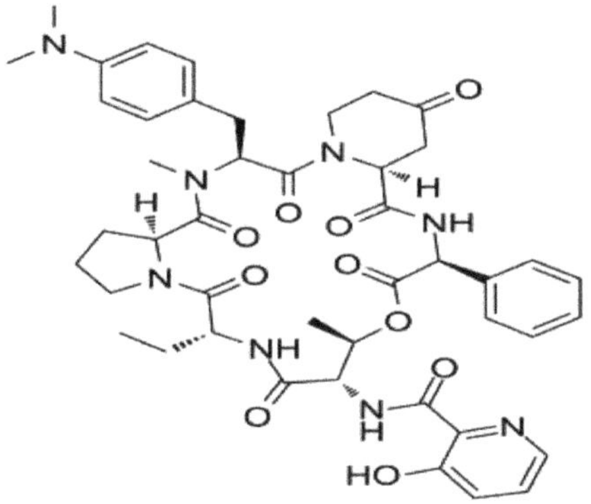

(The above structure has been copied from the Ph. D. thesis of the main author, drawn with stencils in 1988)

Pristinamycin IIB is isolated from soil and its chemical structure was first determined in 1966.
(27R)-26,27-Dihydrovirginiamycin M1; Ostreogrycin G; Virginiamycin M2; Volpristin

Mikamycin B

C$_{28}$H$_{37}$N$_3$O$_7$
Molar mass
527.618 g·mol^{-1}

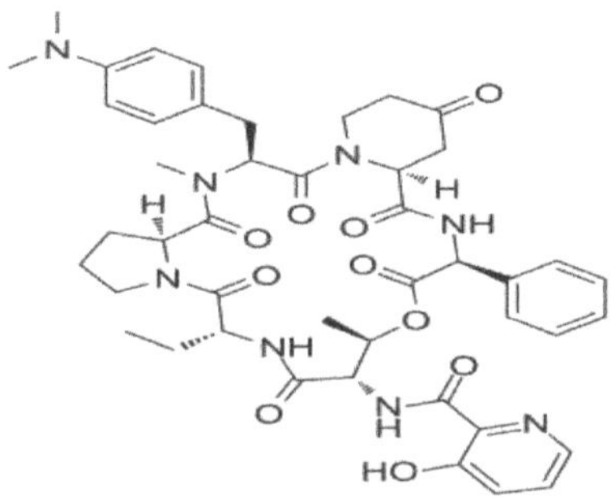

(The above structure has been copied from the Ph. D. thesis of the main author, drawn with stencils in 198

435

REFERENCES

1. Archer JS, Archer DF (2002). "Oral contraceptive efficacy and antibiotic interaction: a myth debunked". J. Am. Acad. Dermatol. 46 (6): 917–23.
2. Watabe, Motoki; Kato, Takahiro A.; Tsuboi, Sho; Ishikawa, Katsuhiko; Hashiya, Kazuhide: Monji, Akira; Utsumi, Hideo; Kanba, Shigenobu (2013-04-18). "Minocycline, a microglial inhibitor, reduces 'honey trap' risk in human economic exchange". Scientific Reports. 3(1).
3. Naeem Hasan Khan, (2010). New HPLC methods for quality control of tetracycline antibiotics. ISBN NO. 978-3-639-26841-6, VDM VERLAG, Germany.
4. Olivia M Dean; et al. (2017). "Adjunctive minocycline treatment for major depressive disorder: A proof of concept trial". Australian & New Zealand Journal of Psychiatry. 51 (8): 829–840.
5. Chatzispyrou IA, Held NM, Mouchiroud L, Auwerx J, Houtkooper RH (2015). "Tetracycline antibiotics impair mitochondria and its experimental use confounds research". Cancer Research. 75 (21): 4446–9.
6. Moullan N, Mouchiroud L, Wang X, Ryu D, Williams EG, Mottis A, Jovaisaite V, Frochaux MV, Quiros PM, Deplancke B, Houtkooper RH, Auwerx J (2015). "Tetracyclines Disturb Mitochondrial Function across Eukaryotic Models: A Call for Caution in Biomedical Research". Celll Reports. 10 (10): 1681–91.
7. Taylor MJ, Makunde WH, McGarry HF, Turner JD, Mand S, Hoerauf A (2005). "Macrofilaricidal activity after doxycycline treatment of Wuchereria bancrofti: a double-blind, randomised placebo-controlled trial". Lancet. 365 (9477): 2116–21.
8. Hoerauf A, Mand S, Fischer K, et al. (2003). "Doxycycline as a novel strategy against bancroftian filariasis-depletion of

Wolbachia endosymbionts from Wuchereria bancrofti and stop of microfilaria production". Med. Microbiol. Immunol. 192 (4): 211–6.

9. Okada T, Morozumi M, Tajima T, Hasegawa M, Sakata H, Ohnari S, Chiba N, Iwata S, Ubukata K (2012). "Rapid effectiveness of minocycline or doxycycline against macrolide-resistant Mycoplasma pneumoniae infection in a 2011 outbreak among Japanese children". Clin Infect Dis. 55 (12): 1642–9.

10. Karlsson M, Hammers-Berggren S, Lindquist L, Stiernstedt G, Svenungsson B (1994). "Comparison of intravenous penicillin G and oral doxycycline for treatment of Lyme neuroborreliosis". Neurologe. 44 (7): 1203–7.

11. Dursun D, Kim MC, Solomon A, Pflugfelder SC (2001). "Treatment of recalcitrant recurrent corneal erosions with inhibitors of matrix metalloproteinase-9, doxycycline and corticosteroids". Am. J. Ophthalmol. 132 (1): 8–13.

12. Moses MA, Harper J, Folkman J (2006). "Doxycycline treatment for lymphangioleio-myomatosis with urinary monitoring for MMPs". N. Engl. J. Med. 354 (24): 2621–2.

13. Raza M, Ballering JG, Hayden JM, Robbins RA, Hoyt JC (2006). "Doxycycline decreasesmonocyte chemoattractant protein-1 in human lung epithelial cells". Exp. Lung Res. 32 (1–2): 15–26.

14. Chung, AM; Reed, MD; Blumer, JL (2002). "Antibiotics and breast-feeding: a critical review of the literature". Paediatric drugs. 4 (12): 817–37.

15. Mylonas, I (January 2011). "Antibiotic chemotherapy during pregnancy and lactation period: aspects for consideration". Archives of gynecology and obstetrics. 283 (1): 7–18.

16. DeRossi SS, Hersh EV (2002). "Antibiotics and oral contraceptives". Dent. Clin. North Am. 46 (4): 653–64.

17. Hagemann RF, Concannon JP (April 1973). "Mechanism of intestinal radiosensitization by actinomycin D". The British Journal of Radiology. 46 (544): 302–8.

18. Gjønnaess H, Holten E (1978). "Doxycycline (Vibramycin) in pelvic inflammatory disease". Acta Obstet Gynecol Scand. 57 (2): 137–9.

19. Nelson, ML; Levy, SB (December 2011). "The history of the tetracyclines". Annals of theNew York Academy of Sciences. 1241: 17–32.

20. Jukes, Thomas H. Some historical notes on chlortetracycline. Reviews of Infectious Diseases 7(5):702-707 (1985).

21. Miyaoka T (October 2008). "Clinical potential of minocycline for schizophrenia". CNS Neurol Disord Drug Targets. 7 (4): 376–81.

22. Bishburg E, Bishburg K (November 2009). "Minocycline--an old drug for a new century: emphasis on methicillin-resistant Staphylococcus aureus (MRSA) and Acinetobacter baumannii". Int. J. Antimicrob. Agents. 34 (5): 395–401.

23. Chen, M; Ona, VO; Li, M; Ferrante, RJ; Fink, KB; Zhu, S; Bian, J; Guo, L; Farrell, LA; Hersch, SM; Hobbs, W; Vonsattel, JP; Cha, JH; Friedlander, RM (July 2000). "Minocycline inhibits caspase-1 and caspase-3 expression and delays mortality in a transgenic mouse model of Huntington disease". Nature Medicine. 6 (7): 797–801.

24. Sadowski, T; Steinmeyer, J (February 2001). "Minocycline inhibits the production of inducible nitric oxide synthase in articular chondrocytes". Journal of Rheumatology. 28 (2): 336–340.

25. Szeto, G.; Brice, A.; Yang, H.; Barber, S.; Siliciano, R.; Clements, J. (2010). "Minocycline attenuates HIV infection and reactivation by suppressing cellular activation in human CD4+ T cells". The Journal of Infectious Diseases. 201 (8): 1132–1140.

26. Song Y, Wei EQ, Zhang WP, Zhang L, Liu JR, Chen Z (2004). "Minocycline protects PC12 cells from ischemic-like injury and inhibits 5-lipoxygenase activation". NeuroReport. 15 (14): 2181–4.

27. Nonaka K, Nakazawa Y, Kotorii T (December 1983). "Effects of antibiotics, minocycline and ampicillin, on human sleep". Brain Res. 288 (1-2): 253–9.

28. Geria AN, Tajirian AL, Kihiczak G, Schwartz RA (2009). "Minocycline-induced skin pigmentation: an update". Acta Dermatovenerol Croat. 17 (2): 123–6.

29. DeRossi SS, Hersh EV (2002). "Antibiotics and oral contraceptives". Dent. Clin. North Am. 46 (4): 653–64.

30. E. Vogel and H. Günther (1967). "Benzene Oxide-Oxepin Valence Tautomerism". Angewandte Chemie International Edition in English. 6 (5): 385–401.

31. Lakshman Mahesh K., Singh Manish K., Parrish Damon, Balachandran Raghavan, Day Billy W. (2010). "Azide–Tetrazole Equilibrium of C-6 Azidopurine Nucleosides and Their Ligation Reactions with Alkynes". The Journal of Organic Chemistry. 75 (8): 2461–2473.

32. Singh, R.; Vince, R. Chem. Rev. 2012, 112 (8), pp 4642–4686."2-Azabicyclo [2.2.1] hept-5-en-3-one: Chemical Profile of a Versatile Synthetic Building Block and its Impact on the Development of Therapeutics"

33. Dalhoff, A.; Janjic, N.; Echols, R. (2006). "Redefining penems". Biochemical Pharmacology. 71 (7): 1085–1095

34. Pichichero ME (April 2005). "A review of evidence supporting the American Academy of Pediatrics recommendation for prescribing cephalosporin antibiotics for penicillin-allergic patients". 115 (4): 1048–57.

35. Fisher, J. F.; Meroueh, S. O.; Mobashery, S. (2005). "Bacterial Resistance to β-Lactam Antibiotics: Compelling Opportunism, Compelling Opportunity†". Chemical Reviews. 105 (2): 395–424.

36. Dalhoff, A.; Janjic, N.; Echols, R. (2006). "Redefining penems". Biochemical Pharmacology. 71 (7): 1085–1095.

37. Townsend, CA; Brown, AM; Nguyen, LT (1983). "Nocardicin A: Stereochemical and biomimetic studies of monocyclic β-lactam formation". Journal of the American Society. 105(4): 919–927.

38. Falagas, M. E.; Grammatikos, A. P.; Michalopoulos, A. (October 2008). "Potential of old-generation antibiotics to address current need for new antibiotics". Expert Review of Anti-infective Therapy. 6 (5): 593–600.

39. Singh, R.; Vince, R. Chem. Rev. 2012, 112 (8), pp 4642–4686."2-Azabicyclo [2.2.1] hept-5-en-3-one: Chemical Profile of a Versatile Synthetic Building Block and its Impact on the Development of Therapeutics"

40. Sutherland R, Elson S, Croydon EA (1972). "Metampicillin. Antibacterial activity and absorption and excretion in man". Chemotherapy. 17 (3): 145–60.

41. Mombelli G (May 1981). "[Aminopenicillin: when, how, what kind?]". Schweiz Med Wochenschr (in German). 111 (18): 641–5.

42. Chanal M, Sirot J, Cluzel M, Joly B, Glanddier Y (June 1983). "[In vitro study of the bacteriostatic and bactericidal activity of temocillin)]". Pathol. Biol. 31 (6): 467–70.

43. Boon RJ, et al. (1985). Antimicrob Agents Chemother. 27 (6): 980–1.

44. Bentley, P. H.; Clayton, J. P.; Boles, M. O.; Girven, R. J. (1979). "Transformations using benzyl 6-isocyanopenicillanate". Journal of the Chemical Society, Perkin Transactions 1: 2455.

45. Livermore DM et al. (2006) Activity of temocillin vs. prevalent ESBL- and AmpC-producing Enterobacteriaceae from SE England. J Antimicrob Chemother. 2006 May; 57(5):1012-4.

46. De Jongh R et al. (2008) Continuous versus intermittent infusion of temocillin, a directed spectrum penicillin for intensive care patients with nosocomial pneumonia: stability, compatibility, population pharmacokinetic studies and breakpoint selection. J Antimicrob Chemother. 2008 Feb;61(2):382-8.

47. Kasten B, Reski R (1997). "β-Lactam antibiotics inhibit chloroplast division in a moss (Physcomitrella patens) but not in tomato (Lycopersicon esculentum)". Journal of Plant Physiology. 150 (1–2): 137–40.

48. Coombes JD (1982). "Metabolism of cefotaxime in animals and humans". Reviews of Infectious Diseases. 4 (Suppl 2): S325–32.

49. Tanphaichitra D, Srimuang S, Chiaprasittigul P, Menday P, Christensen OE (1984). "The combination of pivmecillinam and pivampicillin in the treatment of enteric fever". Infection. 12 (6): 381–3.

50. Holme E, Jodal U, Linstedt S, Nordin I (September 1992). "Effects of pivalic acid-containing prodrugs on carnitine homeostasis and on response to fasting in children". Scand J Clin Lab Invest. 52 (5): 361–72.

51. Makino Y, Sugiura T, Ito T, Sugiyama N, Koyama N (September 2007). "Carnitine-associated encephalopathy caused by long-term treatment with an antibiotic containing pivalic acid". Pediatrics. 120 (3): e739–41.

52. Neu HC (1985). "Amdinocillin: a novel penicillin. Antibacterial activity, pharmacology and clinical use". Pharmacotherapy. 5 (1): 1–10.

53. Geddes AM, Clarke PD (July 1977). "The treatment of enteric fever with mecillinam". J Antimicrob Chemother. 3 Suppl B: 101–2.

54. Goa KL, Noble S (2003). "Panipenem/betamipron". Drugs. 63 (9): 913–25; discussion 926.

55. U.S. Food and Drug Administration. U.S. Department of Health and Human Services. Claforan Sterile (cefotaxime for injection, USP) and Injection (cefotaxime injection, USP). 19 June 2009. Retrieved 2014-04-19.

56. Margolin, L (2004). "Impaired rehabilitation secondary to muscle weakness induced by meropenem". Clinical drug investigation. 24 (1): 61–2.

57. Vardakas, KZ; Tansarli, GS; Rafailidis, PI; Falagas, ME (Dec 2012). "Carbapenems versus alternative antibiotics for the treatment of bacteraemia due to Enterobacteriaceae producing extended-spectrum β-lactamases: a systematic review and meta-analysis". The Journal of antimicrobial chemotherapy. 67 (12): 2793–803.

58. Clissold, SP; Todd, PA; Campoli-Richards, DM (Mar 1987). "Imipenem/cilastatin. A review of its antibacterial activity,

pharmacokinetic properties and therapeutic efficacy". Drugs. 33(3): 183–241.

59. Zhanel, G. G.; Ketter; Rubinstein; Friedland; Redman (2009). "Overview of seizure-inducing potential of doripenem". Drug Safety. 32 (9): 709–16.

60. Mazzei, T (2010). "The pharmacokinetics and pharmacodynamics of the carbapanemes: Focus on doripenem". Journal of Chemotherapy. 22 (4): 219–25.

61. Lund F, Tybring L (April 1972). "6β-amidinopenicillanic acids—a new group of antibiotics". Nature New Biology. 236 (66): 135–7.

62. Naber KG, Schito G, Botto H, Palou J, Mazzei T (May 2008). "Surveillance Study in Europe and Brazil on Clinical Aspects and Antimicrobial Resistance Epidemiology in Females with Cystitis (ARESC): Implications for Empiric Therapy". Eur Urol. 54 (5): 1164–75.

63. Wagenlehner, FME; Schmiemann, G; Hoyme, U; Fünfstück, R; Hummers-Pradier, E; Kaase, M; Kniehl, E; Selbach, I; Sester, U; Vahlensieck, W; Watermann, D; Naber, KG (12 February 2011). "Nationale S3-Leitlinie "Unkomplizierte Harnwegsinfektionen"" [National S3 guideline on uncomplicated urinary tract infection: recommendations for treatment and management of uncomplicated community-acquired bacterial urinary tract infections in adult patients]. 50 (2): 153–169.

64. Y, Ge; Floren L; Redman R; et al. The pharmacokinetics and safety of ceftaroline (PPI-0903) in healthy subjects receiving multiple-dose intravenous infusions. 2006 Interscience Conference on Antimicrobial Agents and Chemotherapy / Infectious Disease Society of America Conference.

65. Hebert A, Sigman E, Levy M (1991). "Serum sickness-like reactions from cefaclor in children". J Am Acad Dermatol. 25 (5 Pt 1): 805–8.

66. Bertels RA, Semmekrot BA, Gerrits GP, Mouton JW (October 2008). "Serum concentrations of cefotaxime and its metabolite

desacetyl-cefotaxime in infants and children during continuous infusion". Infection. 36 (5): 415–20.

67. P, Eckberg; Friedland HD; et al. FOCUS 1 and 2: Randomized, Double-blinded, Multicenter Phase 3 Trials of the Efficacy and Safety of Ceftaroline (CPT) vs. Ceftriaxone (CRO) in Community-acquired pneumonia (CAP). 2009 Interscience Conference on Antimicrobial Agents and Chemotherapy / Infectious Disease Society of America Conference.

68. R, Corey; Wilcox M; Talbot GH; et al. CANVAS-1: Randomized, Double-blinded, Phase 3 Study (P903-06) of the Efficacy and Safety of Ceftaroline vs. Vancomycin plus Aztreonam in Complicated Skin and Skin Structure Infections (cSSSI). 2008 Interscience Conference on Antimicrobial Agents and Chemotherapy / Infectious Disease Society of America Conference.

69. White, N. J.; Dance, D. A.; Chaowagul, W; Wattanagoon, Y; Wuthiekanun, V; Pitakwatchara, N (1989). "Halving of mortality of severe melioidosis by ceftazidime". Lancet. 2 (8665): 697–701.

70. Schichor A; Bernstein B; Weinerman H; Fitzgerald J; Yordan E; Schechter N (January 1994). "Lidocaine as a diluent for ceftriaxone in the treatment of gonorrhea. Does it reduce the pain of the injection?". Arch Pediatr Adolesc Med. 148 (1): 72–5.

71. Parra F, Igea J, Martín J, Alonso M, Lezaun A, Sainz T (1992). "Serum sickness-like syndrome associated with cefaclor therapy". Allergy. 47 (4 Pt 2): 439–40.

72. Drainas D, Kalpaxis DL, Coutsogeorgopoulos C (April 1987). "Inhibition of ribosomal peptidyltransferase by chloramphenicol. Kinetic studies". European Journal of Biochemistry. 164 (1): 53–8.

73. Tenson T, Lovmar M, Ehrenberg M (July 2003). "The mechanism of action of macrolides, lincosamides and streptogramin B reveals the nascent peptide exit path in the ribosome". Journal of Molecular Biology. 330 (5): 1005–14

74. Nguyen M, Chung EP (August 2005). "Telithromycin: the first ketolide antimicrobial". Clinical Therapeutics. 27 (8): 1144–63.

75. Kunze B, Sasse F, Wieczorek H, Huss M (July 2007). "Cruentaren A, a highly cytotoxic benzolactone from Myxobacteria is a novel selective inhibitor of mitochondrial F1-ATPases". FEBS Letters. 581 (18): 3523–7.
76. Abdellatif M, Ghozy S, Kamel MG, Elawady SS, Ghorab MM, Attia AW, Le Huyen TT, Duy DT, Hirayama K, Huy NT (March 2019). "Association between exposure to macrolides and the development of infantile hypertrophic pyloric stenosis: a systematic review and meta-analysis". European Journal of Pediatrics. 178 (3): 301–314.
77. Hansen, Malene Plejdrup; Scott, Anna M; McCullough, Amanda; Thorning, Sarah; Aronson, Jeffrey K; Beller, Elaine M; Glasziou, Paul P; Hoffmann, Tammy C; Clark, Justin; Del Mar, Chris B (18 January 2019). Cochrane Database of Systematic Reviews. 1:
78. Keicho N, Kudoh S (2002). "Diffuse panbronchiolitis: role of macrolides in therapy". American Journal of Respiratory Medicine. 1 (2): 119–31.
79. Schultz MJ (July 2004). "Macrolide activities beyond their antimicrobial effects: macrolides in diffuse panbronchiolitis and cystic fibrosis". The Journal of Antimicrobial Chemotherapy. 54 (1): 21–8.
80. López-Boado YS, Rubin BK (June 2008). "Macrolides as immunomodulatory medications for the therapy of chronic lung diseases". Current Opinion in Pharmacology. 8(3): 286–91.
81. Honein MA, Paulozzi LJ, Himelright IM, Lee B, Cragan JD, Patterson L, Correa A, Hall S, Erickson JD (1999). "Infantile hypertrophic pyloric stenosis after pertussis prophylaxis with erythromcyin: a case review and cohort study". Lancet. 354 (9196): 2101–5.
82. Jones WF, Finland M (September 1957). "Antibiotic combinations; tetracycline, erythromycin, oleandomycin and spiramycin and combinations of tetracycline with each of the other three agents; comparisons of activity in vitro and

antibacterial action of blood after oral administration". The New England Journal of Medicine. 257 (12): 536–47

83. Neff MJ (2004). "AAP, AAFP release guideline on diagnosis and management of acute otitis media". Am Fam Physician. 69 (11): 2713–5.

84. Taylor SP, Sellers E, Taylor BT (2015). "Azithromycin for the Prevention of COPD Exacerbations: The Good, Bad, and Ugly". Am. J. Med. 128 (12): 1362.el–6.

85. Hauk L (2014). "AAP releases guideline on diagnosis and management of acute bacterial sinusitis in children one to 18 years of age". Am Fam Physician. 89 (8): 676–81.

86. Rosenfeld RM, Piccirillo JF, Chandrasekhar SS, Brook I, Ashok Kumar K, Kramper M, Orlandi RR, Palmer JN, Patel ZM, Peters A, Walsh SA, Corrigan MD (2015). "Clinical practice guideline (update): adult sinusitis". Otolaryngol Head Neck Surg. 152 (2 Suppl): S1–S39.

87. Mandell LA, Wunderink RG, Anzueto A, Bartlett JG, Campbell GD, Dean NC, Dowell SF, File TM, Musher DM, Niederman MS, Torres A, Whitney CG (2007). "Infectious Diseases Society of America/American Thoracic Society consensus guidelines on the management of community-acquired pneumonia in adults". Clin. Infect. Dis. 44 Suppl 2: S27–72.

88. Lippincott Illustrated Reviews: Pharmacology Sixth Edition. p. 506.

89. Dart, Richard C. (2004). Medical Toxology. Lippincott Williams & Wilkins. p. 23.

90. Tilelli, John A.; Smith, Kathleen M.; Pettignano, Robert (2006). "Life-Threatening Bradyarrhythmia After Massive Azithromycin Overdose". Pharmacotherapy. 26 (1): 147–50.

91. O'Gorman, MA; Michaels, MG; Kaplan, SL; Otley, A; Kociolek, LK; Hoffenberg, EJ; Kim, KS; Nachman, S; Pfefferkorn, MD; Sentongo, T; Sullivan, JE; Sears, P (Aug 17, 2018). "Safety and Pharmacokinetic Study of Fidaxomicin in Children with Clostridium difficile -Associated Diarrhea: A Phase 2a

Multicenter Clinical Trial". J Pediatric Infect Dis Soc. 7 (3): 210–218.

92.   Golan Y, Mullane KM, Miller MA (September 12–15, 2009). Low recurrence rate among patients with C. difficile infection treated with fidaxomicin. 49th interscience conference on antimicrobial agents and chemotherapy. San Francisco.

93.   Louie, Thomas J.; Miller, Mark A.; Mullane, Kathleen M.; Weiss, Karl; Lentnek, Arnold; Golan, Yoav; Gorbach, Sherwood; Sears, Pamela; Shue, Youe-Kong; Opt-80-003 Clinical Study, Group (2011). "Fidaxomicin versus vancomycin for Clostridium difficile infection". New England Journal of Medicine. 364 (5): 422–31.

94.   Gorbach S, Weiss K, Sears P, et al. (September 12–15, 2009). Safety of fidaxomicin versus vancomycin in treatment of Clostridium difficile infection. 49th interscience conference on antimicrobial agents and chemotherapy. San Francisco.

95.   Revill, P.; Serradell, N.; Bolós, J. (2006). "Tiacumicin B". Drugs of the Future. 31 (6): 494.

96.   Winkel P, Hilden J, Fischer Hansen J, Hildebrandt P, Kastrup J, Kolmos HJ, et al. (2011). "Excess sudden cardiac deaths after short-term clarithromycin administration in the CLARICOR trial: why is this so, and why are statins protective?". Cardiology. 118 (1): 63–7.

97.   The American Society of Health-System Pharmacists. from the original on September 3, 2015. Retrieved September 4,2015.

98.   Yamaguchi S, Kaneko Y, Yamagishi T, et al. [Clarithromycin-induced torsades de pointes]. Nippon Naika Gakkai Zasshi. 2003;92(1):143–5.

99.   Gélisse P, Hillaire-Buys D, Halaili E, Jean-Pastor MJ, Vespignan H, Coubes P, Crespel A (November 2007). "[Carbamazepine and clarithromycin: a clinically relevant drug interaction]". Revue Neurologique. 163 (11): 1096–9.

100.   Kirk, J E; Effersøe, H (1953). "The Effect of Washing with Soap and with a Detergent on the 4-Hour Sebaceous Secretion in the Forehead12". The British Medical Journal. 2(4851): 1421–22.

101. Srinivasan, Dorothy; P.R. Srinivasan (1967). "Studies on the Biosynthesis of Magnamycin". Biochemistry. 6 (10): 3111–18.

102. Ghonaim, S.A.; A.M. Khalil; A.A. Abou-Zeid (March 1980). "Factors affecting fermentative production of magnamycin by Streptomyces halsted II". Agricultural Wastes. 2 (1): 31–36.

103. Baghlaf, A.O.; A.Z.A Abou-Zeid; A.I. El-Diwzny (1981). "Biosynthesis of Carbomycin, its Extraction, Purification and Mode of Action on Bacillus subtilis". Journal of Chemical Technology and Biotechnology. 31 (1): 241–46.

104. Ferrero JL, Bopp BA, Marsh KC, Quigley SC, Johnson MJ, Anderson DJ, et al. (1990). "Metabolism and disposition of clarithromycin in man". Drug Metabolism and Disposition. 18(4): 441–6.

105. Sekar VJ, Spinosa-Guzman S, De Paepe E, De Pauw M, Vangeneugden T, Lefebvre E, Hoetelmans RM (January 2008). "Darunavir/ritonavir pharmacokinetics following coadministration with clarithromycin in healthy volunteers". Journal of Clinical Pharmacology. 48 (1): 60–5.

106. Pringle, Peter (2012). Experiment Eleven: Dark Secrets Behind the Discovery of a Wonder Drug. New York: Walker & Company.

107. Schatz, Albert; Bugle, Elizabeth; Waksman, Selman A. (1944), "Streptomycin, a substance exhibiting antibiotic activity against gram-positive and gram-negative bacteria", Experimental Biology and Medicine, 55: 66–69,

108. Qian H, Li J, Pan X, Sun Z, Ye C, Jin G, Fu Z (March 2012). "Effects of streptomycin on growth of algae Chlorella vulgaris and Microcystis aeruginosa". Environ. Toxicol. 27 (4): 229–37.

109. Metcalfe NH (February 2011). "Sir Geoffrey Marshall (1887-1982): respiratory physician, catalyst for anaesthesia development, doctor to both Prime Minister and King, and World War I Barge Commander". J Med Biogr. 19 (1): 10–4.

110. Waksman SA, Lechevalier HA (March 1949). "Neomycin, a New Antibiotic Active against Streptomycin-Resistant Bacteria, including Tuberculosis Organisms". Science. New York, N.Y. 109 (2830): 305–7.

111. Heidary N, Cohen DE (September 2005). "Hypersensitivity reactions to vaccine components". Dermatitis. 16 (3): 115–20.

112. Kudo F, Fujii T, Kinoshita S, Eguchi T (July 2007). "Unique O-ribosylation in the biosynthesis of butirosin". Bioorganic & Medicinal Chemistry. 15 (13): 4360–8.

113. Gabev E, Kasianowicz J, Abbott T, McLaughlin S (February 1989). "Binding of neomycin to phosphatidylinositol 4,5-bisphosphate (PIP2)". Biochimica et Biophysica Acta. 979 (1): 105–12.

114. Arya DP, Coffee RL, Charles I (November 2001). "Neomycin-induced hybrid triplex formation". Journal of the American Chemical Society. 123 (44): 11093–4.

115. The selection and use of essential medicines: report of the WHO Expert Committee on Selection and Use of Essential Medicines, 2019 (including the 21st WHO Model List of Essential Medicines and the 7th WHO Model List of Essential Medicines for Children). Geneva: World Health Organization.

116. Briggs G (2011). Drugs in Pregnancy and Lactation: A Reference Guide to Fetal and Neonatal Risk. Lippincott Williams & Wilkins. p. 787.

117. Lopez-Novoa JM, Quiros Y, Vicente L, Morales AI, Lopez-Hernandez FJ (January 2011). "New insights into the mechanism of aminoglycoside nephrotoxicity: an integrative point of view". Kidney International. 79 (1): 33–45.

118. Lerner AM, Reyes MP, Cone LA, Blair DC, Jansen W, Wright GE, Lorber RR (May 1983). "Randomised, controlled trial of the comparative efficacy, auditory toxicity, and nephrotoxicity of tobramycin and netilmicin". Lancet. 1 (8334): 1123–6.

119. Yang G, Trylska J, Tor Y, McCammon JA (September 2006). "Binding of aminoglycosidic antibiotics to the oligonucleotide A-site model and 30S ribosomal subunit: Poisson-Boltzmann model, thermal denaturation, and fluorescence studies". Journal of Medicinal Chemistry. 49 (18): 5478–90.

120. Park, Je Won; Ban, Yeon Hee; Nam, Sang-Jip; Cha, Sun-Shin; Yoon, Yeo Joon (1 December 2017). "Biosynthetic pathways

of aminoglycosides and their engineering". Current Opinion in Biotechnology. Chemical biotechnology: Pharmaceutical biotechnology. 48: 33–41.

121. World Health Organization model list of essential medicines: 21st list 2019. Geneva: World Health Organization. WHO/MVP/EMP/IAU/2019.06. License: CC BY-NC-SA 3.0 IGO.

122. Mir LM, Gehl J, Sersa G, Collins CG, Garbay JR, Billard V, Geertsen PF, Rudolf Z, O'Sullivan GC, Marty M (2006). "Standard operating procedures of the electrochemotherapy: Instructions for the use of bleomycin or cisplatin administered either systemically or locally and electric pulses delivered by the Cliniporator™ by means of invasive or non-invasive electrodes". Eur J Cancer Suppl. 4 (11): 14–25.

123. The American Society of Health-System Pharmacists. fom the original on 2015-09-24. Retrieved Sep 6, 2015.

124. Product Information: Humatin(R), paromomycin sulfate capsules. Parke-Davis, Division of Warner-Lambert Company, Morris Plains, NJ, 1999

125. Ben Salah A, Ben Messaoud N, Guedri E, Zaatour A, Ben Alaya N, Bettaieb J, Gharbi A, Belhadj Hamida N, et al. (2013). "Topical Paromomycin with or without Gentamicin for Cutaneous Leishmaniasis". N. Engl. J. Med. 368 (6): 524–32.

126. Hamilton, Richart (2015). Tarascon Pocket Pharmacopoeia 2015 Deluxe Lab-Coat Edition. Jones & Bartlett Learning. p. 54.

127. Davidson RN, den Boer M, Ritmeijer K (2008). "Paromomycin". Transactions of the Royal Society of Tropical Medicine and Hygiene. 103 (7): 653–60.

128. Busby, RW; Townsend, CA (Jul 1996). "A single monomeric iron center in clavaminate synthase catalyzes three nonsuccessive oxidative transformations". Bioorganic & Medicinal Chemistry. 4 (7): 1059–64.

129. Bachmann, BO; Townsend, CA (Sep 19, 2000). "Kinetic mechanism of the beta-lactam synthetase of Streptomyces clavuligerus". Biochemistry. 39 (37): 11187–93.

130. Khaleeli, Nusrat; Li, Rongfeng; Townsend, Craig A. "Origin of the β-Lactam Carbons in Clavulanic Acid from an Unusual Thiamine Pyrophosphate-Mediated Reaction". Journal of the American Chemical Society. 121 (39): 9223–9224.

131. Rodgers GM, Becker PS, Bennett CL, Cella D, Chanan-Khan A, Chesney C, Cleeland C, Coccia PF, Djulbegovic B, Garst JL, Gilreath JA, Kraut EH, Lin WC, Matulonis U, Millenson M, Reinke D, Rosenthal J, Sabbatini P, Schwartz RN, Stein RS, Vij R (July 2008). "Cancer- and chemotherapy-induced anemia". Journal of the National Comprehensive Cancer Network. 6 (6): 536–64.

132. Chen X, Jiang X, Yang M, González U, Lin X, Hua X, Xue S, Zhang M, Bennett C (May 2016). "Systemic antifungal therapy for tinea capitis in children". Cochrane Database Syst Rev (5).

133. Harris, Constance (1976). "Biosynthesis of Griseofulvin". Journal of the American Chemical Society. 98 (17): 5380–5386.

134. Fleece D, Gaughan JP, Aronoff SC (November 2004). "Griseofulvin versus terbinafine in the treatment of tinea capitis: a meta-analysis of randomized, clinical trials". Pediatrics. 114(5): 1312–5.

135. J.F. Grove, D. Ismay, J. Macmillan, T.P.C. Mulholland, M.A.T. Rogers, Chem. Ind. (London), 219 (1951).

136. Grove, J. F.; MacMillan, J.; Mulholland, T. P. C.; Rogers, M. A. T. (1952). "762. Griseofulvin. Part IV. Structure". Journal of the Chemical Society (Resumed): 3977.

137. Pfaller, M; Castaneira, M; Sader, H; Jones, R (2010). "Evaluation of the activity of fusidic acid tested against contemporary Gram-positive clinical isolates from the USA and Canada". International Journal of Antimicrobial Agents. 35 (3): 282–287.

138. Spelman. (1999). "Fusidic acid in skin and soft tissue infections". International Journal of Antimicrobial Agents. 12 Suppl 2: S59–66.

139. Leclercq, R; Bismuth, R; Casin, I; Cavallo, JD; Croize, J; Felten, A; Goldstein, F; Monteil, H; Quentin-Noury, C; Reverdy, M; Vergnaud, M; Roiron, R (2000). "In Vitro Activity of Fusidic

Acid Against Streptococci isolated form Skin and Soft Tissue Infections". J. Antimicrob. Chemother. 45 (1): 27–29.

140. Turnidge J, Collignon P (1999). "Resistance to fusidic acid". Int J Antimicrob Agents. 12(Suppl 2): S35–44.

141. Castanheira M, Mendes RE, Rhomberg PR and Jones RN (2010). Activity of fusidic acid tested against contemporary Staphylococcus aureus collected from United States hospitals. Infectious Diseases Society of America, 48th Annual Meeting, Abstract 226.

142. Lin, Shu-Wen; Lin, Chun-Jung; Yang, Jyh-Chin (August 2017). "Rifamycin SV MMX for the treatment of traveler's diarrhea". Expert Opinion on Pharmacotherapy. 18 (12): 1269–1277.

143. Campbell EA, Korzheva N, Mustaev A, Murakami K, Nair S, Goldfarb A, Darst SA (March 2001). "Structural mechanism for rifampicin inhibition of bacterial rna polymerase". Cell. 104(6): 901–12.

144. Calvori, C.; Frontali, L.; Leoni, L.; Tecce, G. (1965). "Effect of rifamycin on protein synthesis". Nature. 207 (995): 417–8.

145. Floss, H.G.; Yu, T. (2005). "Rifamycin-Mode of Action, Resistance, and Biosynthesis". Chem. Rev. 105 (2): 621–32.

146. Rosenberger A, Tebbe B, Treudler R, Orfanos CE (June 1998). "[Acute generalized exanthematous pustulosis, induced by nystatin]". Der Hautarzt; Zeitschrift Fur Dermatologie, Venerologie, und Verwandte Gebiete (in German). 49 (6): 492–5.

147. Elsner, Zofia; Leszczynska-Bakal, Halina; Pawlak, Elzbieta; Smazynski, Teofil (1976). "Gel with nystatin for treatment of lung mycosis". Polish Journal of Pharmacology and Pharmacy. 28: 49–52.

148. Hilal-Dandan, Randa; Knollmann, Bjorn; Brunton, Laurence (2017-12-05). Goodman & Gilman's the pharmacological basis of therapeutics. Brunton, Laurence L., Knollmann, Björn C., Hilal-Dandan, Randa (Thirteenth ed.). [New York].

149. Akaike N, Harata N (1994). "Nystatin perforated patch recording and its applications to analyses of intracellular mechanisms". The Japanese Journal of Physiology. 44 (5): 433–73.

150. P., Rang, H. (2015-01-21). Rang and Dale's pharmacology. Dale, M. Maureen, Flower, R. J. (Rod J.), 1945-, Henderson, G. (Graeme) (Eighth ed.). [United Kingdom].

151. Steimbach, Laiza M., Fernanda S. Tonin, Suzane Virtuoso, Helena HL Borba, Andréia CC Sanches, Astrid Wiens, Fernando Fernandez-Llimós, and Roberto Pontarolo. "Efficacy and safety of amphotericin B lipid-based formulations—A systematic review and meta-analysis." Mycoses 60, no. 3 (2017): 146-154.

152. J. Czub, M. Baginski. Amphotericin B and Its New Derivatives Mode of action. Department of pharmaceutical Technology and Biochemistry. Faculty of Chemistry, Gdnsk University of Technology. 2009, 10-459-469.

153. Zietse, R.; Zoutendijk, R.; Hoorn, E. J. (2009). "Fluid, electrolyte and acid–base disorders associated with antibiotic therapy". Nature Reviews Nephrology. 5 (4): 193–202.

154. Maertens, J. A. (2004-03-01). "History of the development of azole derivatives". Clinical Microbiology and Infection. 10: 1–10.

155. Xiaochun Chen et al. "Fumagillin and Fumarranol Interact with P. falciparum Methionine Aminopeptidase 2 and Inhibit Malaria Parasite Growth In Vitro and In Vivo". Chemistry & Biology, Vol. 16 Nr. 2 (2009) blz. 193-202. Chen, X.; Xie, S.; Bhat, S.; Kumar, N.; Shapiro, T. A.; Liu, J. O. (2009). "Fumagillin and Fumarranol Interact with P. Falciparum Methionine Aminopeptidase 2 and Inhibit Malaria Parasite Growth in Vitro and in Vivo". Chemistry & Biology. 16 (2): 193–202.

156. Christopher Arico-Muendel et al. "Antiparasitic activities of novel, orally available fumagillin analogs". Bioorganic & Medicinal Chemistry Letters Vol. 19 Nr. 17 (2009), blz. 5128-5131.

157. Yamaguchi, J.; Toyoshima, M.; Shoji, M.; Kakeya, H.; Osada, H.; Hayashi, Y. (2006). "Concise enantio- and diastereoselective total syntheses of fumagillol, RK-805, FR65814, ovalicin, and 5-demethylovalicin". Angewandte Chemie International Edition in English. 45(5): 789–793.

158. Pommier, Y.; Leo, E.; Zhang, H.; Marchand, C. (2010). "DNA topoisomerases and their poisoning by anticancer and antibacterial drugs". Chem. Biol. 17 (5): 421–433.

159. Emmerson AM, Jones AM (May 2003). The Journal of Antimicrobial Chemotherapy. 51 Suppl 1 (Suppl 1): 13–20.

160. Zhanel GG, Fontaine S, Adam H, Schurek K, Mayer M, Noreddin AM, Gin AS, Rubinstein E, Hoban DJ (2006). "A Review of New Fluoroquinolones: Focus on their Use in Respiratory Tract Infections". Treatments in Respiratory Medicine. 5 (6): 437–65.

161. Falagas ME, Matthaiou DK, Vardakas KZ (December 2006). "Fluoroquinolones vs beta-lactams for empirical treatment of immunocompetent patients with skin and soft tissue infections: a meta-analysis of randomized controlled trials". Mayo Clinic Proceedings. 81(12): 1553–66.

162. Solomkin JS, Mazuski JE, Bradley JS, Rodvold KA, Goldstein EJ, Baron EJ, O'Neill PJ, Chow AW, Dellinger EP, Eachempati SR, Hilfiker M, May AK, Nathens AB, Sawyer RG, Bartlett JG (January 2010). "Diagnosis and management of complicated intra-abdominal infection in adults and children: guidelines by the Surgical Infection Society and the Infectious Diseases Society of America". Clinical Infectious Diseases. 50 (2): 133–64.

163. Knottnerus BJ, Grigoryan L, Geerlings SE, Moll van Charante EP, Verheij TJ, Kessels AG, ter Riet G (December 2012). "Comparative effectiveness of antibiotics for uncomplicated urinary tract infections: network meta-analysis of randomized trials". Family Practice. 29 (6): 659–70.

164. Shin HC, Kim JC, Chung MK, Jung YH, Kim JS, Lee MK, Amidon GL (September 2003). "Fetal and maternal tissue distribution of the new fluoroquinolone DW-116 in pregnant rats". Comparative Biochemistry and Physiology. Toxicology & Pharmacology. 136 (1): 95–102.

165. Schaefer C, Amoura-Elefant E, Vial T, Ornoy A, Garbis H, Robert E, Rodriguez-Pinilla E, Pexieder T, Prapas N, Merlob P (November 1996). "Pregnancy outcome after prenatal quinolone

exposure. Evaluation of a case registry of the European Network of Teratology Information Services (ENTIS)". European Journal of Obstetrics, Gynecology, and Reproductive Biology. 69 (2): 83–9.

166. Antimicrobial Agents and Chemotherapy. 42 (6): 1336–9.

167. Arabyat RM, Raisch DW, McKoy JM, Bennett CL (2015). "Fluoroquinolone-associated tendon-rupture: a summary of reports in the Food and Drug Administration's adverse event reporting system". Expert Opin Drug Saf. 14 (11): 1653–60.

168. Vardakas KZ, Konstantelias AA, Loizidis G, Rafailidis PI, Falagas ME (November 2012). "Risk factors for development of Clostridium difficile infection due to BI/NAP1/027 strain: a meta-analysis". Int. J. Infect. Dis. 16 (11): e768–73.

169. Fernández J, Navasa M, Planas R, et al. (2007). "Primary prophylaxis of spontaneous bacterial peritonitis delays hepatorenal syndrome and improves survival in cirrhosis". Gastroenterology. 133 (3): 818–24.

170. Falagas ME, Matthaiou DK, Vardakas KZ (December 2006). "Fluoroquinolones vs beta-lactams for empirical treatment of immunocompetent patients with skin and soft tissue infections: a meta-analysis of randomized controlled trials". Mayo Clin. Proc. 81 (12): 1553–66.

171. Hall, CE; Keegan, H; Rogstad, KE (September 2003). "Psychiatric side effects of ofloxacin used in the treatment of pelvic inflammatory disease". Int J STD AIDS. 14 (9): 636–7.

172. Vardakas KZ, Konstantelias AA, Loizidis G, Rafailidis PI, Falagas ME (November 2012). "Risk factors for development of Clostridium difficile infection due to BI/NAP1/027 strain: a meta-analysis". Int. J. Infect. Dis. 16 (11): e768–73.

173. Flowerdew, A., E. Walker, and S. J. Karran. "Evaluation of biliary pharmacokinetics of oral enoxacin, a new quinolone antibiotic." 14th International Congress of Chemotherapy, Kyoto. 1985.

174. Al-Wabli RI (2017). "Lomefloxacin". Profiles of Drug Substances, Excipients and Related Methodology. Elsevier. pp.

193–240. Lomefloxacin elimination half-life is about 7–8 h and is prolonged in patients with renal impairment.

175. Cluck D, Lewis P, Stayer B, Spivey J, Moorman J (December 2015). "Ceftolozane-tazobactam: A new-generation cephalosporin". American Journal of Health-System Pharmacy. 72 (24): 2135–46.

176. Wooley M, Miller B, Krishna G, Hershberger E, Chandorkar G (2014-04-01). "Impact of renal function on the pharmacokinetics and safety of ceftolozane-tazobactam". Antimicrobial Agents and Chemotherapy. 58 (4): 2249–55.

177. Murano K, Yamanaka T, Toda A, Ohki H, Okuda S, Kawabata K, et al. (March 2008). "Structural requirements for the stability of novel cephalosporins to AmpC beta-lactamase based on 3D-structure". Bioorganic & Medicinal Chemistry. 16 (5): 2261–75.

178. Miller B, Hershberger E, Benziger D, Trinh M, Friedland I (June 2012). "Pharmacokinetics and safety of intravenous ceftolozane-tazobactam in healthy adult subjects following single and multiple ascending doses". Antimicrobial Agents and Chemotherapy. 56 (6): 3086–91.

179. Lanoot B, Vancanneyt M, Cleenwerck I, Wang L, Li W, Liu Z, Swings J (May 2002). "The search for synonyms among streptomycetes by using SDS-PAGE of whole-cell proteins. Emendation of the species Streptomyces aurantiacus, Streptomyces cacaoi subsp. cacaoi, Streptomyces caeruleus and Streptomyces violaceus". International Journal of Systematic and Evolutionary Microbiology. 52 (Pt 3): 823–9.

180. Smith C. G.; Dietz A.; Sokolski W. T.; Savage G. M. (1956). "Streptonivicin, a new antibiotic. I. Discovery and biologic studies". Antibiotics & Chemotherapy. 6: 135–142.

181. Hoeksema H.; Johnson J. L.; Hinman J. W. (1955). "Structural studies on streptonivicin, a new antibiotic". J Am Chem Soc. 77 (24): 6710–6711.

182. Nicolaou K. C.; Mitchell H. J.; Jain N. F.; Winssinger N.; Hughes R.; Bando T. (1999). "Total Synthesis of Vancomycin". Angew. Chem. Int. Ed. 38 (1–2): 240–244.

183. Janata, Jiri; Kamenik, Zdenek; Gazak, Radek; Kadlcik, Stanislav; Najmanova, Lucie (2018). "Biosynthesis and incorporation of an alkylproline-derivative (APD) precursor into complex natural products". Natural Product Reports. 35 (3): 257–289.

184. Birkenmeyer, R. D.; Kagan, F. (1970). "Lincomycin. XI. Synthesis and structure of clindamycin, a potent antibacterial agent". Journal of Medicinal Chemistry. 13 (4): 616–619.

185. Kohli RM, Walsh CT, Burkart MD (August 2002). "Biomimetic synthesis and optimization of cyclic peptide antibiotics". Nature. 418 (6898): 658–61.

186. Stein T, Vater J, Kruft V, et al. (June 1996). "The multiple carrier model of nonribosomal peptide biosynthesis at modular multienzymatic templates". The Journal of Biological Chemistry. 271 (26): 15428–35.

187. Liu, C; Bayer, A; Cosgrove, SE; Daum, RS; Fridkin, SK; Gorwitz, RJ; Kaplan, SL; Karchmer, AW; Levine, DP; Murray, BE; J Rybak, M; Talan, DA; Chambers, HF (February 2011). "Clinical practice guidelines by the infectious diseases society of america for the treatment of methicillin-resistant Staphylococcus aureus infections in adults and children: executive summary". Clinical Infectious Diseases. 52 (3): 285–92.

188. Ribosome-targeting antibiotics and mechanisms of bacterial resistance. Nature Reviews Microbiology. 2014;12(1):35–48.

189. Cunliffe WJ, Holland KT, Bojar R, Levy SF (2002). "A randomized, double-blind comparison of a clindamycin phosphate/benzoyl peroxide gel formulation and a matching clindamycin gel with respect to microbiologic activity and clinical efficacy in the topical treatment of acne vulgaris". Clin Ther. 24 (7): 1117–33.

190. Gemmell CG, O'Dowd A (1983). "Regulation of protein A biosynthesis in Staphylococcus aureus by certain antibiotics: its

effect on phagocytosis by leukocytes". J Antimicrob Chemother. 12 (6): 587–97.

191. Beauduy CE, Winston LG. Tetracyclines, Macrolides, Clindamycin, Chloramphenicol, Streptogramins, & Oxazolidinones. In: Katzung BG. eds. Basic & Clinical Pharmacology, 14e New York, NY: McGraw-Hill.

192. Sharma SV, Jothivasan VK, Newton GL, Upton H, Wakabayashi JI, Kane MG, Roberts AA, Rawat M, La Clair JJ, Hamilton CJ (Jul 2011). "Chemical and Chemoenzymatic syntheses of bacillithiol: a unique low-molecular-weight thiol amongst low G + C Gram-positive bacteria". Angewandte Chemie. 50 (31): 7101–7104.

193. Patel SS, Balfour JA, Bryson HM (Apr 1997). "Fosfomycin tromethamine. A review of its antibacterial activity, pharmacokinetic properties and therapeutic efficacy as a single-dose oral treatment for acute uncomplicated lower urinary tract infections". Drugs. 53 (4): 637–656.

194. Falagas ME, Giannopoulou KP, Kokolakis GN, Rafailidis PI (Apr 2008). "Fosfomycin: use beyond urinary tract and gastrointestinal infections". Clinical Infectious Diseases. 46 (7): 1069–77.

195. Starck SR, Green HM, Alberola-Ila J, Roberts RW (2004). "A general approach to detect protein expression in vivo using fluorescent puromycin conjugates". Chem. Biol. 11 (7): 999–1008.

196. Qin C, Bu X, Wu X, Guo Z (2003). "A chemical approach to generate molecular diversity based on the scaffold of cyclic decapeptide antibiotic tyrocidine A". J Comb Chem. 5 (4): 353–5.

197. Sarges R, Bernhard W (1964). "gramicidin A. IV. Primary sequence of valine and isoleucine gramicidin A". Journal of the American Chemical Society. 86 (9): 1862–1863.

198. Tran AX, Lester ME, Stead CM, et al. (August 2005). "Resistance to the antimicrobial peptide polymyxin requires myristoylation of Escherichia coli and Salmonella typhimurium lipid A". J. Biol. Chem. 280 (31): 28186–28194.

199. B. W. Bycroft (1972). "The crystal structure of viomycin, a tuberculostatic antibiotic". Chem. Commun. (11): 660.

200. Preud'Homme, J; Tarridec, P; Belloc, A (1968). "90. Isolation, characterization and identification of the components of pristinamycin". Bulletin de la Société Chimique de France. 2: 585–91.

201. Kingston, D. G.; Sarin, P. S.; Todd, L; Williams, D. H. (1966). "Antibiotics of the ostreogrycin complex. IV. The structure of ostreogrycin G". Journal of the Chemical Society, Perkin Transactions 1. 20: 1856–60.

202. Uberti EM, Fajardo M, Ferreira SV, Pereira MV, Seger RC, Moreira MA, et al. (December 2009). "Reproductive outcome after discharge of patients with high-risk hydatidiform mole with or without use of one bolus dose of actinomycin D, as prophylactic chemotherapy, during the uterine evacuation of molar pregnancy". Gynecologic Oncology. 115 (3): 476–81.

203. Fornari FA, Randolph JK, Yalowich JC, Ritke MK, Gewirtz DA (April 1994). "Interference by doxorubicin with DNA unwinding in MCF-7 breast tumor cells". 45 (4): 649–56.

204. Pang B, de Jong J, Qiao X, Wessels LF, Neefjes J (2015). "Chemical profiling of the genome with anti-cancer drugs defines target specificities". Nature Chemical Biology. 11 (7): 472–80.

205. Weiss RB (December 1992). "The anthracyclines: will we ever find a better doxorubicin?". Seminars in Oncology. 19 (6): 670–86.

206. Baruffa G (1966). "Clinical trials in Plasmodium falciparum malaria with a long-acting sulphonamide". Trans. R. Soc. Trop. Med. Hyg. 60 (2): 222–4.

207. Katzung, Bertram G., editor. (2017-11-30). Basic & clinical pharmacology.

208. Siitonen, V. et al. Identification of Late-Stage Glycosylation Steps in the Biosynthetic Pathway of the Anthracycline Nogalamycin. ChemBioChem 13, 120–128 (2011).

209. Torkkell, S. et al. The entire nogalamycin biosynthetic gene cluster of Streptomyces nogalater: characterization of a 20-kb DNA region and generation of hybrid structures. Mol Gen Genomics 266, 276–288 (2001).

210. Räty, K. et al. Cloning and characterization of Streptomyces galilaeus aclacinomycins polyketide synthase (PKS) cluster. Gene 293, 115–122 (2002).

211. Metsä-Ketelä, M., Palmu, K., Kunnari, T., Ylihonko, K. & Mäntsälä, P. Engineering Anthracycline Biosynthesis toward Angucyclines. Antimicrob. Agents Chemother. 47, 1291–1296 (2003).

212. Moore DF Jr; Brown TD; LeBlanc M; Dahlberg S; Miller TP; McClure S; Fisher RI. (1999). "Phase II trial of menogaril in non-Hodgkin's lymphomas: a Southwest Oncology Group trial". Invest New Drugs. 17 (2): 169–72.

213. Frederick CA, Williams LD, Ughetto G, van der Marel GA, van Boom JH, Rich A, Wang AH (March 1990). "Structural comparison of anticancer drug-DNA complexes: adriamycin and daunomycin". Biochemistry. 29 (10): 2538–49.

214. Vejpongsa P, Yeh ET (January 2014). "Topoisomerase 2β: a promising molecular target for primary prevention of anthracycline-induced cardiotoxicity". Clinical Pharmacology and Therapeutics. 95 (1): 45–52.

215. Perez EA (March 2009). "Impact, mechanisms, and novel chemotherapy strategies for overcoming resistance to anthracyclines and taxanes in metastatic breast cancer". Breast Cancer Research and Treatment. 114 (2): 195–201.

216. Roness H, Kalich-Philosoph L, Meirow D (2014). "Prevention of chemotherapy-induced ovarian damage: possible roles for hormonal and non-hormonal attenuating agents". Human Reproduction Update. 20 (5): 759–74.

217. Sanders JE, Hawley J, Levy W, Gooley T, Buckner CD, Deeg HJ, Doney K, Storb R, Sullivan K, Witherspoon R, Appelbaum FR (April 1996). "Pregnancies following high-dose cyclophosphamide with or without high-dose busulfan or

total-body irradiation and bone marrow transplantation". Blood. 87 (7): 3045–52.

218. Goodsell DS (2002). "The molecular perspective: DNA topoisomerases". Stem Cells. 20(5): 470–1.

219. Davila ML (January 2006). "Neutropenic enterocolitis". Current Opinion in Gastroenterology. 22 (1): 44–7.

ABOUT THE AUTHOR

NAEEM HASAN KHAN

Professor, Department of Pharmaceutical Chemistry, AIMST University, Malaysia.

He holds Ph.D. from Katholieke Universiteit Leuven, Belgium in the grade of GREAT DISTINCTION. He enjoys about 53 years of his academic, research and professional carrier around globe. He has 50 original research publications in The U.S.A., The U.K., France, Belgium, The Netherlands, Singapore, India and Malaysia. As a key-note speaker, he has participated in many conferences in The U.K., Spain, France, Philippines, Belgium, Malaysia and Singapore.

NABILA PERVEEN

As a co-author, she holds a Ph.D. degree from U.S.M, Malaysia. Presently she is serving as   lecturer at Faculty of Pharmacy, AIMST University, Malaysia. She has about 12 years of professional experience with numerous research publications of International repute.

Lightning Source UK Ltd.
Milton Keynes UK
UKHW010109100223
416722UK00001B/72